Current Topics in Microbiology and Immunology

Volume 387

More information about this series at http://www.springer.com/series/82

Ben Adler

Editor

Leptospira and Leptospirosis

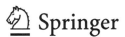 Springer

Editor
Ben Adler
Australian Research Council Centre
of Excellence in Structural and
Functional Microbial Genomics
Monash University
Clayton, VIC
Australia

ISSN 0070-217X   ISSN 2196-9965   (electronic)
ISBN 978-3-662-45058-1   ISBN 978-3-662-45059-8   (eBook)
DOI 10.1007/978-3-662-45059-8

Library of Congress Control Number: 2014954598

Springer Heidelberg New York Dordrecht London

Preface

It is appropriate that this volume should appear on the 100th anniversary of the isolation of *Leptospira* and its discovery as the causative agent of Weil's disease. The last 10 years have seen a resurgence of research activity on *Leptospira*, probably as a result of the availability of whole genome sequences and the development of genetic tools for the manipulation of pathogenic leptospires. The previous decade has seen double the number of papers published on *Leptospira* or leptospirosis than in any previous decade and more than all the publications in the first 50 years of leptospirosis research. It is gratifying that this activity has been accompanied by an increased awareness of the serious disease caused in humans and animals by this global pathogen.

In the years since the publication of "*Leptospira* and Leptospirosis" by Faine et al. (1999, MediSci, Melbourne) it became apparent that it was unlikely that a single person, or even a small group of authors, would be able to find the time to write an updated version. However, although much of the information in that book remains relevant, large parts have become so out of date as to be misleading. The solution to both these problems was to assemble a group of world experts on leptospirosis to contribute to this present volume, which brings together just such a group. There is of necessity some overlap between chapters. This is unavoidable; for example, how can one write about the leptospiral outer membrane without discussing proteins and LPS, which are also key players in pathogenesis and in interactions with the host immune system? The overlap is also desirable, in that each chapter can be read on a stand-alone basis, with reference to other chapters where appropriate.

There are many people to whom I wish to express my heartfelt thanks. First and foremost, I am grateful to the chapter authors in this volume for the alacrity and enthusiasm with which they accepted the invitation to contribute. To my many colleagues and associates over the past decades (too numerous to detail here), I appreciate your willingness to collaborate and to share your wisdom and insight. Many of you are contributors to this volume. However, I would like to express my particular gratitude to Solly Faine, who has been a mentor, colleague and friend for over 44 years, and who first introduced me to that fascinating organism, the leptospire. Finally, my grateful thanks to my wife Stephanie for her love, patience and forbearance during the preparation of this volume and over the last 40 years.

Melbourne, Australia, October 2014   Ben Adler

Contents

History of Leptospirosis and *Leptospira*

Ben Adler

Abstract *Leptospira* was isolated and identified as the causative agent of the severe human syndrome Weil's disease about 100 years ago almost simultaneously, but independently, by workers in Japan and Europe. Since that time leptospires have been isolated from almost all mammalian species on every continent except Antarctica, with leptospirosis now recognized as the most widespread zoonosis worldwide and also a major cause of disease in many domestic animal species. Recent advances in molecular taxonomy have facilitated the development of a rational classification system, while the availability of genome sequences and the development of mutagenesis systems have begun to shed light on mechanisms of pathogenesis that appear to be unique to *Leptospira*.

Contents

1 History of Weil's Disease

The modern history of leptospirosis began in 1886 when Adolph Weil (Fig. 1) described a particular type of jaundice accompanied by splenomegaly, renal dys-

B. Adler (✉)
Department of Microbiology, Australian Research Council Centre of Excellence in Structural
and Functional Microbial Genomics, Monash University, Clayton, VIC 3800, Australia
e-mail: Ben.Adler@monash.edu

© Springer-Verlag Berlin Heidelberg 2015
B. Adler (ed.), *Leptospira and Leptospirosis*, Current Topics in Microbiology
and Immunology 387, DOI 10.1007/978-3-662-45059-8_1

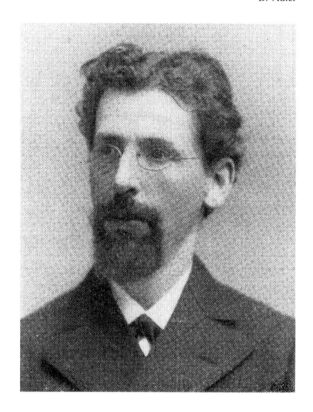

function, conjunctivitis, and skin rashes (Weil 1886). It was subsequently named
Weil's disease. Although the etiology of the disease was unknown, it appeared to be
infectious in nature and was often associated with outdoor occupations in which
persons came into contact with water. Epidemics were common among sewer
workers, rice-field workers, and coal miners.

However, it is apparent that leptospirosis had existed for millennia. Although it
is difficult to draw firm conclusions from records before the advent of modern
medical and scientific literature, it seems clear that at least some of the early disease
outbreaks described in ancient texts were leptospirosis. For example, ancient
Chinese texts carry accounts of "rice field jaundice", while in Japan syndromes
clearly recognizable today as leptospirosis were termed "autumn fever" or "seven-
day fever" (Kitamura and Hara 1918). In Europe, Australia and elsewhere, asso-
ciations were recognized between febrile illness and particular occupations, giving
rise to syndromes such as "cane-cutter's disease", "swine-herd's disease", and
"Schlammfieber (mud fever)", well before the common etiology was recognized
and identified (Alston and Broom 1958; van Thiel 1948). For a more detailed
description of the early accounts of what were almost certainly large-scale outbreaks of leptospirosis, the reader is referred to Chapter 1 of Faine et al. (1999).

2 A Spirochete as the Causative Agent

Although *Leptospira* was first isolated independently and almost simultaneously in Japan and in Europe (see below), it is clear that the first demonstration of lepto-spires was made some years earlier by Stimson (1907), who used the recently described Levaditi silver deposition staining technique to observe spirochetes in kidney tissue sections of a patient described as having died of yellow fever (Figs. 2 and 3). It is probable that the patient was convalescing from Weil's disease when he contracted fatal yellow fever; spirochetes were observed in kidney, but not liver or heart, tissues. Stimson called the organism *Spirocheta interrogans*; the species name, which survives to this day, was suggested by the resemblance of the bacterial cells to a question mark, a feature that we now know to be due to the characteristic hooked ends of leptospires.

The first isolation of *Leptospira* followed just a few years later. In Japan, where Weil's disease was common in coal miners, Inada et al. (Fig. 4) injected guinea-pigs intraperitoneally with the blood of Weil's disease patients and succeeded in reproducing typical, acute leptospirosis in the animals (Inada et al. 1916). This and subsequent papers constituted a *tour de force* for the period; they defined trans-missibility, routes of infection, pathological changes, tissue distribution, urinary excretion, leptospiral filterability, morphology, and motility. Signs in infected guinea-pigs included jaundice, conjunctivitis, inappetence, anemia, hemorrhages, and albuminuria. Disease was transferred in guinea-pigs for up to 50 generations. Spirochetes were observed in most tissues, with liver and kidneys containing the greatest numbers. These observations were extended to postmortem tissues from human cases, which revealed similar findings. These workers also showed that rabbits, mice, and rats were comparatively resistant to acute disease, even when injected with very large volumes of infected guinea-pig tissues.

Within a few months Inada and colleagues had succeeded in propagating the spirochetes in vitro in a medium made from emulsified guinea-pig kidney, and showed a preference for growth at 25 °C, with loss of viability at 37 °C.

Fig. 2 Stimson's original observation of spirochetes in kidney tissue. Reproduced from (Noguchi 1928), with permission from the publishers, University of Chicago Press

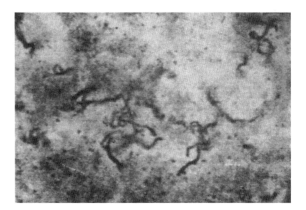

PUBLIC HEALTH REPORTS.

UNITED STATES.

NOTE ON AN ORGANISM FOUND IN YELLOW-FEVER TISSUE.

[By Asst. Surg. A. M. Stimson, Hygienic Laboratory, Public Health and Marine-Hospital Service.]

The spirochætal origin of yellow fever has been suggested by Schaudinn and by Novy, but so far as I know no organism belonging to the genus *Spirochæta* has been reported as having been found in yellow-fever tissues. I have examined some tissues for this class of organisms, using the method of Levaditi, as employed for the demonstration of *Treponema pallidum* in syphilis. The available yellow-fever material was unfortunately limited to the tissues from one case, all other specimens having been fixed otherwise than in formalin, which is required by Levaditi's method. The brain, liver, heart, and kidneys were examined. Nothing of special interest was observed in the first three, but in the kidney a very definite organism was found, having the following characters: Color, opaque black, in sharp contrast to the surrounding tissues; general appearance strongly suggesting a *spirochæte;* often irregularly curved, but some individuals having a regular series of alternate curves, no other indication of segments being observed; one or both extremities often bent back in the form of a hook; entire length variable up to 14 μ or more; width estimated at $\frac{1}{4}$ μ; length of short curves, $1\frac{1}{2}$ to 2 μ. It was confined to the cells and lumina of the tubules of the kidney, none being observed in the blood vessels, glomeruli, or interstitial tissue. While in some fields no organisms were present, in others large numbers were crowded together or scattered individuals were observed. The kidney from another case of yellow fever, where the tissue had been fixed in bichloride of mercury and acetic acid, was examined, and while no stained organisms were found, structures resembling those described were present in an unstained condition. The organisms were not found in kidney tissue from a patient dying of malaria, although the tissue was properly fixed and stained.

The object of this report is simply to invite attention to the findings in a single case, since no opinion as to the significance of this organism can be formed from such meager data. For convenience of reference I would suggest that the organism be called (*?Spirochæta*) *interrogans*, the specific name being suggested by the form, somewhat resembling a question mark, which the organism frequently assumed in my preparations.

Fig. 3 Copy of Stimsom's (1907) article in Public Health Reports. US Public Domain

The organism was named *Spirochaeta icterohaemorrhagiae*. One of the first isolates survives to this day and Ictero No. 1 was accepted by the Subcommittee on the Taxonomy of *Leptospira* in 1990 as the Type Strain of *Leptospira interrogans* (Marshall 1992).

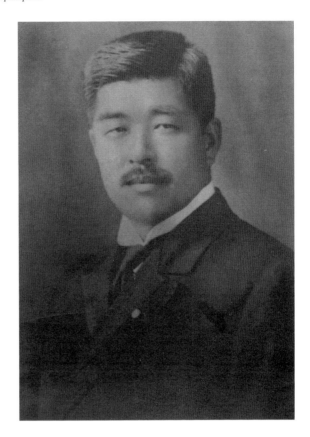

Fig. 4 Portrait of Ryokichi Inada (1874–1950). Kindly provided by Prof. Shin-ichi Yoshida, Kyushu University

Remarkably, the Japanese group also conducted the first vaccination studies. It is worth quoting verbatim.

Guinea pigs were immunized with repeated injections of liver emulsion of the infected animal and later with a pure culture of the spirochete, which had been killed by carbolic acid [Author's note, phenol]. The animals thus immunized did not develop the disease on the injection of the spirochete, which, it was known, would produce the disease in healthy animals. Hence this method seems promising for the prevention of the disease in man. Our conclusion is that the flea and mosquito have no share in the infection.

Of course, in the absence of quantitative data it is impossible to assess the degree of protection.

Finally, Inada and colleagues demonstrated immune lysis of leptospires by patient serum within the guinea-pig peritoneal cavity (the so-called Pfeiffer's method) and showed passive protection of guinea-pigs by convalescent patient serum or immune goat serum, but only if it was administered before the onset of jaundice. The importance of early treatment before the onset of organ failure remains relevant today (see the chapters by D.A. Haake and P.N. Levett and W.A. Ellis, this volume).

The 1916 paper of Inada et al. extended data that were first published in the Japanese literature in early 1915 which described their observation in November 1914 of leptospires in the liver of a guinea-pig injected with the blood of a Weil's disease patient. Of course, this work was not known in Europe where trench warfare in World War I resulted in large numbers of Weil's disease cases. Two German groups independently and almost simultaneously (October 1915) succeeded in transmitting the infection to guinea-pigs and demonstrating the leptospires in guinea-pig tissues (Hubener 1915; Uhlenhuth and Fromme 1915). The groups named the organism *Spirochaeta nodosa* and *Spirochaeta icterogenes* respectively. Some controversy followed about priority, but it is clear that the Japanese discovery predates the European ones by about a year, a fact recognized by the Subcommittee on the Taxonomy of *Leptospira* in specifying Ictero No. 1 as the type strain.

3 Rats as Carriers of *Leptospira*

The key finding that rats were renal carriers of *Leptospira* followed within 2 years, also reported by the Japanese group (Ido et al. 1917). The investigation was prompted by the serendipitous findings of spirochetes in the kidneys of field mice by colleagues working on tstutsugamushi (now *Orientia tstutsugamushi*). Ido and colleagues observed and cultured spirochetes from the kidneys and urine of a range of species of house and wild rats and identified them as *S. icterohaemorrhagiae* based on specific Pfeiffer reactivity with immune serum. They also made the key observation that leptospires were restricted to the kidneys and that the rats appeared healthy, the first observation of the asymptomatic carrier state. The connection between rats and Weil's disease was clearly established, as in coal mines which were frequently infested with rats, and also with the following epithet: "Cooks working in kitchens frequented by rats often became ill with spirochetosis icterohaemorrhagica." Interestingly, the group also observed spirochetes in mouse kidneys, but they were much less virulent when injected into guinea-pigs. It is probable that they observed one of the several serovars that we now know to be carried by mice. The Japanese findings were quickly confirmed in Europe and the U.S.A (Noguchi 1917; Stokes et al. 1917).

The Japanese group also reported some interesting epidemiological observations. Weil's disease in Japan showed a clear increased incidence in spring and autumn, but in coal mines where there was no temperature fluctuation the prevalence was the same year round. While this difference may be explained partly by season-specific human activities, the point was noted that higher incidence corresponded to temperatures of 22–25 °C. In addition, the incidence in coal mines with neutral or alkaline soil and water was high, whereas in mines with acidic soil and water infection was rare, despite equally high levels of rat infestation.

4 Recognition of Leptospirosis in Animals and the Expansion of Serovars and Syndromes

The following decades saw major advances in the understanding of leptospirosis. Arguably, one of the more important was the recognition of leptospirosis as an infectious disease of almost all mammalian species, especially in an increasing range of rodent species, and the importance of domestic animals as a source of human infection (Alston and Broom 1958; van Thiel 1948). For example, Dutch workers reported the isolation of a canine strain, Hond Utrecht IV (Klarenbeek and Schuffner 1933), which remains the type strain for serovar Canicola. The disease in cattle was first reported in Russia in 1940, then referred to as "infectious yellow fever of cattle" (Semskov 1940). By the 1950s the range of serovars and host animals had expanded substantially (Alston and Broom 1958) and by the 1980s leptospirosis was well documented as a veterinary disease of major economic importance in dogs, cattle, swine, horses, and perhaps sheep (Ellis 1990). Current aspects of leptospirosis in animals are detailed in the chapter by W.A. Ellis, this volume.

At the same time as more and more serovars were isolated, it became apparent that severe Weil's disease was not the most common presentation of leptospiral infection. This perhaps should not have come as a surprise. In fact, even the very early accounts described milder, anicteric cases of leptospirosis (Uhlenhuth and Fromme 1915). Thus, over the next few decades it became clear that leptospirosis in humans and animals varied from a mild febrile illness (so-called "influenza-like") through to severe, often fatal infections characterized by liver and kidney failure and severe pulmonary hemorrhage (Bharti et al. 2003; Gouveia et al. 2008). It is clear that the infecting serovar is an important factor that determines the outcome of infection. For example, serovar Hardjo never causes fatal human infections. However, it is also clear that the host and other factors also play a role; even serovars most commonly associated with severe fatal disease commonly cause mild infections (Gouveia et al. 2008).

5 Nomenclature and Classification

The genus name *Leptospira* was first proposed by Noguchi (1918) in order to differentiate the Weil's disease spirochete from others known at the time, especially *Treponema pallidum*, *Spirochaeta* and *Spironema* (later *Borrelia*) *recurrentis*; the differentiation was based almost entirely on morphological characteristics. As new serovars were isolated they were given species status, e.g. *Leptospira pomona*, *Leptospira canicola*, *Leptospira hardjo*, *Leptospira copenhageni*, and so on. Species (serovars) with related antigens were grouped together in serogroups. Even with the limited taxonomic tools available for *Leptospira* at the time, it was apparent that there were not >200 species and so in 1982 the subcommittee on the

Taxonomy of *Leptospira* adopted the notion of two species of *Leptospira*, with *L. interrogans* containing the pathogenic serovars and *Leptospira biflexa* containing the saprophytic serovars (Faine and Stallman 1982). Interestingly, the saprophytic *L. biflexa* had actually been described before the first isolation of pathogenic leptospires (Wolbach and Binger 1914). The family *Leptospiraceae* was formally proposed in 1979 (Hovind-Hougen 1979), although Pillot had suggested this grouping in 1965, but without a valid publication. Hovind-Hougen (1979) also placed *Leptospira illini* in a new genus *Leptonema*. *Leptospira parva* was reclassified as the genus *Turneriella* in 2005 (Levett et al. 2005).

The advent of much more objective and rational molecular taxonomy brought major changes to the classification of *Leptospira*. Based on DNA–DNA relatedness, the former single species *L. interrogans* was divided into seven species (Yasuda et al. 1987). Subsequent new isolations and analyses have added several additional species of both pathogenic and saprophytic *Leptospira* (Adler and de la Peña Moctezuma 2010). The systematics of *Leptospira* is described in detail in the chapter by P.N. Levett, this volume, while a listing and description of leptospiral species and serovars is available at: http://www.kit.nl/net/leptospirosis.

6 Recent Developments

The last 10 years have seen a resurgence of activity into research on *Leptospira* and leptospirosis. The number of publications in this field in the last decade was double that of any previous decade and about the same as the total in the 50 years following the discovery of *Leptospira*. Major changes were made in taxonomy and identification, with the addition of several new species and the development of molecular typing tools such as MLST. Significant advances have been made in the understanding of the biology of *Leptospira* and the mechanisms of interaction of leptospires with the mammalian host at the cellular and molecular levels. Progress has been facilitated by the availability of whole genome sequences concomitant with improvements in bioinformatics, genome analysis, proteomics methods and in particular the development of mutagenesis systems for pathogenic *Leptospira*. All of these areas are explored in detail in the ensuing chapters of this volume.

References

Adler B, de la Peña Moctezuma A (2010) *Leptospira* and leptospirosis. Vet Microbiol 140:287–296
Alston JM, Broom JC (1958) Leptospirosis in man and animals. E & S Linvingstone, Edinburgh
Bharti AR, Nally JE, Ricaldi JN, Matthias MA, Diaz MM, Lovett MA, Levett PN, Gilman RH, Willig MR, Gotuzzo E, Vinetz JM (2003) Leptospirosis: a zoonotic disease of global importance. Lancet Infect Dis 3:757–771
Ellis WA (1990) Leptospirosis; a review of veterinary aspects. Ir Vet News 12:6–12

Faine S, Stallman ND (1982) Amended descriptions of the genus *Leptospira* Noguchi 1917 and the species *L. interrogans* (Stimson 1907) Wenyon 1926 and *L. biflexa* (Wolbach and Binger 1914) Noguchi 1918. Int J Syst Bacteriol 32:461–463

Faine S, Adler B, Bolin C, Perolat P (1999) *Leptospira* and leptospirosis. Medisci, Melbourne

Gouveia EL, Metcalfe J, de Carvalho AL, Aires TS, Villasboas-Bisneto JC, Queirroz A, Santos AC, Salgado K, Reis MG, Ko AI (2008) Leptospirosis-associated severe pulmonary hemorrhagic syndrome, Salvador, Brazil. Emerg Infect Dis 14:505–508

Hovind-Hougen K (1979) *Leptospiraceae*, a new family to include *Leptospira* Noguchi 1917 and *Leptonema* gen. nov. Int J Syst Bacteriol 29:245–251

Hubener R (1915) Beitrage zur Aetiologie der Weischen Krankheit. Mitt I. Deut Med Wochenschr 41:1275

Ido Y, Hoki R, Ito H, Wani H (1917) The rat as a carrier of *Spirochaeta icterohaemorrhagiae*, the causative agent of Spirochaetosis icterohaemorrhagica. J Exp Med 26:341–353

Inada R, Ido Y, Hoki R, Kaneko R, Ito H (1916) The etiology, mode of infection, and specific therapy of Weil's disease (Spirochaetosis Icterohaemorrhagica). J Exp Med 23:377–402

Kitamura H, Hara H (1918) Ueber den Erreger von "Akiyami". Tokyo Med J 2056/57

Klarenbeek A, Schuffner W (1933) Het verkomen van een afwijkend *Leptospira*-ras in Nederland. Ned Tijdschr Geneeskd 77:4271–4276

Levett PN, Morey RE, Galloway R, Steigerwalt AG, Ellis WA (2005) Reclassification of *Leptospira parva* Hovind-Hougen et al 1982 as *Turneriella parva* gen nov. comb. nov. Int J Syst Evol Microbiol 55:1497–1499

Marshall RB (1992) International committee on systematic bacteriology subcommittee on the taxonomy of *Leptospira*: minutes of the meetings, 13 and 15 September 1990, Osaka, Japan. Int J Syst Bacteriol 42:330–334

Noguchi H (1917) *Spirochaeta icterohaemorrhagiae* in American wild rats and its relation to the Japanese and European strains: first paper. J Exp Med 25:755–763

Noguchi H (1918) Morphological characteristics and nomenclature of *Leptospira* (*Spirochaeta*) *icterohaemorrhagiae* (Inada and Ido). J Exp Med 27:575–592

Noguchi H (1928) The spirochetes. In: Jordan EO, Falk IS (eds) The newer knowledge of bacteriology and immunology. University of Chicago Press, Chicago, pp 452–497

Semskov MV (1940) To the materials on etiology of infectious yellow fever of cattle. Sovet Vet 6:22–23

Stimson AM (1907) Note on an organism found in yellow-fever tissue. Pub Health Rep (Washington) 22:541

Stokes A, Ryle JA, Tytler WH (1917) Weil's disease (Spirochaetosis ictero-haemorrhagica) in the British army in Flanders. The Lancet 189:142–153

Uhlenhuth P, Fromme W (1915) Experimentelle Untersuchen uber die sogenannte Weilsche Krankheit. Med Klin (Munchen) 44:1202

van Thiel PH (1948) The leptospiroses. Universitaire Pers Leiden, Leiden

Weil A (1886) Ueber einer eigenhuemliche, mit Milztumor, Icterus un Nephritis einhergehende, acute Infektionskrankheit. Deutsch Arch Klin Med 39:209

Wolbach SC, Binger CAL (1914) Notes on a filterable spirochete from frech water. *Spirochaeta biflexa* (new species). J Med Res 30:23–25

Yasuda PH, Steigerwalt AG, Sulzer KR, Kaufmann AF, Rogers F, Brenner DJ (1987) Deoxyribonucleic acid relatedness between serogroups and serovars in the family *Leptospiraceae* with proposals for seven new *Leptospira* species. Int J Syst Bacteriol 37:407–415

Systematics of *Leptospiraceae*

Paul N. Levett

Abstract Leptospires are spirochetes that may be free-living saprophytes found in freshwater or may cause acute or chronic infection of animals. The family *Leptospiraceae* comprises three genera: *Leptospira*, *Leptonema*, and *Turneriella*. Within the genus *Leptospira*, three clades can be distinguished, of pathogens, nonpathogens, and an intermediate group. Leptospires are further divided into serovars; antigenically related serovars are clustered into serogroups for convenience.

Contents

1 Systematics of *Leptospiraceae*

1.1 Taxonomy

Leptospires are spirochaetes that may be free-living saprophytes found in freshwater or may cause acute or chronic infections of animals (Zuerner 2010). The family *Leptospiraceae* was defined in 1979 to include the genera *Leptospira* and

P.N. Levett (✉)
Saskatchewan Disease Control Laboratory, 5, Research Drive,
Regina, SK S4S 0A4, Canada
e-mail: Plevett@health.gov.sk.ca

© Springer-Verlag Berlin Heidelberg 2015
B. Adler (ed.), *Leptospira and Leptospirosis*, Current Topics in Microbiology
and Immunology 387, DOI 10.1007/978-3-662-45059-8_2

Leptonema (Hovind-Hougen 1979), and was included in the Approved Lists of Bacterial Names (Skerman et al. 1980). It now contains three genera of spirochaetes: *Leptospira*, *Leptonema*, and *Turneriella* (Levett et al. 2005). The type genus is *Leptospira* Noguchi (1917).

The three genera are defined by differences in G + C content, DNA–DNA relatedness, and 16S rRNA gene sequences. The G + C contents of the genera *Leptospira*, *Leptonema*, and *Turneriella* are 33–43, 54, and 53.6 mol%, respectively (Stackebrandt et al. 2013; Yasuda et al. 1987). Other characteristics are described in detail elsewhere (Hovind-Hougen 1979; Johnson and Faine 1984; Zuerner 2010).

1.2 Nomenclature

The species of *Leptospira* are divided into a large number of serovars, defined by agglutination after cross-absorption of rabbit antisera with heterologous antigen (Dikken and Kmety 1978; Kmety and Dikken 1993). If more than 10 % of the homologous titre remains in at least one of the two antisera on repeated testing, two strains are said to belong to different serovars (Wolff and Broom 1954). 193 serovars were cataloged within the species *Leptospira interrogans* sensu lato (Kmety and Dikken 1993), and over 60 serovars of *Leptospira biflexa* sensu lato were recorded (Faine and Stallman 1982). Many additional serovars have been isolated and characterized, and after confirmation in at least one international reference laboratory, are recognized by the Taxonomic Subcommittee.

Serovar names should be written with an initial capital letter and should not be italicized. It is incorrect to write the serovar name after *Leptospira* (Levett and Smythe 2006). An example of the correct nomenclature for a serovar is *L. interrogans* serovar Icterohaemorrhagiae.

Serovars that are antigenically related have traditionally been grouped into serogroups (Kmety and Dikken 1993; Wolff and Broom 1954) for convenience. Serogroups have no taxonomic standing, but they have proved useful for initial serological diagnosis and for epidemiological understanding at the regional or population level.

2 Classification of *Leptospiraceae*

2.1 Historical Classification

The isolation of leptospires was first reported from freshwater in 1914 by Wolbach and Binger (1914), who named the organism *Spirocheta biflexa*. Similar organisms were isolated from the blood of miners suffering from Weil's disease in Japan by

Inada and Ido (1915). The announcement of this discovery was made in January 1915 at the Kyushu University Medical School in Fukuoka, Japan, and the first publication appeared in February 1915 (Kobayashi 2001). Inada and Ido initially named this organism *Spirochaeta icterohaemorrhagica japonica,* but this was changed to *Spirochaeta icterohaemorrhagiae* before the first publication in English (Inada et al. 1916). This finding was rapidly confirmed by studies of soldiers fighting in the trenches in Western Europe (Hübener and Reiter 1915; Uhlenhuth and Fromme 1915). The genus name *Leptospira* was proposed by Noguchi (1917) after study of isolates from Japan, Europe and the USA. See the chapter by B. Adler, this volume for a more detailed description of the history of the discovery of pathogenic *Leptospira.*

In subsequent years, isolates from many different locations were named. Differentiation between strains was by achieved by a variety of agglutination tests and antigenically distinct strains were assigned the status of species. By 1948, four species, *L. icterohaemorrhagiae, Leptospira hebdomadis, L. biflexa,* and *Leptospira canicola* were recognized in Bergey's Manual (Robinson 1948). A further 23 species with inadequate descriptions were listed, with the caution that many were probably synonyms of the four recognized species. Concern about the proliferation of new "species" and the relative difficulty in differentiating the newly described strains from existing strains, led Wolff and Broom (1954) to propose a standardized approach to maintenance of cultures and serological characterization based upon the methods established in Wolff's laboratory in Amsterdam. Wolff and Broom considered that assigning species names for serologically distinct strains was unjustified and suggested the use of the term serotype for the basic taxonomic unit of a serological classification. Using the Amsterdam system, "two strains are considered to belong to different serotypes if, after cross-absorption with adequate amounts of heterologous antigen, 10 % or more of the homologous titre regularly remains in each of the two antisera" (Wolff and Broom 1954); as a result, 32 distinct serotypes were recognized. Wolff and Broom further suggested that closely related serotypes could be clustered into serogroups for convenience.

The definition of a serotype was the subject of discussion at several meetings of the Taxonomic Subcommittee on *Leptospira.* At the 1966 meeting, the definition was modified to state "Two strains are considered to belong to different serotypes if, after cross-absorption with adequate amounts of heterologous antigen, 10 % or more of the homologous titer regularly remains in at least one of the two antisera in repeated tests" (Turner 1971). A further modification was made at the 1986 meeting: "Two strains are said to belong to different serovars if after cross-absorption with adequate amounts of heterologous antigen more than 10 % of the homologous titer regularly remains in at least one of the two antisera in repeated tests" (Stallman 1987). These small changes to the definition of a serovar have unfortunate consequences, in that several serovars defined using the historical definition would no longer be considered distinct from each other using the more recent definition (Hartskeerl et al. 2004). This inconsistency may well be resolved by whole genome sequencing.

In the 7th edition of Bergey's Manual (Wolff and Broom 1957), the genus *Leptospira* was divided into two species, *L. icterohaemorrhagiae*, comprising all pathogenic strains, and *L. biflexa*, containing saprophytic strains isolated from water. *L. icterohaemorrhagiae* was further subdivided into serotypes, but *L. biflexa* was not. At a meeting in 1962, the Taxonomic Subcommittee on *Leptospira* recommended that the pathogenic strains should be named *L. interrogans* and the saprophytic strains *L. biflexa* (Wolff and Turner 1963). At this time, the species were differentiated by growth in the presence of divalent copper ions. In the 1984 edition of Bergey's Manual, the species were differentiated by several phenotypic characteristics: *L. biflexa* was capable of growth at 13 °C and of growth in the presence of 8-azaguanine (225 µg/ml) and failed to form spherical cells in 1 M NaCl (Johnson and Faine 1984).

2.2 Genetic Basis for Classification

The phenotypic classification of leptospires has been replaced by a genotypic one, in which a number of so-called genomospecies includes all serovars of both *L. interrogans* sensu lato and *L. biflexa* sensu lato. Genetic heterogeneity among leptospiral serovars was demonstrated over 40 years ago, when pathogenic and nonpathogenic "complexes" were shown to have little DNA homology (Haapala et al. 1969). Based on base pair ratios, there were at least two groups within the pathogenic strains. Further work expanded the number of homology groups to six (Brendle et al. 1974). In addition, serovar Illini was shown to be genetically distinct from other leptospires (Brendle et al. 1974), leading to the definition of the monospecific genus *Leptonema* (Hovind-Hougen 1979). A further strain was found to be serologically and genetically distinct both from other leptospires and from *Leptonema illini*, and was named *Leptospira parva* (Hovind-Hougen et al. 1981). This species was later transferred to a new genus, *Turneriella* (Levett et al. 2005). Subsequent DNA–DNA hybridization studies led to the definition of 10 species of *Leptospira* (Yasuda et al. 1987). Heterogeneity within the species *L. biflexa* was confirmed independently (Ramadass et al. 1990). An additional species, *L. kirschneri*, was added soon after (Ramadass et al. 1992). After an extensive study of several hundred strains, five new species were described (Brenner et al. 1999), one of which was named *L. alexanderi*. Unfortunately, Brenner et al. did not assign names to four of the new genomospecies that were each represented by only one or two isolates. This led to confusion in the literature, which has been resolved only recently (Smythe et al. 2013).

A number of other species have been described: *Leptospira fainei* (Pérolat et al. 1998), *Leptospira broomii* (Levett et al. 2006), *Leptospira wolffii* (Slack et al. 2008), *Leptospira licerasiae* (Matthias et al. 2008), *Leptospira kmetyi* (Slack et al. 2009b), and *Leptospira idonii* (Saito et al. 2013). There are currently 21 species of *Leptospira* (Table 1).

Table 1 Species within the family *Leptospiraceae*

Species	Valid publication
L. alexanderi	Brenner et al. (1999)
L. alstonii	Smythe et al. (2013)
L. biflexa	Faine and Stallman (1982)
L. borgpetersenii	Yasuda et al. (1987)
L. broomii	Levett et al. (2006)
L. fainei	Pérolat et al. (1998)
L. idonii	Saito et al. (2013)
L. inadai	Yasuda et al. (1987)
L. interrogans	Faine and Stallman (1982)
L. kirschneri	Ramadass et al. (1992)
L. kmetyi	Slack et al. (2009b)
L. licerasiae	Matthias et al. (2008)
L. meyeri	Yasuda et al. (1987)
L. noguchii	Yasuda et al. (1987)
L. santarosai	Yasuda et al. (1987)
L. terpstrae	Smythe et al. (2013)
L. vanthielii	Smythe et al. (2013)
L. weilii	Yasuda et al. (1987)
L. wolbachii	Yasuda et al. (1987)
L. wolffii	Slack et al. (2008)
L. yanagawae	Smythe et al. (2013)
Turneriella parva	Levett et al. (2005)
Leptonema illini	Hovind-Hougen (1979)

2.3 Phylogenetic Classification

The species of *Leptospira* cluster into three groups, comprising pathogens, non-pathogens and an intermediate group (Fig. 1). Similar phylogenies can be produced using several housekeeping genes, including *rrs* (Morey et al. 2006), *rpoB* (La Scola et al. 2006), and *gyrB* (Slack et al. 2006).

The species of *Leptospira* currently recognized do not correspond to the previous two species (*L. interrogans* sensu lato and *L. biflexa* sensu lato). Interestingly, both pathogenic and nonpathogenic serovars occur within several species (Table 2). However, it is also clear that some reference strains have been mislabeled, leading to erroneous classification (Slack et al. 2009a). It is likely that some of the serovars listed in Table 2 will in the future be re-classified into a single species. Genetic heterogeneity within serovars has been demonstrated (Brenner et al. 1999; Bulach et al. 2000; Feresu et al. 1999). The presence of the same LPS biosynthetic genes in strains of different species implies genetic transfer; evidence of inter-species transfer has been detected (Haake et al. 2004). Thus, neither serogroup nor serovar

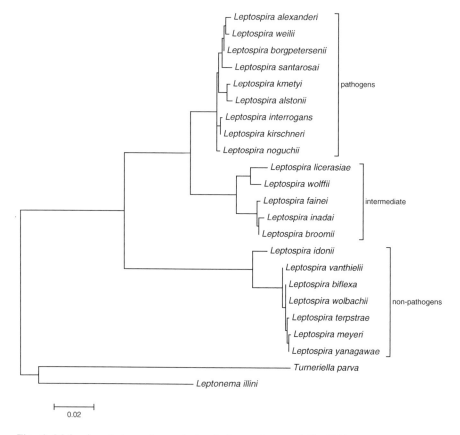

Fig. 1 Molecular phylogenetic analysis of *Leptospiraceae* 16S rRNA gene sequences by maximum likelihood method, based on the Tamura-Nei model, using MEGA5 (Tamura et al. 2011). The tree with the highest log likelihood is shown. The tree is drawn to scale, with branch lengths measured in the number of substitutions per site. All positions containing gaps and missing data were eliminated. There was a total of 1,230 positions in the final dataset

of an isolate currently predicts the species of *Leptospira*. In addition, the phenotypic characteristics formerly used to differentiate *L. interrogans* sensu lato from *L. biflexa* sensu lato do not differentiate the genomospecies (Brenner et al. 1999; Yasuda et al. 1987).

Characterization of leptospiral isolates requires both identification of species and serovar. In addition to sequence-based identification, a wide range of molecular approaches has been applied to species identification (Ahmed et al. 2012). The first leptospiral genome was sequenced over 10 years ago (Xue et al. 2009). The sequencing of 200 further strains has recently been completed through the *Leptospira* Genomics and Human Health Project (http://gsc.jcvi.org/projects/gsc/leptospira/) and the genomes of *L. illini* and *Turneriella parva* have also been

Table 2 Leptospiral serovars found in multiple species

Serovar	Species
Bataviae	*L. interrogans, L. santarosai*
Bulgarica	*L. interrogans, L. kirschneri*
Grippotyphosa	*L. interrogans, L. kirschneri*
Hardjo	*L. borgpetersenii, L. interrogans, L. meyeri*
Icterohaemorrhagiae	*L. interrogans, L. inadai*
Kremastos	*L. interrogans, L. santarosai*
Mwogolo	*L. interrogans, L. kirschneri*
Paidjan	*L. interrogans, L. kirschneri*
Pomona	*L. interrogans, L. noguchii*
Pyrogenes	*L. interrogans, L. santarosai*
Szwajizak	*L. interrogans, L. santarosai*
Valbuzzi	*L. interrogans, L. kirschneri*

It is probable that some of the serovars listed above were actually mislabeled in reference collections. Future examination of reference strains may result in revisions to this list

sequenced recently (Huntemann et al. 2013; Stackebrandt et al. 2013). The analysis of these sequences will further understanding of the taxonomy of the *Leptospiraceae* and will provide molecular tools for species identification and for serovar characterization.

References

Ahmed A, Grobusch MP, Klatser PR, Hartskeerl RA (2012) Molecular approaches in the detection and characterization of *Leptospira*. J Bacteriol Parasitol 3:1000133

Brendle JJ, Rogul M, Alexander AD (1974) Deoxyribonucleic acid hybridization among selected leptospiral serotypes. Int J Syst Bacteriol 24:205–214

Brenner DJ, Kaufmann AF, Sulzer KR, Steigerwalt AG, Rogers FC, Weyant RS (1999) Further determination of DNA relatedness between serogroups and serovars in the family *Leptospiraceae* with a proposal for *Leptospira alexanderi* sp. nov. and four new *Leptospira* genomospecies. Int J Syst Bacteriol 49:839–858

Bulach DM, Kalambaheti T, de La Peña-Moctezuma A, Adler B (2000) Lipopolysaccharide biosynthesis in *Leptospira*. J Mol Microbiol Biotechnol 2:375–380

Dikken H, Kmety E (1978) Serological typing methods of leptospires. In: Bergan T, Norris JR (eds) Methods in microbiology. Academic Press, London, pp 259–307

Faine S, Stallman ND (1982) Amended descriptions of the genus *Leptospira* Noguchi 1917 and the species *L.interrogans* (Stimson 1907) Wenyon 1926 and *L.biflexa* (Wolbach and Binger 1914) Noguchi 1918. Int J Syst Bacteriol 32:461–463

Feresu SB, Bolin CA, van de Kemp H, Korver H (1999) Identification of a serogroup Bataviae *Leptospira* strain isolated from an ox in Zimbabwe. Zentralbl Bakteriol 289:19–29

Haake DA, Suchard MA, Kelley MM, Dundoo M, Alt DP, Zuerner RL (2004) Molecular evolution and mosaicism of leptospiral outer membrane proteins involves horizontal DNA transfer. J Bacteriol 186:2818–2828

Haapala DK, Rogul M, Evans LB, Alexander AD (1969) Deoxyribonucleic acid base composition and homology studies of *Leptospira*. J Bacteriol 98:421–428

Hartskeerl RA, Goris MG, Brem S, Meyer P, Kopp H, Gerhards H, Wollanke B (2004) Classification of *Leptospira* from the eyes of horses suffering from recurrent uveitis. J Vet Med B 51:110–115

Hovind-Hougen K (1979) *Leptospiraceae*, a new family to include *Leptospira* Noguchi 1917 and *Leptonema* gen. nov. Int J Syst Bacteriol 29:245–251

Hovind-Hougen K, Ellis WA, Birch-Andersen A (1981) *Leptospira parva* sp.nov.: some morphological and biological characters. Zentralbl Bakteriol Mikrobiol Hyg A 250:343–354

Hübener EA, Reiter H (1915) Beiträge zur Aetiologie der Weilschen Krankheit. Dtsch Med Wochenschr 41:1275–1277

Huntemann M, Stackebrandt E, Held B, Nolan M, Lucas S, Hammon N, Deshpande S, Cheng JF, Tapia R, Goodwin LA, Pitluck S, Liolios K, Pagani I, Ivanova N, Mavromatis K, Mikhailova N, Pati A, Chen A, Palaniappan K, Land M, Rohde M, Gronow S, Goker M, Detter JC, Bristow J, Eisen JA, Markowitz V, Woyke T, Hugenholtz P, Kyrpides NC, Klenk HP, Lapidus A (2013) Genome sequence of the phylogenetically isolated spirochete *Leptonema illini* type strain (3055^T). Stand Genomic Sci 8:177–187

Inada R, Ido Y (1915) Preliminary report on the identification of a causative spirochete (a new species) of Weil's disease (in Japanese). Fukuoka Acta Medica 8:368–369

Inada R, Ido Y, Hoki R, Kaneko R, Ito H (1916) The etiology, mode of infection, and specific therapy of Weil's disease (spirochaetosis icterohaemorrhagica). J Exp Med 23:377–402

Johnson RC, Faine S (1984) *Leptospira*. In: Krieg NR, Holt JG (eds) Bergey's manual of systematic bacteriology. Williams & Wilkins, Baltimore, pp 62–67

Kmety E, Dikken H (1993) Classification of the species *Leptospira interrogans* and history of its serovars. University Press Groningen, Groningen

Kobayashi Y (2001) Discovery of the causative organism of Weil's disease: historical view. J Infect Chemother 7:10–15

La Scola B, Bui LTM, Baranton G, Khamis A, Raoult D (2006) Partial *rpoB* gene sequencing for identification of *Leptospira* species. FEMS Microbiol Lett 263:142–147

Levett PN, Morey RE, Galloway R, Steigerwalt AG, Ellis WA (2005) Reclassification of *Leptospira parva* Hovind-Hougen et al., 1982 as *Turneriella parva* gen. nov., comb. nov. Int J Syst Evol Microbiol 55:1497–1499

Levett PN, Morey RE, Galloway RL, Steigerwalt AG (2006) *Leptospira broomii* sp. nov., isolated from humans with leptospirosis. Int J Syst Evol Microbiol 56:671–673

Levett PN, Smythe L (2006) International committee on systematics of prokaryotes. Subcommittee on the taxonomy of *Leptospiraceae*. Minutes of the closed meeting, 12 and 13 November 2005, Chiang Mai. Thailand. Int J Syst Evol Microbiol 56:2019–2020

Matthias MA, Ricaldi JN, Cespedes M, Diaz MM, Galloway RL, Saito M, Steigerwalt AG, Patra KP, Ore CV, Gotuzzo E, Gilman RH, Levett PN, Vinetz JM (2008) Human leptospirosis caused by a new, antigenically unique *Leptospira* associated with a *Rattus* species reservoir in the Peruvian Amazon. PLoS Negl Trop Dis 2:e213

Morey RE, Galloway RL, Bragg SL, Steigerwalt AG, Mayer LW, Levett PN (2006) Species-specific identification of *Leptospiraceae* by 16S rRNA gene sequencing. J Clin Microbiol 44:3510–3516

Noguchi H (1917) *Spirochaeta icterohaemorrhagiae* in American wild rats and its relation to the Japanese and European strains: first paper. J Exp Med 25:755–763

Pérolat P, Chappel RJ, Adler B, Baranton G, Bulach DM, Billinghurst ML, Letocart M, Merien F, Serrano MS (1998) *Leptospira fainei* sp. nov., isolated from pigs in Australia. Int J Syst Bacteriol 48:851–858

Ramadass P, Jarvis BDW, Corner RJ, Cinco M, Marshall RB (1990) DNA relatedness among strains of *Leptospira biflexa*. Int J Syst Bacteriol 40:231–235

Ramadass P, Jarvis BDW, Corner RJ, Penny D, Marshall RB (1992) Genetic characterization of pathogenic *Leptospira* species by DNA hybridization. Int J Syst Bacteriol 42:215–219

Robinson GH (1948) *Leptospira*. In: Breed RS, Murray EGD, Hitchens AP (eds) Bergey's manual of determinative bacteriology. Williams & Wilkins, Baltimore, pp 1076–1079

Saito M, Villanueva SY, Kawamura Y, Iida KI, Tomida J, Kanemaru T, Kohno E, Miyahara S, Umeda A, Amako K, Gloriani NG, Yoshida SI (2013) *Leptospira idonii* sp. nov., isolated from environmental water. Int J Syst Evol Microbiol 63:2457–2462

Skerman VBD, McGowan V, Sneath PHA (1980) Approved lists of bacterial names. Int J Syst Bacteriol 30:225–420

Slack AT, Symonds ML, Dohnt MF, Smythe LD (2006) Identification of pathogenic *Leptospira* species by conventional or real-time PCR and sequencing of the DNA gyrase subunit B encoding gene. BMC Microbiol 6:95

Slack AT, Kalambaheti T, Symonds ML, Dohnt MF, Galloway RL, Steigerwalt AG, Chaicumpa W, Bunyaraksyotin G, Craig S, Harrower BJ, Smythe LD (2008) *Leptospira wolffii* sp. nov., isolated from a human with suspected leptospirosis in Thailand. Int J Syst Evol Microbiol 58:2305–2308

Slack AT, Galloway RL, Symonds ML, Dohnt MF, Smythe LD (2009a) Reclassification of *Leptospira meyeri* serovar Perameles to *Leptospira interrogans* serovar Perameles through serological and molecular analysis: evidence of a need for changes to current procedures in *Leptospira* taxonomy. Int J Syst Evol Microbiol 59:1199–1203

Slack AT, Khairani-Bejo S, Symonds ML, Dohnt MF, Galloway RL, Steigerwalt AG, Bahaman AR, Craig S, Harrower BJ, Smythe LD (2009b) *Leptospira kmetyi* sp. nov., isolated from an environmental source in Malaysia. Int J Syst Evol Microbiol 59:705–708

Smythe L, Adler B, Hartskeerl RA, Galloway RL, Turenne CY, Levett PN (2013) Classification of *Leptospira* genomospecies 1, 3, 4 and 5 as *Leptospira alstonii* sp. nov., *Leptospira vanthielii* sp. nov., *Leptospira terpstrae* sp. nov. and *Leptospira yanagawae* sp. nov., respectively. Int J Syst Evol Microbiol 63:1859–1862

Stackebrandt E, Chertkov O, Lapidus A, Nolan M, Lucas S, Hammon N, Deshpande S, Cheng JF, Tapia R, Goodwin LA, Pitluck S, Liolios K, Pagani I, Ivanova N, Mavromatis K, Mikhailova N, Huntemann M, Pati A, Chen A, Palaniappan K, Land M, Pan C, Rohde M, Gronow S, Goker M, Detter JC, Bristow J, Eisen JA, Markowitz V, Hugenholtz P, Woyke T, Kyrpides NC, Klenk HP (2013) Genome sequence of the free-living aerobic spirochete *Turneriella parva* type strain (H^T), and emendation of the species *Turneriella parva*. Stand Genomic Sci 8:228–238

Stallman ND (1987) International committee on systematic bacteriology subcommittee on the taxonomy of Leptospira. Int J Syst Bacteriol 37:472–473. Minutes of the meeting, 5 and 6 Sept 1986, Manchester, England.

Tamura K, Peterson D, Peterson N, Stecher G, Nei M, Kumar S (2011) MEGA5: molecular evolutionary genetics analysis using maximum likelihood, evolutionary distance, and maximum parsimony methods. Mol Biol Evol 28:2731–2739

Turner LH (1971) Statements and recommendations of the ICNB subcommittee on the taxonomy of *Leptospira*. Int J Syst Bacteriol 21:142–146

Uhlenhuth P, Fromme W (1915) Experimentelle Untersuchungen über die sogenannte Weilsche Krankheit (ansteckende Gelbsucht). Med Klin 44:1202–1203

Wolbach SB, Binger CAL (1914) Notes on a filterable spirochete from fresh water. *Spirocheta biflexa* (new species). J Med Res 30:23–25

Wolff JW, Broom JC (1954) The genus *Leptospira* Noguchi, 1917; problems of classification and a suggested system based on antigenic analysis. Doc Med Geogr Trop 6:78–95

Wolff JW, Broom JC (1957). Leptospira *Noguchii* 1957. In: Breed RS, Murray EGD, Smith NR (eds) Bergey's manual of determinative bacteriology. Williams & Wilkins, Baltimore, pp 907–913

Wolff JW, Turner LH (1963) Report of a meeting of the taxonomic subcommittee on *Leptospira* Montreal, 16–17 August 1962. Int Bull Bacteriol Nomencl Taxon 13:161–165

Xue F, Yan J, Picardeau M (2009) Evolution and pathogenesis of *Leptospira* spp.: lessons learned from the genomes. Microbes Infect 11:328–333

Yasuda PH, Steigerwalt AG, Sulzer KR, Kaufmann AF, Rogers F, Brenner DJ (1987) Deoxyribonucleic acid relatedness between serogroups and serovars in the family *Leptospiraceae* with proposals for seven new *Leptospira* species. Int J Syst Bacteriol 37:407–415

Zuerner RL (2010) Family IV. *Leptospiraceae* Hovind-Hougen 1979, 245[AL] emend. Levett, Morey, Galloway, Steigerwalt and Ellis 2005, 1499. In: Krieg NR, Staley JT, Brown DR, Hedlund BP, Paster BJ, Ward NL, Ludwig W, Whitman WB (eds) Bergey's manual of systematic bacteriology. Springer, New York, pp 546–563

Leptospiral Structure, Physiology, and Metabolism

Caroline E. Cameron

Abstract Members of the family *Leptospiraceae* are thin, spiral, highly motile bacteria that are best visualized by darkfield microscopy. These characteristics are shared with other members of the Order Spirochaetales, but few additional parallels exist among spirochetes. This chapter describes basal features of *Leptospira* that are central to survival and, in the case of pathogenic leptospiral species, intimately linked with pathogenesis, including its morphology, characteristic motility, and unusual metabolism. This chapter also describes the general methodology and critical requirements for in vitro cultivation and storage of *Leptospira* within a laboratory setting.

Contents

C.E. Cameron (✉)
Department of Biochemistry and Microbiology, University of Victoria,
Victoria BC V8W 3P6, Canada
e-mail: caroc@uvic.ca

© Springer-Verlag Berlin Heidelberg 2015
B. Adler (ed.), *Leptospira and Leptospirosis*, Current Topics in Microbiology
and Immunology 387, DOI 10.1007/978-3-662-45059-8_3

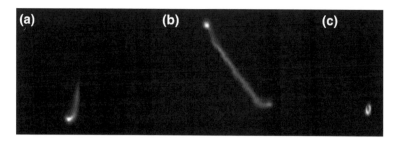

Fig. 1 Darkfield image of three distinct states of laboratory-grown *L. interrogans* cultures, taken using a 100x oil immersion lens: **a** hooked, motile; **b** elongated, semi-motile; **c** spherical

1 General Morphological Features

1.1 Size and Appearance

Members of the family *Leptospiraceae* are long, thin, highly motile, spiral-shaped bacteria that comprise both saprophytic and pathogenic species, with the latter demonstrating the capacity to infect a broad range of hosts and survive within both marine environments and mammalian host settings. Despite exhibiting these diverse lifestyles, *Leptospira* spp. maintain general consistency in, among other things, shape, size, motility, and ultrastructure. Due to its slender morphology and rapid motility, normal light microscopy is problematic for viewing *Leptospira* and instead the bacterium is best visualized using darkfield microscopy. *Leptospira* has a spiral shape with an average diameter of approximately 0.1 μm, length range of 6–20 μm, helical amplitude of 0.1–0.15 μm, and wavelength of 0.5 μm (Carleton et al. 1979; Faine et al. 1999; Goldstein and Charon 1988, 1990). Pathogenic *Leptospira* species that have been freshly isolated from a mammalian host are routinely shorter and more tightly coiled than laboratory strains that have undergone repeated serial passage and saprophytic strains (Ellis et al. 1983). Leptospires that have been grown in the laboratory under nutrition-limiting conditions can become extremely elongated, a morphology that often corresponds with decreased motility and poor cell health. Further deterioration of cell health frequently results in an increased proportion of spherical bodies within laboratory-grown *Leptospira* cultures. Figure 1 provides a visual representation of the morphology of highly motile *Leptospira* (a), elongated *Leptospira* with limited motility (b) and nonmotile, spherical *Leptospira* (c).

1.2 Cell Envelope

The general ultrastructure of *Leptospira* is similar to that of Gram-negative bacteria, with an outer membrane in which lipopolysaccharide (LPS) is embedded in the outer leaflet, an inner membrane, and an intervening, peptidoglycan-containing

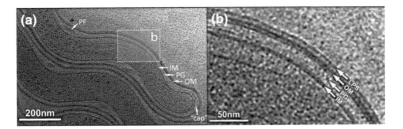

Fig. 2 *L. interrogans* ultrastructure: **a** outer membrane (*OM*), inner membrane (*IM*), peptidoglycan layer (*PG*), periplasmic flagellum (*PF*), and the "cap" at the cell end **b** magnified image showing the structural details of the cell envelope (Adapted with permission from Raddi et al. 2012)

periplasmic space (Fig. 2). Beyond this basal similarity few parallels exist, and in fact *Leptospira* possesses features that are unique even among the Order Spirochaetales.

1.2.1 Outer Envelope

Unlike other major spirochete genera such as *Treponema* or *Borrelia*, *Leptospira* possesses LPS on its surface. In fact, divergent leptospiral LPS structures form the basis for the categorization of *Leptospira* into 24 serogroups and at least 250 serovars (Evangelista and Coburn 2010) and LPS plays a key role in leptospiral virulence (Murray et al. 2010; Nahori et al. 2005; Werts et al. 2001). As shown by cryo-electron tomography, the leptospiral outer membrane consists of three distinct density layers. The first two layers exhibit a spacing of approximately 5 nm and correspond to the inner and outer leaflets of the outer membrane. The third layer, corresponding to the LPS, exhibits differential thickness between pathogenic and saprophytic leptospiral species, with LPS from pathogenic *L. interrogans* extending 9.2 nm from the outer leaflet of the outer membrane and saprophytic *L. biflexa* exhibiting a thinner LPS layer of 6.0 nm. Cryo-electron tomography revealed the presence of a "cap"-like structure of unknown function at the polar ends of the bacterium (Fig. 2) (Raddi et al. 2012). The outer envelope also contains numerous lipoproteins and transmembrane proteins. A description of the outer membrane and its components is beyond the scope of this chapter, but a detailed description of this subject can be found in the chapter by David A. Haake and Wolfram R. Zücker, this volume.

1.2.2 Periplasm

Similar to Gram-negative bacteria, leptospires derive their rigidity, shape, and strength from the peptidoglycan layer (Fig. 2). However, unlike Gram-negative bacteria, in *Leptospira* the peptidoglycan layer is found in closer proximity to the cytoplasmic membrane than the outer membrane (Holt 1978), a phenomenon that leads to a fluid outer membrane that is loosely connected to the cell body (Charon et al. 1981; Raddi et al. 2012). The major components of peptidoglycan have been studied in the saprophytic species *L. biflexa* and consist of the disaccharide tripeptide GlucNAc-MurNAc-L-Ala-D-Glu-(*meso*)-DAP and the cross-linked dimer GlucNAc-MurNAc-L-Ala-D-Glu-(*meso*)-DAP-D-Ala→(*meso*)-DAP-D-Glu-L-Ala-MurNAc-GlucNAc. A series of shorter peptidoglycan fragments, derived from the cross-linked dimer peptidoglycan species, have been detected and have been suggested to represent fragments formed during peptidoglycan remodeling. In comparison, a pathogenic *L. interrogans* strain demonstrated a similar overall peptidoglycan composition, but with an apparent lower proportion of the cross-linked peptidoglycan dimer. It has been suggested that this adaptation is suited to the physiological osmolarity encountered by pathogenic *Leptospira* within hosts (Slamti et al. 2011).

Consistent with other spirochetes, leptospires have endoflagella that reside within the periplasm and are responsible for their characteristic corkscrew motility (Charon and Goldstein 2002; Wolgemuth et al. 2006) (Fig. 2). However, the location of anchorage of the *Leptospira* motility machinery and range of cell coverage differs from other spirochetes, thus providing *Leptospira* with a distinctive shape among spirochetes. *Leptospira* possesses two single flagella that are anchored approximately 0.18 nm from the ends of the cell (one per pole) (Faine et al. 1999; Hovind-Hougen 1976), wrap around the cell in a right-handed coiling fashion (Carleton et al. 1979; Kayser and Adrian 1978; Yoshii 1978), and do not overlap or cover the entirety of the cell length (Bromley and Charon 1979; Goldstein and Charon 1988). This combination of subterminal tethering, incomplete cell coverage, and directional rotation provides the bacterium with its signature hooks that appear at one or both cell ends (Fig. 3) (Charon and Goldstein 2002; Faine et al. 1999; Hovind-Hougen 1976).

1.3 Spiral Shape

In contrast with *Borrelia burgdorferi*, the spirochete that causes Lyme disease (Motaleb et al. 2000), the spiral shape of *Leptospira* has been demonstrated to be independent of the periplasmic flagella. In studies conducted within the saprophyte *L. biflexa*, which was the first leptospire to be described (Wolbach and Binger 1914), inactivation of the gene encoding the *flaB* flagellar core protein produced mutants that were nonmotile but still retained their helical shape (Picardeau et al. 2001). Subsequent studies have demonstrated that the peptidoglycan layer and cytoskeletal proteins are key contributors to the spiral shape of *Leptospira* (Slamti et al. 2011). Interestingly, cryo-electron tomography performed on *Leptospira* has identified flagella-independent periplasmic filaments that wrap around the cell body

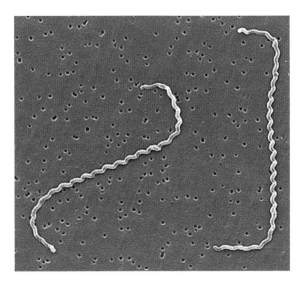

Fig. 3 Scanning electron micrograph of *Leptospira interrogans* strain RGA isolated in 1915 from the blood of a soldier in Belgium clearly demonstrating the signature hooked ends (*Image* obtained from the Public Health Image Library at the Centers for Disease Control and Prevention; content provider CDC/NCID/Rob Weyant)

in a right-handed fashion (Fig. 4). These filaments are particularly concentrated within the middle of the bacterium where flagellar filaments are lacking, leading to the hypothesis that these novel filaments may also partly contribute to the spiral shape of the bacterium (Raddi et al. 2012).

2 Motility

Due to its relative ease of culture (compared to other spirochetes), *Leptospira* has functioned as the model organism for elucidating the molecular mechanisms of spirochete motility. *Leptospira* displays rapid translational motility, travelling approximately 20 μm in 2–3 s in ordinary media (Faine et al. 1999). The most accepted theory as to how *Leptospira* accomplishes motility is that the rigid, coiled periplasmic flagellum rotates at the leading end, generating a gyrating helical wave which propels the cell along the flagellum by rolling in an opposite direction from the flagellar gyration (Goldstein and Charon 1988). Consistent with this theory, the outer envelope of the bacterium has been shown to behave as a fluid mosaic in studies where latex particles are linked to the leptospiral surface via antibodies (Charon et al. 1981).

Fig. 4 Periplasmic filaments (*PFil*) are located in the middle of elongated organisms while periplasmic flagella (*PF*) are located near the pole (Adapted with permission from Raddi et al. 2012)

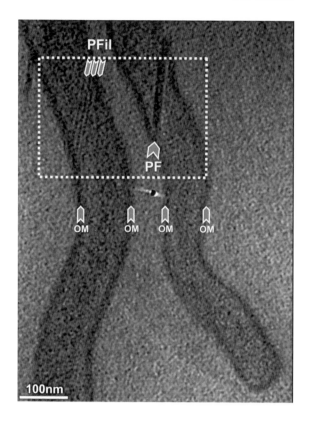

2.1 Leptospiral Flagellar Machinery

Cryo-electron tomography and subsequent three-dimensional reconstruction of the collected data have shown that the flagellar motor consists of the hook, rod, rod-associated L and P rings, MS (membrane and supramembrane)-ring, stator ring, C ring, and export apparatus (Fig. 5) (Raddi et al. 2012). The latter two components are more complex than any bacterial motor complexes characterized to date, and the portion of the export apparatus that is embedded in the cytoplasmic membrane has a larger diameter than those present in other bacteria, including other spirochetes (Raddi et al. 2012). The leptospiral flagellar filaments are similarly complex and consist of a flagellar FlaB core surrounded by a flagellar sheath, presumed to be composed of FlaA (Li et al. 2008). Two *flaA* genes and four *flaB* genes can be found within the *L. interrogans* genome (Ren et al. 2003), all of which are expressed (Malmstrom et al. 2009). Mutation experiments conducted with the *L. biflexa flaB* gene produced nonmotile bacteria that lacked flagella, and in fact this study represented the first example of gene inactivation within *Leptospira* (Picardeau et al. 2001). Subsequent mutation experiments performed in *L. interrogans* that targeted the FlaA proteins have demonstrated that a *flaA1* mutant, which

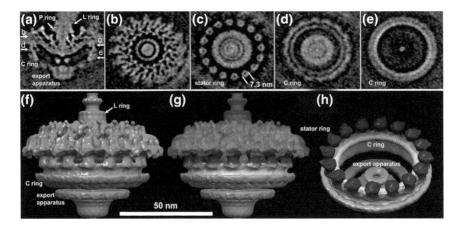

Fig. 5 Components of the leptospiral flagellar motor: **a** centered section parallel to the direction of the flagellar filament, **b–e** horizontal cross-sections, **f–h** surface rendering of the flagellar motor (Adapted with permission from Raddi et al. 2012)

continues to express FlaA2, exhibits decreased motility, while a *flaA2* mutant expresses neither FlaA protein and exhibits altered morphology, lacks motility, and is non-virulent in an animal infection model. Interestingly, the *flaA2* mutant, despite expressing neither FlaA1 nor FlaA2, displayed flagella of the same thickness as wild-type flagella, suggesting the flagellar sheath is composed of additional components that are independent of FlaA (Lambert et al. 2012).

2.2 Mechanics of Directional Motility

With regard to the directional motility displayed by *Leptospira*, counterclockwise rotation of the flagellum results in a spiral-shaped end and clockwise rotation creates a hook-shaped end (Wolgemuth et al. 2006). Thus leptospires that are translating (displaying directional movement or swimming) rotate their flagella in opposite directions, and thereby exhibit either a hook–spiral or spiral–hook shape, with the bacteria moving in the direction of the spiral end (Fig. 6). In contrast, leptospires that are non-translating have flagella that are rotating in the same direction and thus exhibit either a hook–hook or spiral–spiral shape (Charon and Goldstein 2002; Li et al. 2000; Wolgemuth et al. 2006). Mutation of the FlaA2 flagellar sheath protein prevents formation of the hook–spiral shape and eliminates motility, reinforcing the importance of the spiral end for directional movement (Lambert et al. 2012).

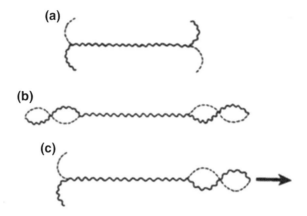

Fig. 6 Leptospiral motility: **a**, **b** non-translating forms with either hook–hook (**a**) or spiral–spiral (**b**) ends, **c** translating forms, with one hooked end and one spiral end, move in the direction of the spiral end. Reprinted with permission from (Goldstein and Charon 1990)

2.3 Connection to Infectivity

In contrast to externally flagellated bacteria, and similar to other spirochetes, *Leptospira* species exhibit increased swimming speeds under conditions of high viscosity (Charon and Goldstein 2002; Kaiser and Doetsch 1975; Petrino and Doetsch 1978; Takabe et al. 2013). One experimental study showed the average velocity of *L. biflexa* increased from 5–6 μm/s at approximately 10 centipoise (cP) to 25–30 μm/s at 200–500 cP (Kaiser and Doetsch 1975). This capability has been suggested to increase survival of the bacterium within natural environments and invasion of tissues by pathogenic leptospiral species (Goldstein and Charon 1988; Takabe et al. 2013). Pathogenic *L. interrogans* spp., which survive within the substantially different environments of water and mammalian hosts, maintain motility upon exposure to physiological osmolarity (approximately 150 mM NaCl) while motility of the saprophyte *L. biflexa* is lost under these conditions (Takabe et al. 2013). The fact that the motility of pathogenic *Leptospira* species can withstand osmotic change, while the motility of saprophytic *Leptospira* species cannot, highlights the essential link between motility and leptospiral virulence. Indeed, mutants constructed in the FlaA2 flagellar protein (Lambert et al. 2012) have reduced or no motility and, accordingly, lack virulence in an animal infection model. Similarly, inactivation of the gene encoding a putative flagellar motor switch protein (*fliY*) produced a mutant that displayed decreased rotative motion and migration in liquid and semisolid media, respectively, and also demonstrated decreased lethality in the guinea pig infection model (Liao et al. 2009).

3 Metabolism

The leptospiral genome encodes complete pathways for amino acid and nucleic acid biosynthesis (Faine et al. 1999; Ren et al. 2003), in direct contrast to the spirochetes *B. burgdorferi* and *T. pallidum*. *L. biflexa*, but not *L. interrogans*, can synthesize purines and pyrimidines and is able to grow in the presence of the purine analog 8-azaguanine. The addition of 8-azaguanine to leptospiral cultivation medium thus provides a means of differentiating pathogenic and saprophytic leptospires (Johnson and Rogers 1964). *Leptospira* species are unusual in that they derive their major energy and carbon sources through beta-oxidation of long chain (>C15) fatty acids (Henneberry and Cox 1970), and accordingly *Leptospira* possesses a complete beta-oxidation pathway (Nascimento et al. 2004a). Surprisingly, the lack of utilization of glucose as a primary energy source by *Leptospira* is not due to lack of a glucose utilization pathway, since genome sequencing has revealed a complete pathway within *Leptospira*, with two notable differences; there is substitution of pyrophosphate-fructose-6-phosphage 1-phosphotransferase for the usual phospho-fructokinase and a glucose kinase has been proposed to serve as a replacement for hexokinase (Nascimento et al. 2004a; Picardeau et al. 2008; Zhang et al. 2011). Instead, the lack of usage of glucose as an energy source has been proposed to stem from a limited glucose transport system (Nascimento et al. 2004a). *Leptospira* is unable to synthesize long chain fatty acids from pyruvate or acetate (Johnson et al. 1970; Stern et al. 1969), and instead must obtain these fatty acids from the growth medium (for in vitro cultured organisms) or from fatty acids located at solid–liquid interfaces (for *Leptospira* occurring in natural environments) (Kefford and Marshall 1984).

   Leptospira spp. grow in aerobic or microaerophilic environments, and thus the genome possesses a complete set of genes encoding tricarboxylic acid cycle and respiratory electron transport chain components. Accordingly, *Leptospira* generates ATP by oxidative phosphorylation, using an F_0F_1-type ATPase (Nascimento et al. 2004a; Ren et al. 2003). *L. interrogans* uses O_2 as the final electron acceptor, and it has been proposed that H_2O_2 can act as an alternative final electron acceptor (Nascimento et al. 2004a). *Leptospira* displays cytochrome c, oxidase, and catalase activity (Baseman and Cox 1969; Corin et al. 1978), with the latter enzyme being required for in vivo leptospiral survival, presumably by mediating protection against reactive oxygen species (Eshghi et al. 2012). Growth of *Leptospira* requires a nitrogen source which is frequently supplied in the form of ammonia (Faine et al. 1999), although some leptospiral species produce a urease which allows substitution of ammonia with urea (Kadis and Pugh 1974). Microarray analyses have revealed that genes involved in oxidative phosphorylation, the tricarboxylic acid cycle, and fatty acid metabolism are down-regulated upon interaction with macrophage cell lines of murine and human origin, while the gene encoding catalase and genes involved in nitrogen metabolism are up-regulated under these conditions (Xue et al. 2010). Studies comparing the protein expression levels of high laboratory passage, virulence-attenuated, and pathogenic *L. interrogans* serovar Lai strains have demonstrated that proteins involved in lipid metabolism are up-regulated in the virulence-attenuated strain (Zhong et al. 2011).

Genome sequencing has demonstrated that pathogenic leptospiral species possess the complete repertoire of genes necessary for protoheme and vitamin B_{12} biosynthesis, while the genes encoding these pathways are absent in the spirochetes *B. burgdorferi* and *T. pallidum* (Nascimento et al. 2004b; Ricaldi et al. 2012). The genome of a leptospiral species of intermediary pathogenicity that causes mild disease in humans, *L. licerasiae*, encodes proteins involved in nitrogen, amino acid, and carbohydrate metabolism that are missing from pathogenic leptospiral species, likely accounting for the ease of growth of this species in vitro (Ricaldi et al. 2012). Also of interest is the observation that *L. borgpetersenii*, a pathogenic leptospiral species that is proposed to be transmitted host-to-host rather than via the contaminated surface water route more commonly used by *L. interrogans*, has a reduced genome size. In particular, compared to *L. interrogans*, *L. borgpetersenii* has fewer metabolic transporter functions, a genomic tailoring that has been suggested to reflect the differing metabolic requirements of *L. borgpetersenii* during direct host-to-host transmission (Bulach et al. 2006).

4 Nutritional Requirements, Growth, and Cultivation

4.1 Nutritional Requirements

The primary nutritional requirements for growth of *Leptospira* are sources of carbon and nitrogen and the presence of select vitamins and nutritional supplements. Long chain fatty acids represent an essential carbon source for growth of leptospires, with growth of *L. biflexa* supported on long or short chain, saturated or unsaturated fatty acids. In contrast, growth of *L. interrogans* requires the presence of long chain unsaturated fatty acids; only in the presence of unsaturated fatty acids is *L. interrogans* able to metabolize saturated fatty acids (Faine et al. 1999; Johnson et al. 1969; Khisamov and Morozova 1988). These essential fatty acids are also toxic, and thus growth of *Leptospira* in vitro requires the addition of detoxicants such as albumin-containing serum or sorbitol-complexed fatty acids (Tweens) to the medium (Faine et al. 1999; Stalheim and Wilson 1964b). Albumin can also be extracted from serum and used in serum-free defined medium (Ellinghausen and McCullough 1965). Albumin functions by absorbing large quantities of fatty acids and promoting their slow release into the medium at concentrations that are nontoxic (Faine et al. 1999). Tweens (polyoxyethylene sorbitan ester) present fatty acids in a nontoxic form, although impurities such as polyethylene glycol, unesterified fatty acids, and other contaminants must be avoided to prevent growth inhibition (Ellinghausen and McCullough 1965; Faine et al. 1999; Staneck et al. 1973). Glycerol as an additional carbon source augments the growth of some leptospires (Faine et al. 1999; Staneck et al. 1973). Ammonium ions are the only recognized nitrogen source and can be supplied as either ammonium salts or by the deamination of amino acids (Faine et al. 1999; Shenberg 1967). Required nutritional supplements include thiamin, biotin (for some strains), phosphate, calcium, magnesium, and iron and additional compounds that are routinely added to the culture medium, particularly for isolation and maintenance of pathogenic leptospires, include copper, manganese, and sulfate (Faine 1959; Faine et al. 1999; Shenberg 1967; Stalheim and Wilson 1964a; Staneck et al. 1973). Vitamin B_{12} has historically been deemed an essential nutrient for growth of pathogenic *Leptospira* at 37 °C (Stalheim and Wilson 1964a). However, as outlined above, genome sequencing has revealed the presence of a complete vitamin B_{12} biosynthesis operon within pathogenic leptospires, and thus the addition of this nutrient to in vitro culture media may in fact be unnecessary (Nascimento et al. 2004b).

4.2 Growth

Saprophytic and pathogenic leptospires both grow under aerobic conditions but they differ in the range of temperatures at which they will grow. Saprophytes have an optimum growth range in vitro of 28–30 °C and will exhibit growth at low temperatures (11–13 °C). Pathogenic leptospires also exhibit optimum growth in vitro at 28–30 °C and will grow at 37 °C, but in contrast they do not exhibit growth at low temperatures. The optimal pH range for growth is 7.2–7.6. Bacterial growth rates in vitro vary depending upon the species being grown, the extent of prior adaptation to laboratory growth, and the inoculum used to initiate culture. The doubling times for pathogenic leptospires in vivo and in vitro (provided they have had prior adaptation to in vitro culture) is estimated at 6–8 h, while the doubling time for pathogenic species freshly isolated from their host and introduced into culture is estimated at 14–18 h, with a lag time for initiation of growth of days to weeks. In vitro growth of saprophytic strains is faster, with an estimated doubling time of 4.5 h. The lag time for initiation of growth of laboratory-adapted strains depends on the size of the inoculum, with use of a smaller inoculum resulting in longer lag periods. Use of a stationary phase seed culture consisting of 1–10 % of the volume of fresh medium typically results in attainment of maximal growth of pathogenic leptospires in 4–7 days and saprophytic leptospires in 2–3 days (Faine et al. 1999). Achieved final densities in vitro are routinely 10^7-10^8 bacteria/ml for well-adapted laboratory strains, and the yield can be increased by providing aeration during culturing (Faine et al. 1999; Zuerner 2005). Growth of cultures is best monitored via darkfield microscopy, with cell counting accomplished using a Petroff-Hausser counting chamber. A hemocytometer is not suitable, due to the depth of the chamber. Occasional rapid lysis of late log to early stationary phase cultures can occur as a result of lipases produced by leptospires which eliminate the detoxicant capacity of the culture media (Faine et al. 1999).

4.3 Cultivation

This section provides the salient features of in vitro leptospiral cultivation and pertinent recipes for successful leptospiral growth using information primarily derived from Faine et al. (1999) and Zuerner (2005). For highly informative, detailed methodologies and culture conditions for the laboratory maintenance of *Leptospira* and in vivo growth of *Leptospira* in laboratory animals the reader is directed to the classic book by Faine et al. (1999) and the Current Protocols in Microbiology articles written by Zuerner (2005) and Haake (2006). A description of leptospirosis in laboratory animals can also be found in the chapter by William A. Ellis, this volume.

Onc of the essential requirements for the preparation of *all* solutions and media needed for the cultivation of *Leptospira* is the use of glass-distilled or double-deionized water that has been sterilized by autoclaving (routinely 20 min at 121 °C) and then cooled. Sterilization is necessary to eliminate saprophytic leptospires which are ubiquitous in water sources. One should also note that filter-sterilization cannot be used in place of autoclaving, since saprophytic *Leptospira* can pass through microbiological filters. The other critical factor in the successful propagation of pathogenic leptospires is the source and quality of the serum albumin supplement added to the medium to serve as a fatty acid detoxicant. The most frequent form of albumin used is bovine serum albumin (BSA). Analysis of different BSA lots for their suitability for successful leptospiral cultivation, especially for isolation of leptospires from clinical samples, is essential. Upon identification of a suitable BSA lot, purchase of a large quantity of that particular lot is recommended to provide sufficient material for successful cultivation in the future. BSA can also be delipidated by extraction of the dry powder with chloroform/methanol (2:1, vol/vol). A 0.22 μm filter, instead of autoclaving, must be used as a final sterilization step for prepared media that contains albumin, as albumin is heat-labile. Alternatively, leptospiral growth media may be commercially purchased. All media should be heated at 56 °C for 30 min to ensure killing of saprophytic leptospires. It should also be noted that pathogenic *Leptospira* species constitute Biosafety Level 2 (BSL-2) pathogens and thus appropriate biosafety guidelines should be followed.

4.3.1 Growth in Liquid Media

The success of leptospiral growth in liquid media depends upon the nature of the seed inoculum. Well-adapted laboratory strains can be directly passaged as liquid cultures, using 1–10 % of the volume of the fresh medium as the seed inoculum. Three different types of media commonly used for liquid culture of *Leptospira* are described. In all cases reagents should be added in the specified order.

EMJH medium The most frequently used liquid medium for culturing *Leptospira* is the Johnson and Harris (Johnson and Harris 1967) modification of

Ellinghuasen McCullough medium (Ellinghausen and McCullough 1965) (EMJH). Rabbit serum can be added to this medium; if serum is to be added it must be collected from a sero-negative rabbit and heat-inactivated by incubation for 30 min at 56 °C. EMJH supplemented with albumin is prepared from a series of stock solutions (all prepared in sterile, distilled water) as outlined below.

Basal Salt Stock Solution (Zuerner 2005):

1 g Na_2HPO_4
0.3 g KH_2PO_4
1 g NaCl
1 ml of ammonium chloride stock solution (25 g NH_4Cl/100 ml water)
1 ml of thiamine stock solution (0.5 g thiamine/100 ml water)
1 ml of glycerol stock solution (10 ml glycerol/100 ml water)

- Add components to ∼800 ml sterile, distilled water with stirring.
- Adjust pH to 7.4 with dilute solutions of NaOH or HCl.
- Bring volume to 1 liter with sterile, distilled water.
- Sterilize by autoclaving.
- Store up to 1 month at 4 °C.

BSA Stock Solution (Zuerner 2005):

Add 10 g bovine serum albumin, fraction V, to 50 ml sterile, distilled water with constant, slow stirring (avoid foaming). To facilitate dissolving of the BSA, this solution can either be gently heated to <50 °C or left at 4 °C overnight. Use immediately to prepare the BSA Supplement (see recipe below).

BSA Supplement (Zuerner 2005):

To 50 ml BSA Stock Solution (see recipe above) add the following stock solutions with constant stirring:

1 ml of calcium chloride stock solution (1 g $CaCl_2 \cdot 2H_2O$/100 ml water)
1 ml of magnesium chloride stock solution (1 g $MgCl_2 \cdot 2H_2O$/100 ml water)
1 ml of zinc sulfate stock solution (0.4 g $ZnSO_4 \cdot 7H_2O$/100 ml water)
0.1 ml of copper sulfate stock solution (0.3 g $CuSO_4 \cdot 5H_2O$/100 ml water)
10 ml of ferrous sulfate stock solution (0.5 g $FeSO_4 \cdot 7H_2O$/100 ml water)
1 ml of vitamin B_{12} stock solution (0.02 g/100 ml water)
12.5 ml of Tween 80 stock solution (10 ml/100 ml water)

- Adjust pH to 7.4 using approximately 0.4 ml of 2 N NaOH.
- Bring the final volume to 100 ml with sterile, distilled water.
- Sterilize by filtration through a 0.22 μm filter.
- Store indefinitely at −20 °C.

Complete EMJH Medium (Zuerner 2005):

Start with 100 ml of the BSA Supplement (see recipe above) and add the following components using aseptic technique. To further reduce the incidence of contaminants, which is particularly important during primary isolation of pathogenic *Leptospira*, add 10 ml of 5-fluorouracil stock solution (1 g/100 ml water) to 890 ml Basal Salt Stock Solution (see recipe above). If rabbit serum is added, reduce the volume of Basal Salt Stock Solution to maintain a final volume of 1 liter. Store up to 1 month at room temperature.

Modified Complete EMJH Medium for growth of *Leptospira* at 37 °C (Ellis and Thiermann 1986; Bolin unpublished):

As mentioned previously, optimal growth of *Leptospira* in vitro is accomplished at a temperature range of 28–30 °C, although *Leptospira* can be successfully grown at 37 °C using a version of the Complete EMJH Medium that is modified as outlined below:

- Best growth is achieved by preparing all solutions using commercially purchased sterile, distilled water (e.g. Gibco #15230-204). Sterile, double glass distilled water prepared in-house may also be suitable.
- To the BSA Supplement add 0.1 ml of manganese sulfate stock solution (0.3 g $MnSO_4 \cdot H_2O$/100 ml water) in place of the 0.1 ml of copper sulfate stock solution.
- To 100 ml of the BSA Supplement, add 1 g of lactalbumin hydrolysate, 100 μl of 10 mg/ml superoxide dismutase and 0.04 g sodium pyruvate. Allow the solids to dissolve without swirling the bottle.
- Vacuum-filter the Complete EMJH Medium using a 1 liter, 0.22 μm filter apparatus.
- The observed growth rate for *L. interrogans* serovar Copenhageni is enhanced in this modified version of the Complete EMJH Medium. Final densities of $\sim 10^9$ bacteria/ml are achieved within 3 days at 37 °C using a seed inoculum of 2 % of the final volume.
- It has been our observation that the modified version of the Complete EMJH Medium has a shorter half-life than the conventional Complete EMJH Medium. If sustained maximal leptospiral growth is desired, the modified medium version must be prepared at approximately 2-week intervals and stored at 4 °C.

Stuart's medium (Zuerner 2005) This medium was originally formulated by Stuart (1946) and subsequently modified by Faine (1994). It is rich in rabbit serum, which fosters leptospiral growth, but also has a propensity to precipitate phosphates present in the medium. Such precipitates can obscure viewing of bacteria upon darkfield analysis of cultures.

1.93 g NaCl
0.34 g NH_4Cl
0.19 g $MgCl_2$ $6H_2O$

   0.13 g L-asparagine
   0.67 g Na$_2$HPO$_4$
   0.087 g KH$_2$PO$_4$

- Dissolve components in distilled water to make a final volume of 1 liter.
- Adjust pH to 7.5 with dilute solutions of NaOH or HCl.
- Sterilize by autoclaving for 20 min at 121 °C, cool.
- Store for up to 1 year at room temperature.
- Prior to use, aseptically add sterile rabbit serum to 10 % final concentration.

Korthof's medium (Faine et al. 1999; Korthof 1932) This is another commonly used serum-containing medium that, similar to Stuart's medium, enhances leptospiral growth, but can complicate darkfield viewing of bacteria if phosphate precipitates form.

   0.8 g peptone
   1.4 g NaCl
   0.02 g NaHCO$_3$
   0.04 g KCl
   0.04 g CaCl$_2$
   0.24 g KH$_2$PO$_4$
   0.88 g Na$_2$HPO$_4$

- Dissolve components, one at a time, in distilled water to make a final volume of 1 liter.
- Steam the solution at 100 °C for 20 min (boiling can be used in place of steaming). Cool overnight at 4 °C.
- Filter off the resulting precipitate through Whatman No. 1 filter paper.
- Dispense into working aliquots.
- Sterilize by autoclaving for 20 min at 121 °C, cool.
- Aseptically add sterile rabbit serum to 10 % final concentration.
- The final pH of the medium should be 7.2–7.6.

Isolation of *Leptospira* from contaminated samples The simplest way to eliminate contamination from *Leptospira* cultures is to filter the culture using a 0.22 μm sterile filter; leptospires will pass through and the filtrate can be incubated and subcultured (Faine et al. 1999). Alternatively, successful isolation of *Leptospira* from samples contaminated with common clinical and environmental microorganisms has been achieved using a combination of the antimicrobial agents sulfamethoxazole (40 μg/ml), trimethoprim (20 μg/ml), amphotericin B (5 μg/ml), fosfomycin (400 μg/ml), and 5-fluorouracil (100 μg/ml) (Chakraborty et al. 2011). Leptospires may also be recovered from contaminated cultures by animal inoculation. The culture is injected intraperitoneally and blood is taken aseptically under anesthesia after 10–30 min. Hamsters, mice, and guinea-pigs have been used.

4.3.2 Growth in Semisolid Media

Pathogenic *Leptospira*, and particularly leptospires recently isolated from clinical samples, grow well in a semisolid medium where they form a dense zone of growth referred to as a Dinger's disk (Lawrence 1951). To facilitate growth in a semisolid medium, aseptically transfer $\sim$100–250 µl of culture to a tube containing 6–8 ml of semisolid medium (see recipe below). Transfer the Dinger's disk to a tube containing fresh semisolid medium when a disk forms that has visible density. The timing of transfer depends upon the leptospiral strain being grown, with some strains requiring weekly transfer and others taking up to 6 months to attain sufficient growth to allow transfer.

Semisolid EMJH medium (Zuerner 2005):

- Add 1.5 g agar to 900 ml of Basal Salt Stock Solution (see recipe above).
- Sterilize by autoclaving for 20 min at 121 °C.
- When the Basal Salt Stock Solution/agar mixture has cooled to $\sim$50 °C add 100 ml BSA Supplement (see recipe above) per liter.
- Store in 1 liter bottles for up to 1 year at room temperature.

4.3.3 Growth on Solid Media

Growth of isolated colonies of *Leptospira* on solid media is often difficult and, for some fastidious pathogenic leptospiral strains, unachievable. To isolate individual leptospiral colonies, streak cultures or spread limiting dilutions on solid EMJH medium (see recipe below). Minimize potential contamination by working in a sterile fashion, sealing the plates with Parafilm, and placing the Parfilmed plates in a sealed plastic bag. Invert the plates, incubate, and monitor for growth at weekly intervals. The time to development of isolated colonies depends on the strain, with some exhibiting growth within 10 days of plating and others taking up to 6 weeks to arise. Colonies appear embedded just below the agar surface, are white in color and typically have a diameter of 1–2 and 2–3 mm for pathogenic and saprophytic leptospires, respectively. Isolation of colonies is achieved by gently aspirating the colony into the tip of a sterile filter tip or Pasteur pipette, followed by introduction of the colony into semisolid or liquid medium and incubation until growth appears.

Solid EMJH Medium (Zuerner 2005):

- Add 8 g agar to 900 ml Basal Salt Stock Solution (see recipe above).
- Sterilize by autoclaving for 20 min at 121 °C.
- When the Basal Salt Stock Solution/agar mixture has cooled to $\sim$50 °C add 100 ml BSA Supplement (see recipe above) per liter.
- Pour into individual Petri plates with $\sim$40 ml/plate, preferably in a biological safety cabinet to decrease the chances of plate contamination.
- Store solidified plates in the original Petri plate bag, inverted, at 4 °C.

4.3.4 Isolation of Pathogenic Leptospires from Clinical Samples

Urine (Zuerner 2005) Pathogenic *Leptospira* spp. are shed into the environment within the urine of infected animals, and thus *Leptospira* can be isolated by collecting urine using a clean catch method into a sterile container. Add 1 ml of urine to 9 ml of *Leptospira* storage medium (see recipe below) in a sealable tube, vortex the sample for 10 s, add 1 ml of the diluted sample to an additional 9 ml of storage medium, vortex again, and then add 0.3 ml of the 10^{-2} dilution to 6 ml semisolid EMJH medium. Samples are checked for growth at weekly intervals for up to 6 months.

Leptospira storage medium (Zuerner 2005):

- Add 10 g BSA to 90 ml phosphate buffer (see recipe below). Dissolve overnight at 4 °C.
- Adjust pH to 7.4 using 2 N NaOH.
- Bring the final volume to 100 ml with phosphate buffer.
- Sterilize by filtration through a 0.22 µm filter.
- Store in 10 ml aliquots at 4 °C for up to 1 month.

Phosphate buffer (Zuerner 2005):

0.087 g KH_2PO_4
0.664 g Na_2HPO_4

- Bring the final volume to 1 liter with distilled, sterile water with stirring.
- Prepare fresh.

Tissues (Zuerner 2005) Pathogenic *Leptospira* can be isolated from the kidneys and liver of infected animals postmortem. To reduce the chances of growth of contaminants from tissues collected in the field, spray surfaces (both animal surface prior to necropsy and tissue surface during necropsy) with 70 % (vol/vol) ethanol. Approximately 1 g of tissue sample is placed into 9 ml *Leptospira* storage medium (see recipe above) and homogenized. The tissue homogenate sample is processed out to a 10^{-3} dilution, introduced to semisolid medium and monitored for growth as described above for the urine samples.

Blood (Wuthiekanun et al. 2007) The standard method for isolation of *Leptospira* from blood samples is to inoculate 100–200 µl of whole blood into 5–10 ml of semisolid or liquid EMJH medium. Too much blood can inhibit the growth of leptospires. Optimal yield of *Leptospira* from human clinical blood samples has been achieved by first centrifuging 3 ml of plasma, collecting the approximately 200 µl pellet that forms, adding 100 µl of whole blood to this pellet, and inoculating semisolid or liquid EMJH medium supplemented with 3 % rabbit serum with this whole blood/plasma pellet combination. Blood culture must be taken before the initiation of antibiotic therapy.

5 Storage

Leptospira can be stored long-term in semisolid media at room temperature. However, under these storage conditions pathogenic *Leptospira* may have reduced viability and demonstrate loss of virulence. Long-term storage is best achieved by mixing equal volumes of fresh culture in late logarithmic growth at a minimum density of 1×10^8 bacteria/ml with *Leptospira* storage medium (see recipe above) (Zuerner 2005). Alternatively, cultures can be frozen in EMJH liquid medium (Samir and Wasfy 2013). Two milliliter aliquots are prepared in sterile cryogenic vials, and the tubes are pre-cooled at −70 °C for 4 h prior to freezing in liquid nitrogen (Zuerner 2005). Long-term leptospiral viability is best maintained by the addition of the cryoprotectant dimethylsulphoxide (DMSO; 5 % vol/vol) prior to freezing (Palit et al. 1986). The viability of the samples should be checked within a month of freezing by thawing and re-inoculating into liquid media (for laboratory-adapted strains) or semisolid media (for fastidious strains) (Zuerner 2005).

Acknowledgments   The author thanks Rebecca Hof and Dr. Timothy Witchell for critical reading of the chapter and for assistance with figure preparation.

References

Baseman JB, Cox CD (1969) Terminal electron transport in *Leptospira*. J Bacteriol 97:1001–1004
Bolin C Unpublished observations
Bromley DB, Charon NW (1979) Axial filament involvement in the motility of *Leptospira interrogans*. J Bacteriol 137:1406–1412
Bulach DM, Zuerner RL, Wilson P et al (2006) Genome reduction in *Leptospira borgpetersenii* reflects limited transmission potential. Proc Natl Acad Sci USA 103:14560–14565
Carleton O, Charon NW, Allender P et al (1979) Helix handedness of *Leptospira interrogans* as determined by scanning electron microscopy. J Bacteriol 137:1413–1416
Chakraborty A, Miyahara S, Villanueva SY et al (2011) A novel combination of selective agents for isolation of *Leptospira* species. Microbiol Immunol 55:494–501
Charon NW, Goldstein SF (2002) Genetics of motility and chemotaxis of a fascinating group of bacteria: the spirochetes. Ann Rev Genet 36:47–73
Charon NW, Lawrence CW, O'Brien S (1981) Movement of antibody-coated latex beads attached to the spirochete *Leptospira interrogans*. Proc Natl Acad Sci USA 78:7166–7170
Corin RE, Boggs E, Cox CD (1978) Enzymatic degradation of H_2O_2 by *Leptospira*. Infect Immun 22:672–675
Ellinghausen HC Jr, McCullough WG (1965) Nutrition of *Leptospira pomona* and growth of 13 other serotypes: fractionation of oleic albumin complex and a medium of bovine albumin and polysorbate 80. Am J Vet Res 26:45–51
Ellis WA, Hovind-Hougen K, Moller S et al (1983) Morphological changes upon subculturing of freshly isolated strains of *Leptospira interrogans* serovar Hardjo. Zentralbl Bakteriol Mikrobiol Hyg A 255:323–335
Ellis WA, Thiermann AB (1986) Isolation of *Leptospira interrogans* serovar bratislava from sows in Iowa. Am J Vet Res 47:1458–1460
Eshghi A, Lourdault K, Murray GL et al (2012) *Leptospira interrogans* catalase is required for resistance to H_2O_2 and for virulence. Infect Immun 80:3892–3899

Evangelista KV, Coburn J (2010) *Leptospira* as an emerging pathogen: a review of its biology, pathogenesis and host immune responses. Future Microbiol 5:1413–1425

Faine S (1959) Iron as a growth requirement for pathogenic *Leptospira*. J Gen Microbiol 20:246–251

Faine S (1994) *Leptospira* and *leptospirosis*. CRC Press, Boca Raton

Faine S, Adler B, Bolin C et al (1999) *Leptospira* and *leptospirosis*. MedSci, Melbourne

Goldstein SF, Charon NW (1988) Motility of the spirochete *Leptospira*. Cell Motil Cytoskelet 9:101–110

Goldstein SF, Charon NW (1990) Multiple-exposure photographic analysis of a motile spirochete. Proc Natl Acad Sci USA 87:4895–4899

Haake DA (2006). The hamster model of leptospirosis. Current protocol microbiology chapter 12, unit 12E.2

Henneberry RC, Cox CD (1970) Beta-oxidation of fatty acids by *Leptospira*. Can J Microbiol 16:41–45

Holt SC (1978) Anatomy and chemistry of spirochetes. Microbiol Rev 42:114–160

Hovind-Hougen K (1976) Determination by means of electron microscopy of morphological criteria of value for classification of some spirochetes, in particular treponemes. Acta Pathol Microbiol Scand Suppl 255:1–41

Johnson RC, Harris VG (1967) Differentiation of pathogenic and saprophytic leptospires. I. Growth at low temperatures. J Bacteriol 94:27–31

Johnson RC, Harris VG, Walby JK (1969) Characterization of leptospires according to fatty acid requirements. J Gen Microbiol 55:399–407

Johnson RC, Livermore BP, Walby JK et al (1970) Lipids of parasitic and saprophytic leptospires. Infect Immun 2:286–291

Johnson RC, Rogers P (1964) Differentiation of pathogenic and saprophytic leptospires with 8-azaguanine. J Bacteriol 88:1618–1623

Kadis S, Pugh WL (1974) Urea utilization by *Leptospira*. Infect Immun 10:793–801

Kaiser GE, Doetsch RN (1975) Letter: enhanced translational motion of *Leptospira* in viscous environments. Nature 255:656–657

Kayser A, Adrian M (1978) Spirochetes: coiling direction. Ann Microbiol (Paris) 129:351–360

Kefford B, Marshall KC (1984) Adhesion of *Leptospira* at a solid-liquid interface: a model. Arch Microbiol 138:84–88

Khisamov GZ, Morozova NK (1988) Fatty acids as resource of carbon for leptospirae. J Hyg Epidemiol Microbiol Immunol 32:87–93

Korthof G (1932) Experimentelles Schlammfieber beim Menschen. Zentralbl Bakteriol, Parasitenkunde Hyg Abt I 125:429–434

Lambert A, Picardeau M, Haake DA et al (2012) FlaA proteins in *Leptospira interrogans* are essential for motility and virulence but are not required for formation of the flagellum sheath. Infect Immun 80:2019–2025

Lawrence JJ (1951) The growth of *Leptospirae* in semi-solid media. Aust J Exp Biol Med Sci 29:195–199

Li C, Motaleb A, Sal M et al (2000) Spirochete periplasmic flagella and motility. J Mol Microbiol Biotechnol 2:345–354

Li C, Wolgemuth CW, Marko M et al (2008) Genetic analysis of spirochete flagellin proteins and their involvement in motility, filament assembly, and flagellar morphology. J Bacteriol 190:5607–5615

Liao S, Sun A, Ojcius DM et al (2009) Inactivation of the *fliY* gene encoding a flagellar motor switch protein attenuates mobility and virulence of *Leptospira interrogans* strain Lai. BMC Microbiol 9:253

Malmstrom J, Beck M, Schmidt A et al (2009) Proteome-wide cellular protein concentrations of the human pathogen *Leptospira interrogans*. Nature 460:762–765

Motaleb MA, Corum L, Bono JL et al (2000) *Borrelia burgdorferi* periplasmic flagella have both skeletal and motility functions. Proc Natl Acad Sci USA 97:10899–10904

Murray GL, Srikram A, Henry R et al (2010) Mutations affecting *Leptospira interrogans* lipopolysaccharide attenuate virulence. Mol Microbiol 78:701–709

Nahori MA, Fournie-Amazouz E, Que-Gewirth NS et al (2005) Differential TLR recognition of leptospiral lipid A and lipopolysaccharide in murine and human cells. J Immunol 175:6022–6031

Nascimento AL, Ko AI, Martins EA et al (2004a) Comparative genomics of two *Leptospira interrogans* serovars reveals novel insights into physiology and pathogenesis. J Bacteriol 186:2164–2172

Nascimento AL, Verjovski-Almeida S, Van Sluys MA et al (2004b) Genome features of *Leptospira interrogans* serovar Copenhageni. Braz J Med Biol Res 37:459–477

Palit A, Haylock LM, Cox JC (1986) Storage of pathogenic leptospires in liquid nitrogen. J Appl Bacteriol 61:407–411

Petrino MG, Doetsch RN (1978) 'Viscotaxis', a new behavioural response of *Leptospira interrogans* (*biflexa*). strain B16. J Gen Microbiol 109:113–117

Picardeau M, Brenot A, Saint Girons I (2001) First evidence for gene replacement in Leptospira spp. Inactivation of L. biflexa flaB results in non-motile mutants deficient in endoflagella. Mol Microbiol 40:189–199

Picardeau M, Bulach DM, Bouchier C et al (2008) Genome sequence of the saprophyte *Leptospira biflexa* provides insights into the evolution of *Leptospira* and the pathogenesis of leptospirosis. PLoS ONE 3:e1607

Raddi G, Morado DR, Yan J et al (2012) Three-dimensional structures of pathogenic and saprophytic *Leptospira* species revealed by cryo-electron tomography. J Bacteriol 194:1299–1306

Ren SX, Fu G, Jiang XG et al (2003) Unique physiological and pathogenic features of *Leptospira interrogans* revealed by whole-genome sequencing. Nature 422:888–893

Ricaldi JN, Fouts DE, Selengut JD et al (2012) Whole genome analysis of *Leptospira licerasiae* provides insight into leptospiral evolution and pathogenicity. PLoS Negl Trop Dis 6:e1853

Samir A, Wasfy MO (2013) A simple technique for long-term preservation of leptospires. J Basic Microbiol 53:299–301

Shenberg E (1967) Growth of pathogenic *Leptospira* in chemically defined media. J Bacteriol 93:1598–1606

Slamti L, de Pedro MA, Guichet E et al (2011) Deciphering morphological determinants of the helix-shaped *Leptospira*. J Bacteriol 193:6266–6275

Stalheim OH, Wilson JB (1964a) Cultivation of *Leptosirae*. I. Nutrition of Leptospira canicola. J Bacteriol 88:48–54

Stalheim OH, Wilson JB (1964b) Cultivation of Leptospirae. II. Growth and lysis in synthetic medium. J Bacteriol 88:55–59

Staneck JL, Henneberry RC, Cox CD (1973) Growth requirements of pathogenic *Leptospira*. Infect Immun 7:886–897

Stern N, Shenberg E, Tietz A (1969) Studies on the metabolism of fatty acids in *Leptospira*: the biosynthesis of delta 9- and delta 11-monounsaturated acids. Eur J Biochem 8:101–108

Stuart RD (1946) The preparation and use of a simple culture medium for leptospirae. J Pathol Bacteriol 58:343–349

Takabe K, Nakamura S, Ashihara M et al (2013) Effect of osmolarity and viscosity on the motility of pathogenic and saprophytic *Leptospira*. Microbiol Immunol 57:236–239

Werts C, Tapping RI, Mathison JC et al (2001) Leptospiral lipopolysaccharide activates cells through a TLR2-dependent mechanism. Nat Immunol 2:346–352

Wolbach SB, Binger CA (1914) Notes on a filterable Spirochete from fresh Water. *Spirocheta biflexa* (new species). J Med Res 30:23–26

Wolgemuth CW, Charon NW, Goldstein SF et al (2006) The flagellar cytoskeleton of the spirochetes. J Mol Microbiol Biotechnol 11:221–227

Wuthiekanun V, Chierakul W, Limmathurotsakul D et al (2007) Optimization of culture of *Leptospira* from humans with leptospirosis. J Clin Microbiol 45:1363–1365

Xue F, Dong H, Wu J et al (2010) Transcriptional responses of *Leptospira interrogans* to host innate immunity: significant changes in metabolism, oxygen tolerance, and outer membrane. PLoS Negl Trop Dis 4:e857

Yoshii Z (1978) Studies on the spatial direction of the *Leptospira* cell body. Proc Jap Acad Series B 54(B):200–205

Zhang Q, Zhang Y, Zhong Y et al (2011) *Leptospira interrogans* encodes an ROK family glucokinase involved in a cryptic glucose utilization pathway. Acta Biochim Biophys Sin (Shanghai) 43:618–629

Zhong Y, Chang X, Cao XJ et al (2011) Comparative proteogenomic analysis of the *Leptospira interrogans* virulence-attenuated strain IPAV against the pathogenic strain 56601. Cell Res 21:1210–1229

Zuerner RL (2005) Laboratory maintenance of pathogenic *Leptospira*. Current protocol microbiology chapter 12, unit 12E.1

Genomics, Proteomics, and Genetics of *Leptospira*

Mathieu Picardeau

Abstract Recent advances in molecular genetics, such as the ability to construct defined mutants, have allowed the study of virulence factors and more generally the biology in *Leptospira*. However, pathogenic leptospires remain much less easily transformable than the saprophyte *L. biflexa* and further development and improvement of genetic tools are required. Here, we review tools that have been used to genetically manipulate *Leptospira*. We also describe the major advances achieved in both genomics and postgenomics technologies, including transcriptomics and proteomics.

Contents

M. Picardeau (✉)
"Biology of Spirochetes" Unit, Institut Pasteur, 28 Rue Du Docteur Roux,
75724 Paris Cedex 15, France
e-mail: mathieu.picardeau@pasteur.fr

© Springer-Verlag Berlin Heidelberg 2015   43
B. Adler (ed.), *Leptospira and Leptospirosis*, Current Topics in Microbiology
and Immunology 387, DOI 10.1007/978-3-662-45059-8_4

1 Genomics

1.1 Genome Organization

The first nucleotide sequences of *Leptospira*, consisting of genes involved in amino acid biosynthesis and ribosomal DNA, were published in the 1980s (Fukunaga et al. 1989; Yelton and Cohen 1986). In 2003 and 2004, *L. interrogans* serovars Lai (Ren et al. 2003) and Copenhageni (Nascimento et al. 2004) were the first two *Leptospira* genomes to be sequenced. Both strains, which are representatives of the most predominant pathogenic *Leptospira* strains in China (Zhang et al. 2012a) and Brazil (Ko et al. 1999), respectively, belong to the serogroup Icterohaemorrhagiae. The two genomes exhibit 95 % identity at the nucleotide level and consist of a large circular chromosome (4,277 kb, 35 mol% GC) and a smaller replicon (350 kb, 35 mol% GC). The majority of the *L. interrogans* chromosomes are collinear except for a few gaps and a large inversion in the large chromosome (Nascimento et al. 2004). The availability of complete genome sequences of the saprophyte *L. biflexa* (Picardeau et al. 2008), the intermediate *L. licerasiae* (Ricaldi et al. 2012a) and pathogenic species other than *L. interrogans* (Bulach et al. 2006; Chou et al. 2012) provide insight into genome features in the three phylogenetic groups (Table 1). This picture will be completed soon with the release of whole genome sequences for additional *Leptospira* species as well as a diverse and representative set of pathogenic *Leptospira* strains (www.jcvi.com).

Leptospira spp. have a relatively large genome (>3.9 Mb) when compared to other spirochetes, such as *Treponema pallidum* (1.1 Mb) (Fraser et al. 1998) and *Borrelia burgdorferi* (1.5 Mb) (Fraser et al. 1997). All members of the *Leptospira* genus that have been analyzed carry at least two circular replicons (Zuerner 1991). The large circular chromosomes (cI, >3.6 Mb) have a gene density of 75–92 % and encode largely housekeeping functions. The small second replicon, also called cII, ranges in size from 278 to 350 kb and carries essential genes such as *metF* (encoding methylene tetrahydrofolate reductase) and *asd* (encoding aspartate semialdehyde dehydrogenase) (Bourhy and Saint Girons 2000; Zuerner et al. 1993). Contrary to the typical replication origin of bacterial circular chromosomes consisting of the *dnaA-dnaN-recF-gyrA-gyrB* locus, leptospiral small replicons have plasmid or phage replication and partitioning systems. A third circular replicon, called p74 (74 kb, 36 mol% GC), has been identified by whole genome sequencing only in *L. biflexa*. These secondary replicons (p74 and cII) can be considered as "chromids" (Harrison et al. 2010) for two reasons; first, these replicons carry core genes located on the large chromosomes in other *Leptospira* species (Picardeau et al. 2008) and secondly, they have nucleotide compositions and codon usage that are very similar to those of the large chromosomes with which they are associated. Plasmids or prophages may become chromids as a result of the acquisition of core genes from the large chromosome into the smaller replicons. Complete (nondraft) genome sequences will be necessary to further determine the presence of extra-chromosomal elements in the *Leptospira* genus.

Table 1 Summary of genome features of pathogenic, intermediate, and saprophytic *Leptospira* spp

Leptospira spp. (strain)	Pathogenicity	Host or source	Genome size (Mbp)	Sequence	G +C (%)	CDS[a]	rRNA (5S, 16S, 23S)	Transposases	References
L. borgpetersenii (L550)	Strict pathogen	Human (Australia)	~3.9	Complete	40.2	2,842	5	121	(Bulach et al. 2006)
L. borgpetersenii (JB197)	Strict pathogen	Cattle (USA)	~3.9	Complete	40.2	2,770	5	126	(Bulach et al. 2006)
L. interrogans (Fiocruz L1-130)	Pathogen	Human (Brazil)	~4.6	Complete	35.1	3,379	5	26	(Nascimento et al. 2004)
L. interrogans (Lai 56601)	Pathogen	Human (China)	~4.7	Complete	35.1	3,663	5	55	(Ren et al. 2003; Zhong et al. 2011)
L. santarosai (LT821)	Pathogen	Human (Taiwan)	~3.9	Draft	41.8	3,990	5	43	(Chou et al. 2012)
L. biflexa (Paris)	Non pathogen	Water (Italy)	~4.0	Complete	38.9	3,590	6	10	(Picardeau et al. 2008)
L. licerasiae (VAR010)	Intermediate	Human (Peru)	~4.2	Draft	41.6	3,931	4	1	(Ricaldi et al. 2012a)

[a] Excluding transposases and pseudogenes

1.2 General Features of the Genomes

The genome of *Leptospira* is characterized by a G+C content of 35–42 mol%, depending on the species, with a genome size ranging between 3.9 and 4.6 Mbp (Table 1). There are between one and two of each of the rRNA genes in *Leptospira*. In contrast to the situation in many other bacteria where the 16S (*rrs*), 23S (*rrl*), and 5S (*rrf*) rRNA genes are clustered and co-transcribed, those in *Leptospira* are widely scattered on the large chromosome (Baril et al. 1992a; Saint Girons et al. 1992). Slow-growing pathogenic species *L. interrogans* and *L. borgpetersenii* and the faster growing intermediate *L. liceraasiae* and saprophyte *L. biflexa* have a similar number (35–37) of transfer RNA (tRNA) genes (Picardeau et al. 2008; Ricaldi et al. 2012a).

Several insertion sequences such as IS*1500* (Boursaux–Eude et al. 1995), IS*1502* (Zuerner and Huang 2002), and IS*1533* (Zuerner 1994) have been identified in *Leptospira*. The copy number of these IS elements varies considerably between serovars and between the isolates of a given serovar. The recent sequencing of *Leptospira* genomes allowed the identification of several other IS elements, one example being IS*lin1* (Nascimento et al. 2004). These IS elements belong to a diverse range of IS families, including IS*110*, IS*3*, and IS*4* (Cerqueira and Picardeau 2009; Nascimento et al. 2004). The number of insertion sequences in *L. borgpetersenii* (mostly from the IS*110* family) is much higher than those in *L. biflexa*, *L. liceraasiae*, and *L. interrogans* (Bulach et al. 2006) (Table 1). Genome reduction in *L. borgpetersenii* serovar Hardjo (see below) may be the result of genomic deletions or rearrangements mediated by IS elements.

A few phage related genomic islands have been characterized in *L. interrogans* and *L. liceraasiae* (Bourhy et al. 2007; Qin et al. 2008; Ricaldi et al. 2012a), but many more laterally acquired regions can been detected in the genomes of *Leptospira*. Although nothing is known about phages that may infect pathogenic *Leptospira*, it was shown previously that one of these genomic islands can excise from the *L. interrogans* chromosome and form a circular intermediate (Bourhy et al. 2007). In the saprophytes, the genome of the temperate leptophage LE1, with morphology similar to group A1 in the family *Myoviridae* (Saint Girons et al. 1990) (Fig. 1), was fully sequenced (Bourhy et al. 2005a). The 74 kb LE1 prophage, which can replicate as a circular replicon in *L. biflexa* (Saint Girons et al. 2000), has a GC content of 36 %, similar to that of *Leptospira* spp. Most of the 79 predicted coding sequences (CDS) display no similarity to known CDS, but 21 CDS appeared to be organized in clusters that might encode head and tail structural proteins and immunity repressor proteins (Bourhy et al. 2005a).

1.3 Gene Content and Evolution of Leptospira Species

The original genome annotation of *L. interrogans* serovar Lai strain 56601 (Ren et al. 2003) revealed 4,727 CDS. However, after re-sequencing, reannotation and proteomic analysis, 1,088 CDS have been removed from the previous version,

Fig. 1 *Leptophage*. Electron micrograph of phages of the saprophyte *L. biflexa* negatively stained with uranyl acetate (courtesy of Isabelle Saint Girons, Institut Pasteur, Paris, France). The bar represents 200 nm

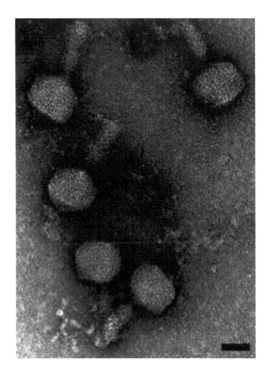

mostly due to the short (30 codons) cutoff value used initially; 79 CDS have been added, resulting in a total of 3,718 CDS (Zhong et al. 2011). A high-passage, virulence-attenuated isolate of serovar Lai was also sequenced, revealing extensive conservation of gene content and gene order with the virulent isolate. Mutations (insertions, deletions, and single-nucleotide variations) were detected in 101 genes (2.7 % of total gene content) (Zhong et al. 2011). DNA microarray hybridization also revealed a high similarity in the gene content among 11 *L. interrogans* strains from different serovars (He et al. 2007). Gene redundancy is more common in *L. interrogans* in comparison to the saprophytes (Picardeau et al. 2008). Family members within a genome, the paralogs, are believed to be products of gene duplication. For example, *L. interrogans* has an expanded repertoire of approximately 20 genes encoding proteins with Leucine Rich Repeat (LRR) domains. Some of these genes are present in clusters, suggesting that they originally arose from duplication events. The presence of conserved repeat sequences makes them naturally prone to recombination, and may be at the origin of their diversity.

The *L. borgpetersenii* serovar Hardjo genomes contain about 2,800 CDS and are 700 kb smaller than that of *L. interrogans*. Gene content analyses also showed that the Hardjo genomes carry numerous pseudogenes and mobile elements (approximately

12 % of the CDS encode transposases or are pseudogenes). Genome size reduction and ongoing gene and function decay in serovar Hardjo correlate with the restricted niche of the sequenced strains, which are responsible for chronic infections in cattle, and their inability to survive outside of the host (Bulach et al. 2006).

The genome sequences of *L. biflexa*, *L. interrogans*, *L. borgpetersenii*, *L. santarosai*, and *L. licerasiae* contain approximately 35 % putative protein coding genes with no assigned function (Bulach et al. 2006; Chou et al. 2012; Nascimento et al. 2004; Picardeau et al. 2008; Ren et al. 2003; Ricaldi et al. 2012a). Comparison of the proteins across the genomes has revealed a common backbone of 1,547 proteins for this genus (Ricaldi et al. 2012a). Most of the core genes with assigned functions are housekeeping genes (DNA replication, repair, cell division, transcription, translation, energy metabolism, etc.); others include ATP-binding cassettes (ABC) transporters ($\approx$80 genes), lipoproteins ($\approx$150 genes), and flagellum and chemotaxis genes ($\approx$80 genes). The genome of *Leptospira* spp., unlike most other spirochetes, contains a locus including the genes necessary for the biosynthesis of the lipolysaccharide (LPS) (de la Peña Moctezuma et al. 2001). Comparison with other spirochetes (*T. pallidum*, *T. denticola*, and *B. burgdorferi*) revealed a common backbone of 618 CDS conserved in all spirochetes but not found in other phyla. This subset includes genes involved in the biosynthesis of the periplasmic flagellum which has a unique structure in bacteria (Seshadri et al. 2004).

The saprophyte *L. biflexa* has many more genes encoding environmental sensing and metabolic proteins when compared to pathogenic species, reflecting its capacity to survive in diverse environments (Picardeau et al. 2008). The pathogenic species *L. interrogans* and *L. borgpetersenii* display sequence similarity in 2,708 genes and sequence similarity in 2,100 genes with the saprophyte *L. biflexa* (Picardeau et al. 2008). Essentially, no synteny (conservation of gene order) exists between the *L. biflexa* and *L. interrogans* genomes (Picardeau et al. 2008). Comparative genomics of the pathogens *L. interrogans* and *L. borgpetersenii* and the saprophyte *L. biflexa* has allowed the identification of 893 pathogen-specific genes. In this subset of pathogen-specific genes, the genes encoding proteins of unknown function are over-represented. Thus of the 655 proteins unique to *L. interrogans*, 78 % have no known function, suggesting the presence of pathogenic mechanisms unique to *Leptospira* (Adler et al. 2011; Picardeau et al. 2008). The intermediate *L. licerasiae* shares 2,237 genes with *L. interrogans*, 2,077 genes with *L. borgpetersenii*, and 1,898 genes with *L. biflexa* (Ricaldi et al. 2012a). *L. licerasiae* also has the highest average protein identity with the pathogens and genes encoding putative virulence factors such as LipL32 and LigB are found in the intermediate species. These data suggest that *L. licerasiae*, which occupies an intermediate position between the pathogens and saprophytes based on 16S rRNA phylogeny, is more closely related to the pathogenic *Leptospira* species than to the saprophytes (Ricaldi et al. 2012a).

1.4 Gene Regulation

Multiple reports using both microarray and quantitative reverse transcriptase (RT)-PCR approaches have shown that *Leptospira* responds to altered environmental conditions at the RNA level.

The identification of over 200 genes encoding signal transduction proteins (not including chemotaxis proteins) in each *Leptospira* genome in the Microbial Signal Transduction database (MiSTDB2) (Ulrich and Zhulin 2010) suggests that *Leptospira* is capable of responding to a diverse array of environmental signals. For example, the genome of *L. biflexa* serovar Patoc possesses 95 two-component systems, encoding either the sensor histidine kinase, response regulators, or both. One of these two-component systems in *L. biflexa* has been demonstrated to be involved in the regulation of the heme biosynthetic pathway (Louvel et al. 2008; Morero et al. 2014). A total of 140 and 86 DNA-binding domains have been identified among proteins of *L. biflexa* serovar Patoc and *L. interrogans* serovar Copenhageni, respectively. For example, four regulatory proteins of the ferric uptake regulator (FUR) family were identified in the *Leptospira* genomes (Louvel et al. 2006), including a PerR homolog which was shown to act as a regulator of the oxidative stress response following transcriptome analysis of a *perR* mutant (Lo et al. 2010). The KdpE sensor was shown to be an activator of the KdpABC potassium transporter (Matsunaga and Coutinho 2012) and the *L. interrogans* LexA repressor binds the palindrome TTTGN(5)CAAA found in the *recA* promoter (Cuñé et al. 2005).

Sigma factors allow sequence-specific binding of RNA polymerase to bacterial promoters. The *Leptospira* genomes carry genes for sigma-54 (RpoN) and sigma-70 (RpoD) and a variable number of alternative sigma factors. For example, the genomes of *L. biflexa* serovar Patoc and *L. interrogans* serovar Copenhageni have 10 ECF sigma factors (Ulrich and Zhulin 2010). *Leptospira* also possesses anti-sigma factors and antisigma factor antagonists that are regulatory proteins that control sigma factor functions in promoter recognition and initiation of RNA polymerase. Prediction of DNA motifs that are targets of RNA polymerases, sigma factors and transcription factors is a difficult mission, due mainly to undiscovered features in *Leptospira* DNA sequences or structures in leptospiral promoter regions (Ballard et al. 1993). Experimentally proven transcription factor binding sites have not been described in the literature and promoter prediction algorithms and *E. coli* consensus sequences of DNA motifs are not always appropriate for *Leptospira*.

Bacterial small ($\sim$30–500 nt) noncoding RNAs (sRNAs) are an emerging class of posttranscriptional regulators which play a variety of important roles in many biological processes. sRNAs typically function by binding near the translation start site of their target mRNAs and thereby inhibit or activate translation. Studies on sRNA regulation of gene expression in *Leptospira* are currently in their infancy. sRNA-mediated regulation may contribute to the lack of correlation between transcript and protein levels of known temperature-regulated proteins (Lo et al. 2009). High-throughput RNA sequencing allowed the identification of 11 sRNAs in

L. interrogans, five of these are homologous to the tmRNA, RNaseP, PyrR binding site and cobalamin sRNA families, but their functions remains to be determined (Caimano et al. 2014). The cobalamin (vitamin B_{12}) and thiamine pyrophosphate riboswitches have also been described in *L. licerasiae* and other *Leptospira* genomes (Ricaldi et al. 2012a). A temperature-sensing riboswitch was shown to be responsible for the regulation of *ligA* and *ligB* expression in *L. interrogans* (Matsunaga et al. 2013). Genome analysis identified few loci with Clustered Regularly Interspaced Short Palindromic Repeats (CRISPRs) in *L. interrogans* (http://crispr.u-psud.fr/crispr/). These sRNAs have been described as conferring resistance against invading phages and plasmids. *Leptospira* spp. contain one gene encoding the RNA binding protein Hfq which, in other organisms, facilitates base pairing between a class of sRNA, called trans-encoded sRNA, and its target mRNA.

2 Post-genomics and Proteomics

Humans usually get infected by *Leptospira* through contact with environmental water contaminated with the urine of rodents. *Leptospira* therefore undergoes several environmental transitions (changes in temperature, pH, osmolarity, nutrient content, and concentration, etc.). However, in vitro culture conditions are very different from conditions found inside the host or in the environment: the *Leptospira* culture medium, EMJH, is an enriched medium of low osmolarity (67 mOsm, in comparison to the physiological level of 300 mOsm) and the optimal cultivation temperature is 30 °C. To study global changes at the mRNA and protein levels, genome-wide transcriptome and proteome analysis have been recently performed in *Leptospira*.

2.1 Transcriptomics

Whole genome microarrays have been used to determine global changes in transcript levels of *L. interrogans* in response to interaction with phagocytic cells (Xue et al. 2010), temperature (Lo et al. 2006; Qin et al. 2006), osmolarity (Matsunaga et al. 2007), iron depletion (Lo et al. 2010), and serum exposure (Patarakul et al. 2010), which are relevant to changes that occur during acute and chronic disease. High-throughput RNA sequencing has been recently used to study the transcriptome of leptospires cultivated in dialysis membrane chambers implanted into the peritoneal cavities of rats (Caimano et al. 2014). Experiments utilizing RT-PCR have also been used to show that *L. interrogans* differentially regulates gene expression in resistant and susceptible animal models, showing, for example, that *ligB* and *ompL37* are upregulated in the blood of infected animals in comparison to in vitro cultures (Matsui et al. 2012).

2.2 Proteomics

At the protein level, the highest number of proteins reported in a single study to date has been 2,673 proteins in cultures of *L. interrogans* serovar Lai (Cao et al. 2010). It must be noted that in standard leptospiral culture medium (67 mOsm, 30 °C, exponential phase culture), some proteins, including LigA/LigB (Matsunaga et al. 2005), LipL36 (Haake et al. 1998), heat shock proteins (Nally et al. 2001), are not detectable or expressed at low levels. Other comparative proteomic analysis of in vitro cultures of *L. interrogans* provided evidence for differential protein expression in response to temperature, iron limitation, and serum presence (Cullen et al. 2002; Eshghi et al. 2009; Lo et al. 2009).

Several studies have determined the subcellular location for various proteins (Haake and Matsunaga 2010). However, the localization and function of some of them have remained controversial (Pinne and Haake 2013) and several complementary experiments are required to accurately identify the subcellular location of leptospiral proteins (Pinne and Haake 2009).

Nally et al. examined protein expression of intact leptospires in tissues and urine of infected animals and compared with that of in vitro-cultivated leptospires (Monahan et al. 2008; Nally et al. 2005a). In a further study, Nally et al. also examined proteins present in the soluble and membrane-associated fractions of the leptospires in infected tissues by taking advantage of the fact that hydrophobic protein antigens are selectively partitioned to the detergent phase following solubilization in Triton X-114. The proteome is then characterized by standard proteomic methodologies, including two-dimensional gel electrophoresis, immunoblotting and mass spectrometry (Nally et al. 2005b, 2007). In these studies, for example, Loa22 was found to be induced in "acute disease" conditions compared with in vitro-cultivated leptospires, whereas the lipo-polysaccharide content was downregulated during acute infection.

A novel approach combining cryo-electron tomography and quantitative mass spectrometry took advantage of the fact that leptospires are thin bacteria to determine protein abundances per *Leptospira* cell and identified protein complexes localized to specific cellular compartments (Beck et al. 2009; Malmström et al. 2009). This approach provided concentration estimates for $\sim 1,800$ proteins of *L. interrogans,* representing 51 % of the CDS of the genome, and showed, for example, that LipL32 is the most abundant protein of the entire cell at 38,000 copies per cell (Malmström et al. 2009). Visual proteomics also produces 3D snapshots of the cellular distributions of large complexes in responses to heat shock, antibiotic treatment, and starved conditions (Beck et al. 2009).

2.3 Posttranslational Modifications

The current understanding of posttranslational chemical modifications (PTMs) in *Leptospira* is limited. A global proteomic analysis identified 155 methylated, 32 phosphorylated, and 46 acetylated proteins in *L. interrogans* serovar Lai

(Cao et al. 2010). Another study showed the methylation of a surface-exposed protein (Eshghi et al. 2012b). Proteomic analysis also suggests that nonulosonic acids, which includes sialic acids, are synthesized by *L. interrogans* and used for modification of surface-exposed lipoproteins (Ricaldi et al. 2012b). These data suggest that PTMs are common in *L. interrogans* and may have an important role for protein function and/or host cell interactions.

3 Genetics

Knowledge of the genetics of *Leptospira* remains at a very early stage in comparison to that of other bacterial species. Prior to the year 2000, genetic analysis of *Leptospira* had been impeded by the lack of methods for the introduction of DNA into leptospiral cells. In the first genetic studies carried out in the 1990s, several *Leptospira* genes were isolated by the functional complementation of *E. coli* mutants. This method led to the identification of a number of amino acid biosynthesis genes, including *asd*, *aroD*, *dapD*, *metX*, *metY*, *trpE*, *proA* and *leuB* (Baril et al. 1992b; Belfaiza et al. 1998; Richaud et al. 1990; Yelton and Cohen 1986). Similarly, the *L. biflexa recA* gene was found to confer functional complementation of *recA* mutations in *E. coli* (Stamm et al. 1991).

3.1 Replicative Vectors, Markers, and Other Genetic Tools

DNA can be introduced by electroporation (Saint Girons et al. 2000) or conjugation between *E. coli* and *Leptospira* spp. (Fig. 2) using RP4 derivative conjugative plasmids (Picardeau 2008). Transformed *Leptospira* appears on solid medium, forming subsurface colonies, after 1 week (*L. biflexa*) to 4 weeks (*L. interrogans*) of incubation at 30 °C. Saint Girons et al. isolated and characterized three bacteriophages from sewage water, whose replication was limited to the saprophyte *L. biflexa* (Saint Girons et al. 1990). One of these phages, LE1, was shown to replicate as a circular plasmid in *L. biflexa* and was used as the basis for the first *L. biflexa*-*E. coli* plasmid shuttle vector (Saint Girons et al. 2000) (Fig. 3). More recently, cloning of the putative replication origins of the *L. biflexa* replicon p74 (Picardeau et al. 2008) and a phage-related genomic island from *L. interrogans* (Bourhy et al. 2007) have also been used to achieve autonomous replication in *L. biflexa*, but to date, there is no replicative plasmid vector available for pathogenic *Leptospira*. Replicative vectors enable, for example, the heterologous expression of the pathogen-specific genes *ligA* and *ligB* in the saprophyte *L. biflexa* (Figueira et al. 2011). The expression of LigA and LigB on the surface of *L. biflexa* had significant effects on adhesion of *lig*-transformed *L. biflexa* to fibronectin and cultured cells, suggesting the involvement of Lig proteins in cell adhesion. The saprophyte *L. biflexa*, which is a fast-growing leptospire, may therefore represent a

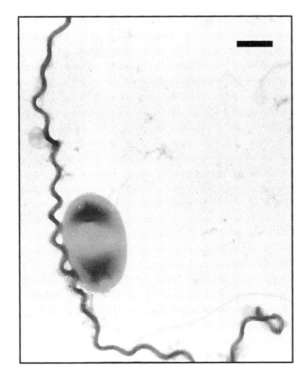

Fig. 2 *Conjugation between E. coli and L. biflexa*. Microscopic analysis of *E. coli* ß2163 and *L. biflexa* after filter mating. Intimate junctions are observed between the *L. biflexa* and *E. coli* membranes, suggesting that the DNA transfer from *E. coli* to *L. biflexa* occurs by a conjugative mechanism requiring close cell-to-cell contact between the donor and recipient cells. Electron microscopy of bacterial cells negatively stained with uranyl acetate. The bar represents 500 nm

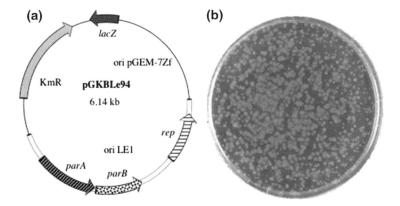

Fig. 3 *Development of shuttle vector in L. biflexa*. **a** Schematic representation of the *E. coli-L. biflexa* shuttle vector pGKBLe94 (Saint Girons et al. 2000). This plasmid vector contains the replication origin of the leptophage LE1, including the *rep* and *par* genes. KmR, kanamycin-resistance cassette. **b** Kanamycin-resistant colonies of *L. biflexa* obtained after transformation with pGKBLe94. EMJH plates supplemented with kanamycin were incubated for 1 week at 30 °C (*Leptospira* cells grow into the solid medium, forming subsurface colonies)

good surrogate host to characterize the role of key virulence factors contributing to leptospirosis.

Selectable markers used in *Leptospira* have included kanamycin (*Enterococcus faecalis* cassette), spectinomycin (*Staphylococcus aureus* cassette), and gentamicin (*Enterobacter cloacae* cassette) (Bauby et al. 2003; Bourhy et al. 2005b; Poggi et al. 2010; Saint Girons et al. 2000). Antibiotics such as penicillin and doxycycline should not be used because they are clinically useful for the treatment of patients with leptospirosis (Hardham and Rosey 2000). The commonly used counterselectable marker *sacB* was found to be unsuitable in *L. biflexa*, but the *rpsL* gene, which encodes the S12 ribosomal protein, was used as an efficient counterselectable marker in a *L. biflexa* streptomycin-resistant strain (Picardeau et al. 2001). The *Photorhabdus luminescens luxCDABE* cassette and *gfp* and *mRFP1* alleles have been transferred into *Leptospira* strains to produce luminescent and fluorescent leptospires, respectively (Aviat et al. 2010; Murray et al. 2010a). While the bacteria expressing the fluorescent and luminescent alleles were not sufficiently bright to be clearly visible from outside the infected animal or recorded with conventional microscopes, the *lux* construct could be used as a viability reporter for cell populations and the *gfp* construct can be used as a reporter gene system (Aviat et al. 2010; Cerqueira et al. 2011). A reporter gene system that enables translational fusion of leptospiral genes directly to the leptospiral chromosomal gene of *bgal* (β-galactosidase) has also been developed (Matsunaga and Coutinho 2012). The *E. coli lac* system is also functional in *Leptospira* and can be used to control the expression of genes (Aviat et al. 2010). For example, by using the LacI repressor-based system, it was possible to generate an *L. biflexa* strain that conditionally expresses the endogenous MreB, encoded by an essential gene involved in cell morphogenesis (Slamti et al. 2011).

3.2 Mutagenesis

Leptospira is difficult to manipulate genetically and development of techniques lags behind those available for other bacterial systems. Targeted mutagenesis was achieved in *L. biflexa* with a suicide plasmid delivering the inactivated allele to the targeted chromosomal gene (Fig. 4). However, in this species, treatment of the DNA used for transformation with UV or NaOH before electroporation is essential for the generation of large numbers of recombinants (Picardeau et al. 2001). Several chromosomal genes, including *flaB, trpE, metY, metX, metW, hemH*, and *recA*, have been disrupted using this approach in saprophytic strains (Louvel and Picardeau 2007). Because of poor efficiency of transformation and/or homologous recombination, there are few published reports of allelic replacement in pathogenic leptospires; they include inactivation of *ligB* (Croda et al. 2008), *mce* (Zhang et al. 2012b), *colA* (Kassegne et al. 2014), and *fliY* (Liao et al. 2009) in *L. interrogans* (Table 2).

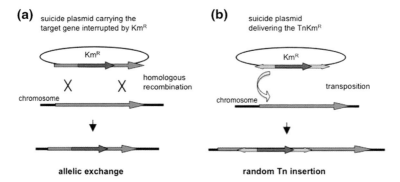

Fig. 4 *Schematic representation of targeted and random mutagenesis.* **a** For targeted mutagenesis, a suicide vector (i.e., not replicating in *Leptospira* spp.) is used to introduce an inactivated allele, which corresponds to the target gene interrupted by a resistance cassette, into the cell, thus replacing the wild-type copy by a double homologous recombination event. However, allelic exchanges are rare events and single crossover events, which usually result in a wild-type phenotype, are more frequent in *Leptospira* spp. **b** The *Himar1* transposon has been used successfully for random mutagenesis in *Leptospira* spp. A suicide plasmid containing the *Himar1* transposon carrying a kanamycin-resistant cassette and, located outside of the transposon, the C9 hyperactive transposase is used to deliver the transposon which randomly inserts into the chromosome

A system for random mutagenesis using the *Himar1 mariner* transposon has been developed in both saprophytic and pathogenic *Leptospira* spp. (Bourhy et al. 2005b; Louvel et al. 2005; Murray et al. 2009a) (Fig. 4). The efficiency of this approach is much higher in the saprophyte, where thousands of random mutants can be readily obtained in *L. biflexa*, thereby generating extensive libraries of mutants that could be screened for phenotypes affecting diverse aspects of metabolism and physiology, such as amino acid biosynthesis and iron acquisition systems (Louvel et al. 2005, 2006). While the *Himar1 mariner* transposon system is applicable to pathogenic *Leptospira* spp., the transformation efficiencies are 2–3 orders of magnitude lower than for *L. biflexa* (Bourhy et al. 2005b). Three years of trans-formation experiments performed simultaneously in two different laboratories, have generated a library of 1,000 distinct *L interrogans* mutants (Murray et al. 2009a). Of the 1,000 insertion sites, 721 of the mutations identified affected the protein coding regions of 551 different genes. Thus, to date, approximately 18 % of the nonessential genes of *L. interrogans* have been inactivated by transposon muta-genesis. A large set of random mutants has been analyzed in *L. interrogans*, including *lipL41* (King et al. 2013), *htpX* (Henry et al. 2013), *katE* (Eshghi et al. 2012a), *flaA1* and *flaA2* (Lambert et al. 2012), *clpB* (Lourdault et al. 2011), *hemO* (Murray et al. 2008), *lipL32* (Murray et al. 2009c), *lruA* (Zhang et al. 2013), *htpG* (King et al. 2014), and *perR* (Lo et al. 2010) (Table 2). A detailed discussion of the importance of the development of mutagenesis systems for elucidating pathogenesis is presented in chapter G.L. Murray.

Table 2 Selected mutants obtained in *Leptospira interrogans*

Inactivated gene	Strain[a]	Method	Virulence[b]	Additional phenotype (s)	References
ligB	Fiocruz L1-130	Allelic exchange	Normal	No attenuation of adherence to epithelial cells	(Croda et al. 2008)
mce	Lai 56601	Allelic exchange	Attenuated	Attenuation of adherence and invasion of macrophages	(Zhang et al. 2012b)
fliY	Lai 56601	Allelic exchange	Attenuated	Attenuation of motility	(Liao et al. 2009)
loa22	Lai 56601	Himar1	Attenuated		(Ristow et al. 2007)
hemO	L495	Himar1	Attenuated	Hemin-growth deficiency	(Murray et al. 2008, 2009b)
lipL32	L495	Himar1	Normal	No attenuation of adhesion to extracellular matrix	(Murray et al. 2009c)
katE	L495	Himar1	Attenuated	Increased susceptibility to oxidative stress	(Eshghi et al. 2012a)
lipL41	LT993	Himar1	Normal		(King et al. 2013)
perR	L495	Himar1	Normal	Increased resistance to peroxide stress	(Lo et al. 2010)
flaA2	L495	Himar1	Attenuated	Attenuation of motility	(Lambert et al. 2012)
clpB	Kito	Himar1	Attenuated	Resistance to stress conditions	(Lourdault et al. 2011)
htpX	Lai 56601	Himar1	Not tested	Production of an iron precipitate and formation of outer membrane vesicles	(Henry et al. 2013)
LA1641	L495	Himar1	Attenuated	Altered LPS	(Murray et al. 2010b)
lruA	L495	Himar1	Attenuated	Increased binding to the mammalian Apo-lipoprotein A-I	(Zhang et al. 2013)

[a] Lai 56601: *L. interrogans* serovar Lai strain Lai 56601, Fiocruz L1-130: *L. interrogans* serovar Copenhageni strain Fiocruz L1-130, L495: *L. interrogans* serovar Manilae strain L495, Kito: *L. interrogans* serogroup Canicola strain Kito, LT993: *L. interrogans* serovar Pomona strain LT993

[b] Virulence is usually tested by intraperitoneal infections in susceptible animal models (hamsters or guinea pigs)

4 Conclusions

Despite over one century of research and the availability of animal models that reproduce disease manifestation in humans, progress in understanding the biology of *Leptospira* has been slow and difficult. The lack of adequate and efficient genetic tools has impeded the application of Koch's molecular postulates to the study of pathogenic *Leptospira* strains. The basic requirement when using Koch's molecular postulates to demonstrate a causal relationship between a bacterial gene, its product and a defined phenotype is the ability to isolate null mutants and complement them by transferring DNA containing the wild-type gene into the mutated bacteria (Falkow 1988). The use of transposon libraries has been pivotal in identifying and characterizing the role of various genes in pathogenic *Leptospira* (Murray et al. 2009a). However, extrachromosomal cloning vectors have yet to be developed for the purpose of genetic complementation. One hypothesis to explain the difficulties encountered transforming leptospires is the presence of a higher number of restriction-modification systems within pathogenic strains when compared to the saprophytic strains, thereby inhibiting the maintenance of foreign DNA. Other crucial points are the low frequency of homologous recombination events in leptospires and the apparent large degree of functional redundancy of virulence-associated gene products. Other factors hindering the genetic analysis of *Leptospira* spp. are the complexity of their culture media, their slow growth and loss of virulence after several in vitro passages. Developing methods for the genetic manipulation of pathogenic strains is therefore still a challenge, as these fastidious bacteria cannot generally benefit from the genetic tools available for Gram-negative or Gram-positive organisms. At present, eight leptospiral genomes have been published, and many more are present in the databases. The new wealth of data generated by ongoing genome projects now has to be deciphered. Comparative genome analysis will provide an opportunity to identify features that are unique to pathogenic species. At the postgenomic level of research, proteomic studies can provide valuable information on the factors involved in the colonization process, leading to an acute or chronic infection in the hosts, and the survival in the environment. Technologies such as transcriptome deep sequencing should also provide insight into the transcriptional landscape of the *Leptospira* genome (transcriptional start sites, operon mapping, etc.) and identify small RNAs, providing a framework for the understanding of leptospiral biology.

Acknowledgments Original work in the author's laboratory was supported by Institut Pasteur and Agence Nationale de la Recherche (05-JCJC-0105 and 08-MIE-018).

References

Adler B, Lo M, Seemann T, Murray GL (2011) Pathogenesis of leptospirosis: the influence of genomics. Vet Microbiol 153:73–81

Aviat F, Slamti L, Cerqueira GM, Lourdault KMP (2010) Expanding the genetic toolbox for Leptospira species by generation of fluorescent bacteria. Appl Environ Microbiol 76:8135–8142

Ballard SA, Segers RP, Bleumink-Pluym N, Fyfe J, Faine S, Adler B (1993) Molecular analysis of the *hsp* (*groE*) operon of *Leptospira interrogans* serovar copenhageni. Mol Microbiol 8:739–751

Baril C, Herrmann JL, Richaud C, Margarita D, Girons IS (1992a) Scattering of the rRNA genes on the physical map of the circular chromosome of *Leptospira interrogans* serovar icterohaemorrhagiae. J Bacteriol 174:7566–7571

Baril C, Richaud C, Fournie E, Baranton G, Saint Girons I (1992b) Cloning of *dapD*, *aroD* and *asd* of *Leptospira interrogans* serovar icterohaemorrhagiae, and nucleotide sequence of the asd gene. J Gen Microbiol 138:47–53

Bauby H, Saint Girons I, Picardeau M (2003) Construction and complementation of the first auxotrophic mutant in the spirochaete *Leptospira meyeri*. Microbiology 149:689–693

Beck M, Malmström JA, Lange V, Schmidt A, Deutsch EW, Aebersold R (2009) Visual proteomics of the human pathogen *Leptospira interrogans*. Nat Methods 6:817–823

Belfaiza J, Martel A, Margarita D, Saint Girons I (1998) Direct sulfhydrylation for methionine biosynthesis in *Leptospira meyeri*. J Bacteriol 180:250–255

Bourhy P, Saint Girons I (2000) Localization of the *Leptospira interrogans metF* gene on the CII secondary chromosome. FEMS Microbiol Lett 191:259–263

Bourhy P, Frangeul L, Couve E, Glaser P, Saint Girons I, Picardeau M (2005a) Complete nucleotide sequence of the LE1 prophage from the spirochete *Leptospira biflexa* and characterization of its replication and partition functions. J Bacteriol 187:3931–3940

Bourhy P, Louvel H, Saint Girons I, Picardeau M (2005b) Random insertional mutagenesis of Leptospira interrogans, the agent of leptospirosis, using a *mariner* transposon. J Bacteriol 187:3255–3258

Bourhy P, Salaün L, Lajus A, Médigue C, Boursaux-Eude C, Picardeau M (2007) A genomic island of the pathogen *Leptospira interrogans* serovar Lai can excise from its chromosome. Infect Immun 75:677–683

Boursaux-Eude C, Saint Girons I, Zuerner RL (1995) IS1500, an IS3-like element from *Leptospira interrogans*. Microbiology 141:2165–2173

Bulach DM, Zuerner RL, Wilson P, Seemann T, McGrath A, Cullen PA, Davis J, Johnson M, Kuczek E, Alt DP, Peterson-Burch B, Coppel RL, Rood JI, Davies JK, Adler B (2006) Genome reduction in *Leptospira borgpetersenii* reflects limited transmission potential. Proc Natl Acad Sci USA 103:14560–14565

Caimano MJ, Sivasankaran SK, Allard A, Hurley D, Hokamp K, Grassmann AA, Hinton JC, Nally JE (2014) A model system for studying the transcriptomic and physiological changes associated with mammalian host-adaptation by *Leptospira interrogans* serovar Copenhageni. PLoS Pathog 13,10(3):e1004004

Cao XJ, Dai J, Xu H, Nie S, Chang X, Hu BY, Sheng QH, Wang LS, Ning ZB, Li YX, Guo XK, Zhao GP, Zeng R (2010) High-coverage proteome analysis reveals the first insight of protein modification systems in the pathogenic spirochete *Leptospira interrogans*. Cell Res 20:197–210

Cerqueira GM, Picardeau M (2009) A century of *Leptospira* strain typing. Infect Genet Evol 9:760–768

Cerqueira GM, Souza NM, Araújo ER, Barros AT, Morais ZM, Vasconcellos SA, Nascimento AL (2011) Development of transcriptional fusions to assess *Leptospira interrogans* promoter activity. PLoS ONE 6:e17409

Chou LF, Chen YT, Lu CW, Ko YC, Tang CY, Pan MJ, Tian YC, Chiu CH, Hung CC, Yang CW (2012) Sequence of *Leptospira santarosai* serovar Shermani genome and prediction of virulence-associated genes. Gene 11:364–370

Croda J, Figueira CP, Wunder EAJ, Santos CS, Reis MG, Ko AI, Picardeau M (2008) Targeted mutagenesis in pathogenic *Leptospira*: disruption of the *ligB* gene does not affect virulence in animal models of leptospirosis. Infect Immun 76:5826–5833

Cullen PA, Cordwell SJ, Bulach DM, Haake DA, Adler B (2002) Global analysis of outer membrane proteins from *Leptospira interrogans* serovar Lai. Infect Immun 70:2311–2318

Cuñé J, Cullen P, Mazon G, Campoy S, Adler B, Barbe J (2005) The *Leptospira interrogans lexA* gene is not autoregulated. J Bacteriol 187:5841–5845

DelaPeña-Moctezuma A, Bulach DM, Kalambaheti T, Adler B (2001) Genetic differences among the LPS biosynthetic loci of serovars of *Leptospira interrogans* and *Leptospira borgpetersenii*. FEMS Immunol Med 31:73–81

Eshghi A, Cullen PA, Cowen L, Zuerner RL, Cameron CE (2009) Global proteome analysis of *Leptospira interrogans*. J Proteome Res 8:4564–4578

Eshghi A, Lourdault K, Murray GL, Bartpho T, Sermswan RW, Picardeau M, Adler B, Snarr B, Zuerner RL, Cameron CE (2012a) *Leptospira interrogans* catalase is required for resistance to H$_2$O$_2$ and for virulence. Infect Imm 80(11):3892-3899

Eshghi A, Pinne M, Haake DA, Zuerner RL, Frank A, Cameron CE (2012b) Methylation and in vivo expression of the surface-exposed *Leptospira interrogans* outer-membrane protein OmpL32. Microbiology 158:622–635

Falkow S (1988) Molecular Koch's postulates applied to microbial pathogenicity. Rev Infect Dis 10:274–276

Figueira CP, Croda J, Choy HA, Haake DA, Reis MG, Ko AI, Picardeau M (2011) Heterologous expression of pathogen-specific genes *ligA* and *ligB* in the saprophyte *Leptospira biflexa* confers enhanced adhesion to cultured cells and fibronectin. BMC Microbiol 11:129

Fraser CM, Casjens S, Huang WM, Sutton GG, Clayton R, Lathigra R, White O, Ketchum KA, Dodson R, Hickey EK, Gwinn M, Dougherty B, Tomb JF, Fleischmann RD, Richardson D, Peterson J, Kerlavage AR, Quackenbush J, Salzberg S, Hanson M, Vanvugt R, Palmer N, Adams MD, Gocayne J, Weidman J et al (1997) Genomic sequence of a lyme disease spirochaete, *Borrelia burgdorferi*. Nature 390:580–586

Fraser CM, Norris SJ, Weinstock CM, White O, Sutton GG, Dodson R, Gwinn M, Hickey EK, Clayton R, Ketchum KA, Sodergren E, Hardham JM, McLeod MP, Salzberg S, Peterson J, Khalak H, Richardson D, Howell JK, Chidambaram M, Utterback T, McDonald L, Artiach P, Bowman C, Cotton MD, Fujii C et al (1998) Complete genome sequence of *Treponema pallidum*, the syphilis spirochete. Science 281:375–388

Fukunaga M, Horie I, Mifuchi I (1989) Nucleotide sequence of a 23S ribosomal RNA gene from *Leptospira interrogans* serovar canicola strain Moulton. Nucleic Acids Res 17:2123

Haake DA, Martinich C, Summers TA, Shang ES, Pruetz JD, McCoy AM, Mazel MK, Bolin CA (1998) Characterization of Leptospiral outer membrane lipoprotein LipL36: downregulation associated with late-log-phase growth and mammalian infection. Infect Immun 66:1579–1587

Haake DA, Matsunaga J (2010) *Leptospira*: a spirochaete with a hybrid outer membrane. Mol Microbiol 77:805-814

Hardham JM, Rosey EL (2000) Antibiotic selective markers and spirochete genetics. J Mol Microbiol Biotechnol 2:425–432

Harrison PW, Lower RP, Kim NK, Young JP (2010) Introducing the bacterial chromid: not a chromosome, not a plasmid. Trends Microbiol 18:141–148

He P, Sheng YY, Shi YZ, Jiang XG, Qin JH, Zhang ZM, Zhao GP, Guo XK (2007) Genetic diversity among major endemic strains of *Leptospira interrogans* in China. BMC Genom 8:204

Henry R, Lo M, Khoo C, Zhang H, Boysen RI, Picardeau M, Murray GL, Bulach DM, Adler B (2013) Iron precipitation on the surface of *Leptospira interrogans* is associated with mutation of the stress-response metalloprotease HtpX. Appl Environ Microbiol 79:4653–4660

Kassegne K, Hu W, Ojcius DM, Sun D, Ge Y, Zhao J, Yang XF, Li L, Yan J (2014) Identification of collagenase as a critical virulence factor for invasiveness and transmission of pathogenic *Leptospira* species. J Infect Dis 209:1105–1115

King AM, Bartpho T, Sermswan RW, Bulach DM, Eshghi A, Picardeau M, Adler B, Murray GL (2013) Leptospiral outer membrane protein LipL41 is not essential for acute leptospirosis, but requires a small chaperone, Lep, for stable expression. Infect Immun 81:2768–2776

King AM, Pretre G, Bartpho T, Sermswan RW, Toma C, Suzuki T, Eshghi A, Picardeau M, Adler B, Murray GL (2014) High temperature protein G (HtpG) is an essential virulence factor of *Leptospira interrogans*. Infect Immun 82:1123–1131

Ko AI, Galvao Reis M, Ribeiro Dourado CM, Johnson WD Jr, Riley LW (1999) Urban epidemic of severe leptospirosis in Brazil. Salvador Leptospirosis Study Group Lancet 354:820–825

Lambert A, Picardeau M, Haake DA, Sermswan RW, Srikram A, Adler B, Murray GA (2012) FlaA proteins in *Leptospira interrogans* are essential for motility and virulence but are not required for formation of the flagellum sheath. Infect Immun 80:2019–2025

Liao S, Sun A, Ojcius DM, Wu S, Zhao J, Yan J (2009) Inactivation of the fliY gene encoding a flagellar motor switch protein attenuates mobility and virulence of *Leptospira interrogans* strain Lai. BMC Microbiol 9:253

Lo M, Bulach DM, Powell DR, Haake DA, Matsunaga J, Paustian ML, Zuerner RL, Adler B (2006) Effects of temperature on gene expression patterns in *Leptospira interrogans* serovar Lai as assessed by whole-genome microarrays. Infect Immun 74:848–859

Lo M, Cordwell SJ, Bulach DM, Adler B (2009) Comparative transcriptional and translational analysis of *leptospiral* outer membrane protein expression in response to temperature. PLoS Negl Trop Dis 3:560

Lo M, Murray GL, Khoo CA, Haake DA, Zuerner RL, Adler B (2010) Transcriptional response of *Leptospira interrogans* to iron limitation and characterization of a PerR homolog. Infect Immun 78:4850–4859

Lourdault K, Cerqueira GM, Wunder EAMP (2011) Inactivation of *clpB* in the pathogen *Leptospira interrogans* reduces virulence and resistance to stress conditions. Infect Immun 79:3711–3717

Louvel H, Saint Girons I, Picardeau M (2005) Isolation and characterization of FecA- and FeoB-mediated iron acquisition systems of the spirochete *Leptospira biflexa* by random insertional mutagenesis. J Bacteriol 187:3249–3254

Louvel H, Bommezzadri S, Zidane N, Boursaux-Eude C, Creno S, Magnier A, Rouy Z, Medigue C, Girons IS, Bouchier C, Picardeau M (2006) Comparative and functional genomic analyses of iron transport and regulation in *Leptospira* spp. J Bacteriol 188:7893–7904

Louvel H, Picardeau M (2007) Genetic manipulation of *Leptospira biflexa*. Wiley, Hoboken

Louvel H, Betton JM, Picardeau M (2008) Heme rescues a two-component system *Leptospira biflexa* mutant. BMC Microbiol 8:25

Malmström J, Beck M, Schmidt A, Lange V, Deutsch EW, Aebersold R (2009) Proteome-wide cellular protein concentrations of the human pathogen *Leptospira interrogans*. Nature 460:762–765

Matsui M, Soupé ME, Becam J, Goarant C (2012) Differential in vivo gene expression of major *Leptospira* proteins in resistant or susceptible animal models. Appl Environ Microbiol 78:6372–6376

Matsunaga J, Sanchez Y, Xu X, Haake DA (2005) Osmolarity, a key environmental signal controlling expression of Leptospiral proteins LigA and LigB and the extracellular release of LigA. Infect Immun 73:70–78

Matsunaga J, Schlax PJ, Haake DA (2013) Role for cis-acting RNA sequences in the temperature-dependent expression of the multiadhesive lig proteins in *Leptospira interrogans*. J Bacteriol 195:5092–5101

Matsunaga J, Lo M, Bulach DM, Zuerner RL, Adler B, Haake DA (2007) Response of *Leptospira interrogans* to physiologic osmolarity: relevance in signaling the environment-to-host transition. Infect Immun 75:2864–2874

Matsunaga J, Coutinho ML (2012) Positive regulation of *Leptospira interrogans* kdp expression by KdpE as demonstrated with a novel β-galactosidase reporter in *Leptospira biflexa*. Appl Environ Microbiol 78:5699–5707

Monahan AM, Callanan JJ, Nally JE (2008) Proteomic analysis of *Leptospira interrogans* shed in urine of chronically infected hosts. Infect Immun 76:4952–4958

Morero NR, Botti H, Nitta KR, Carrión F, Obal G, Picardeau M, Buschiazzo A (2014) HemR is an OmpR/PhoB-like response regulator from Leptospira, which simultaneously effects transcriptional activation and repression of key haem metabolism genes. Mol Microbiol. doi:10.1111/mmi.12763

Murray GL, Ellis KM, Lo M, Adler B (2008) *Leptospira interrogans* requires a functional heme oxygenase to scavenge iron from hemoglobin. Microbes Infect 10:791–797

Murray GL, Morel V, Cerqueira GM, Croda J, Srikram A, Henry R, Ko AI, Dellagostin OA, Bulach DM, Sermswan R, Adler B, Picardeau M (2009a) Genome-wide transposon mutagenesis in pathogenic *Leptospira* spp. Infect Immun 77:810–816

Murray GL, Srikram A, Henry R, Puapairoj A, Sermswan RW, Adler B (2009b) *Leptospira interrogans* requires heme oxygenase for disease pathogenesis. Microbes Infect 11:311–314

Murray GL, Srikram A, Hoke DE, Wunder EAJ, Henry R, Lo M, Zhang K, Sermswan RW, Ko AI, Adler B (2009c) The major surface protein LipL32 is not required for either acute or chronic infection with *Leptospira interrogans*. Infect Immun 77:952–958

Murray GL, King AM, Srikram A, Sermswan RW, Adler B (2010a) Use of luminescent *Leptospira interrogans* for enumeration in biological assays. J Clin Microbiol 48:2037–2042

Murray GL, Srikram A, Henry R, Hartskeerl RA, Sermswan RW, Adler B (2010b) Mutations affecting *Leptospira interrogans* lipopolysaccharide attenuate virulence. Mol Microbiol 78:701–709

Nally JE, Artiushin S, Timoney JF (2001) Molecular characterization of thermoinduced immunogenic proteins Q1p42 and Hsp15 of *Leptospira interrogans*. Infect Immun 69:7616–7624

Nally JE, Chow E, Fishbein MC, Blanco DR, Lovett MA (2005a) Changes in lipopolysaccharide O antigen distinguish acute versus chronic *Leptospira interrogans* infections. Infect Immun 73:3251–3260

Nally JE, Whitelegge JP, Aguilera R, Pereira MM, Blanco DR, Lovett MA (2005b) Purification and proteomic analysis of outer membrane vesicles from a clinical isolate of *Leptospira interrogans* serovar Copenhageni. Proteomics 5:144–152

Nally JE, Whitelegge JP, Bassilian S, Blanco DR, Lovett MA (2007) Characterization of the outer membrane proteome of *Leptospira interrogans* expressed during acute lethal infection. Infect Immun 75:766–773

Nascimento AL, Ko AI, Martins EA, Monteiro-Vitorello CB, Ho PL, Haake DA, Verjovski-Almeida S, Hartskeerl RA, Marques MV, Oliveira MC, Menck CF, Leite LC, Carrer H, Coutinho LL, Degrave WM, Dellagostin OA, El-Dorry H, Ferro ES, Ferro MI, Furlan LR, Gamberini M, Giglioti EA, Goes-Neto A, Goldman GH, Goldman MH, Harakava R, Jeronimo SM, Junqueira-de-Azevedo IL, Kimura ET, Kuramae EE, Lemos EG, Lemos MV, Marino CL, Nunes LR, de Oliveira RC, Pereira GG, Reis MS, Schriefer A, Siqueira WJ, Sommer P, Tsai SM, Simpson AJ, Ferro JA, Camargo LE, Kitajima JP, Setubal JC, Van Sluys MA (2004) Comparative genomics of two *Leptospira interrogans* serovars reveals novel insights into physiology and pathogenesis. J Bacteriol 186:2164–2172

Patarakul K, Lo M, Adler B (2010) Global transcriptomic response of *Leptospira interrogans* serovar Copenhageni upon exposure to serum. BMC Microbiol 10:31

Picardeau M, Brenot A, Saint Girons I (2001) First evidence for gene replacement in *Leptospira* spp. Inactivation of *L. biflexa flaB* results in non-motile mutants deficient in endoflagella. Mol Microbiol 40:189–199

Picardeau M (2008) Conjugative transfer between *Escherichia coli* and *Leptospira* spp. as a new genetic tool. Appl Environ Microbiol 74:319–322

Picardeau M, Bulach DM, Bouchier C, Zuerner RL, Zidane N, Wilson PJ, Creno S, Kuczek ES, Bommezzadri S, Davis JC, McGrath A, Johnson MJ, Boursaux-Eude C, Seemann T, Rouy Z, Coppel RL, Rood JI, Lajus A, Davies JK, Médigue C, Adler B (2008) Genome sequence of the saprophyte *Leptospira biflexa* provides insights into the evolution of *Leptospira* and the pathogenesis of leptospirosis. PLoS ONE 3:1607

Pinne M, Haake DA (2009) A comprehensive approach to identification of surface-exposed, outer membrane-spanning proteins of *Leptospira interrogans*. PLoS ONE 4:6071

Pinne M, Haake DA (2013) LipL32 is a subsurface lipoprotein of *Leptospira interrogans*: presentation of new data and reevaluation of previous studies. PLoS ONE 8:51025

Poggi D, Oliveirade Giuseppe P, Picardeau M (2010) Antibiotic resistance markers for genetic manipulations of *Leptospira* spp. Appl Environ Microbiol 76:4882–4885

Qin JH, Sheng YY, Zhang ZM, Shi YZ, He P, Hu BY, Yang Y, Liu SG, Zhao GP, Guo XK (2006) Genome-wide transcriptional analysis of temperature shift in *L. interrogans* serovar lai strain 5660. BMC Microbiol 6:51

Qin JH, Zhang Q, Zhang ZM, Zhong Y, Yang Y, Hu BY, Zhao GP, Guo XK (2008) Identification of a novel prophage-like gene cluster actively expressed in both virulent and avirulent strains of *Leptospira interrogans* serovar Lai. Infect Immun 76:2411–2419

Ren S, Fu G, Jiang X, Zeng R, Xiong H, Lu G, Jiang HQ, Miao Y, Xu H, Zhang Y, Guo X, Shen Y, Qiang BQ, Danchin A, Saint Girons I, Somerville RL, Weng YM, Shi M, Chen Z, Xu JG, Zhao GP (2003) Unique and physiological and pathogenic features of *Leptospira interrogans* revealed by whole genome sequencing. Nature 422:888–893

Ricaldi JN, Fouts DE, Selengut JD, Harkins DM, Moreno A, Lehmann JS, Purushe J, Sanka R, Torres M, Webster NJ, Vinetz JM, Matthias MA (2012a) Whole genome analysis of *Leptospira licerasiae* provides insight into Leptospiral evolution and pathogenicity. PLoS Negl Trop Dis 6:1853

Ricaldi JN, Matthias MA, Vinetz JM, Lewis AL (2012b) Expression of sialic acids and other nonulosonic acids in *Leptospira*. BMC Microbiol 12:161

Richaud C, Margarita D, Baranton G, Saint Girons I (1990) Cloning of genes required for amino acid biosynthesis from *Leptospira interrogans* serovar icterohaemorrhagiae. J Gen Microbiol 136:651–656

Ristow P, Bourhy P, da Cruz McBride FW, Figueira CP, Huerre M, Ave P, Girons IS, Ko AI, Picardeau M (2007) The OmpA-like protein Loa22 is essential for Leptospiral virulence. PLoS Pathog 3:97

Saint Girons I, Margarita D, Amouriaux P, Baranton G (1990) First isolation of bacteriophages for a spirochaete: potential genetic tools for *Leptospira*. Res Microbiol 141:1131–1138

Saint Girons I, Norris SJ, Gobel U, Meyer J, Walker EM, Zuerner R (1992) Genome structure of spirochetes. Res Microbiol 143:615–621

Saint Girons I, Bourhy P, Ottone C, Picardeau M, Yelton D, Hendrix RW, Glaser P, Charon N (2000) The LE1 bacteriophage replicates as a plasmid within *Leptospira biflexa*: construction of an *L. biflexa-Escherichia coli* shuttle vector. J Bacteriol 182:5700–5705

Seshadri R, Myers GS, Tettelin H, Eisen JA, Heidelberg JF, Dodson RJ, Davidsen TM, DeBoy RT, Fouts DE, Haft DH, Selengut J, Ren Q, Brinkac LM, Madupu R, Kolonay J, Durkin SA, Daugherty SC, Shetty J, Shvartsbeyn A, Gebregeorgis E, Geer K, Tsegaye G, Malek J, Ayodeji B, Shatsman S, McLeod MP, Smajs D, Howell JK, Pal S, Amin A, Vashisth P, McNeill TZ, Xiang Q, Sodergren E, Baca E, Weinstock GM, Norris SJ, Fraser CM, Paulsen IT (2004) Comparison of the genome of the oral pathogen *Treponema denticola* with other spirochete genomes. Proc Natl Acad Sci USA 101:5646–5651

Slamti L, de Pedro MA, Guichet E, Picardeau M (2011) Deciphering morphological determinants of the helix-shaped *Leptospira*. J Bacteriol 193:6266–6275

Stamm LV, Parrish EA, Gherardini FC (1991) Cloning of the *recA* gene from a free-living leptospire and distribution of RecA-like protein among spirochetes. Appl Environ Microbiol 57:183–189

Ulrich LE, Zhulin IB (2010) The MiST2 database: a comprehensive genomics resource on microbial signal transduction. Nucleic Acids Res 38:401–407

Xue F, Dong H, Wu J, Wu Z, Hu W, Sun A, Troxell B, Yang XF, Yan J (2010) Transcriptional responses of *Leptospira interrogans* to host innate immunity: significant changes in metabolism, oxygen tolerance, and outer membrane. PLoS Negl Trop Dis 4(10):e857

Yelton DB, Cohen RA (1986) Analysis of cloned DNA from *Leptospira biflexa* serovar patoc which complements a deletion of the *Escherichia coli trpE* gene. J Bacteriol 165:41–46

Zhang C, Wang H, Yan J (2012a) Leptospirosis prevalence in Chinese populations in the last two decades. Microbes Infect 14:317–323

Zhang K, Murray GL, Seemann T, Srikram A, Bartpho T, Sermswan RW, Adler B, Hoke DE (2013). Leptospiral LruA is required for virulence and modulates an interaction with mammalian Apolipoprotein A-I. Infect Imm 8:3872–3879

Zhang L, Zhang C, Ojcius DM, Sun D, Zhao J, Lin X, Li L, Li L, Yan J (2012b) The mammalian cell entry (Mce) protein of pathogenic *Leptospira* species is responsible for RGD motif-dependent infection of cells and animals. Mol Microbiol 83:1006–1023

Zhong Y, Chang X, Cao XJ, Zhang Y, Zheng H, Zhu YZ, Cai C, Cui Z, Zhang Y, Li YY, Jiang XG, Zhao GP, Wang S, Li Y, Zeng R, Li X, Guo XK (2011) Comparative proteogenomic analysis of the *Leptospira interrogans* virulence-attenuated strain IPAV against the pathogenic strain 56601. Cell Res 21:1210–1229

Zuerner RL (1991) Physical mapping of chromosomal and plasmid DNA comprising the genome of *Leptospira interrogans*. Nucleic Acids Res 19:4857–4860

Zuerner RL, Herrmann JL, Saint Girons I (1993) Comparison of genetic maps for two *Leptospira interrogans* serovars provides evidence for two chromosomes and intraspecies heterogeneity. J Bacteriol 175:5445–5451

Zuerner RL (1994) Nucleotide sequence analysis of IS1533 from *Leptospira borgpetersenii*: identification and expression of two IS-encoded proteins. Plasmid 31:1–11

Zuerner RL, Huang WM (2002) Analysis of a *Leptospira interrogans* locus containing DNA replication genes and a new IS, IS*1502*. FEMS Microbiol Lett 215:175–182

Leptospirosis in Humans

David A. Haake and Paul N. Levett

Abstract Leptospirosis is a widespread and potentially fatal zoonosis that is endemic in many tropical regions and causes large epidemics after heavy rainfall and flooding. Infection results from direct or indirect exposure to infected reservoir host animals that carry the pathogen in their renal tubules and shed pathogenic leptospires in their urine. Although many wild and domestic animals can serve as reservoir hosts, the brown rat (*Rattus norvegicus*) is the most important source of human infections. Individuals living in urban slum environments characterized by inadequate sanitation and poor housing are at high risk of rat exposure and leptospirosis. The global burden of leptospirosis is expected to rise with demographic shifts that favor increases in the number of urban poor in tropical regions subject to worsening storms and urban flooding due to climate change. Data emerging from prospective surveillance studies suggest that most human leptospiral infections in endemic areas are mild or asymptomatic. Development of more severe outcomes likely depends on three factors: epidemiological conditions, host susceptibility, and pathogen virulence (Fig. 1). Mortality increases with age, particularly in patients older than 60 years of age. High levels of bacteremia are associated with poor clinical outcomes and, based on animal model and in vitro studies, are related in part to poor recognition of leptospiral LPS by human TLR4. Patients with severe leptospirosis experience a cytokine storm characterized by high levels of IL-6, TNF-alpha, and IL-10. Patients with the HLA DQ6 allele are at higher risk of disease, suggesting a role for lymphocyte stimulation by a leptospiral superantigen. Leptospirosis typically presents as

D.A. Haake (✉)
Division of Infectious Diseases, VA Greater Los Angeles Healthcare System,
Los Angeles, CA, USA
e-mail: dhaake@ucla.edu

D.A. Haake
Departments of Medicine, Urology, and Microbiology, Immunology,
and Molecular Genetics, The David Geffen School of Medicine at UCLA,
Los Angeles, CA, USA

P.N. Levett
Saskatchewan Disease Control Laboratory, Regina, SK, Canada
e-mail: plevett@health.gov.sk.ca

© Springer-Verlag Berlin Heidelberg 2015
B. Adler (ed.), *Leptospira and Leptospirosis*, Current Topics in Microbiology
and Immunology 387, DOI 10.1007/978-3-662-45059-8_5

a nonspecific, acute febrile illness characterized by fever, myalgia, and headache and may be confused with other entities such as influenza and dengue fever. Newer diagnostic methods facilitate early diagnosis and antibiotic treatment. Patients progressing to multisystem organ failure have widespread hematogenous dissemination of pathogens. Nonoliguric (high output) renal dysfunction should be supported with fluids and electrolytes. When oliguric renal failure occurs, prompt initiation of dialysis can be life saving. Elevated bilirubin levels are due to hepatocellular damage and disruption of intercellular junctions between hepatocytes, resulting in leaking of bilirubin out of bile caniliculi. Hemorrhagic complications are common and are associated with coagulation abnormalities. Severe pulmonary hemorrhage syndrome due to extensive alveolar hemorrhage has a fatality rate of >50 %. Readers are referred to earlier, excellent summaries related to this subject (Adler and de la Peña-Moctezuma 2010; Bharti et al. 2003; Hartskeerl et al. 2011; Ko et al. 2009; Levett 2001; McBride et al. 2005).

Contents

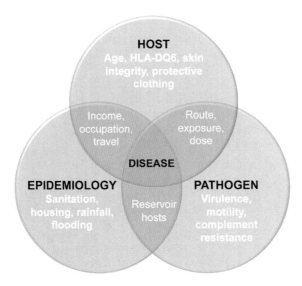

Fig. 1 Factors contributing to leptospirosis. Development of leptospirosis depends on three types of factors (*epidemiology*, *host*, and *pathogen*) and their interactions. Epidemiologic factors include sanitation, housing, rainfall, and whether flooding occurs. Incidence is linked to income level, occupation, and travel, representing epidemiologic factors linked to specific hosts. Hosts vary in susceptibility depending on age, genetic factors (e.g., HLA-DQ6), skin integrity, and whether protective clothing (e.g., gloves and boots) are worn. The ways in which the host and leptospires interact determine the route, exposure, and dose of the pathogen. Leptospiral pathogens differ in their ability to cause disease, a reflection of their virulence, motility, and ability to survive in the host, a reflection (at least in part) of complement resistance. The types of reservoir hosts determine the types of pathogens present in a particular epidemiologic setting

1 Epidemiology and Surveillance

1.1 Sources of Infection

Pathogenic leptospires are widespread in nature, reflecting maintenance in the kidneys of many wild and domestic reservoir hosts. The leptospiral life cycle involves shedding in the urine, persistence in the ambient environment, acquisition of a new host, and hematogenous dissemination to the kidneys through the glomerulus or peritubular capillaries. Once leptospires gain access to the renal tubular lumen of the kidney, they colonize the brush border of the proximal renal tubular epithelium, from which urinary shedding can persist for long periods of time without significant ill effects on the reservoir host. For this reason, leptospiral infection of the reservoir host can be considered a commensal relationship (Fig. 1).

Small mammals are the most important reservoirs, with large herbivores as additional significant sources of infection. Pathogenic *Leptospira* species have been isolated from hundreds of mammalian species, including bats and pinnipeds (see the chapter by W.A. Ellis, this volume). In addition, leptospires have been recovered from poikilothermic animals such as frogs and toads, and it is possible that these animals play a role in the circulation of leptospirosis in the environment, although they may not be significant reservoirs of human infection. Only a few studies have reported isolation of leptospires from amphibians (Babudieri et al. 1973; Everard et al. 1988; Gravekamp et al. 1991). However, the results justify further attempts to understand the role of amphibians in maintaining leptospires in nature (Adler and de la Peña-Moctezuma 2010; Bharti et al. 2003; Hartskeerl et al. 2011; Ko et al. 2009; Levett 2001; McBride et al. 2005; Felzemburgh et al. 2014).

Leptospirosis is primarily a zoonosis, with humans serving as accidental hosts. However, it is worth noting that transient leptospiral shedding does occur during human infection and human-to-human infection, although extremely rare, has occurred through sexual intercourse (Doeleman 1932; Harrison and Fitzgerald 1988) and during lactation (Bolin and Koellner 1988). Transplacental transmission may occur if infection occurs during pregnancy, resulting in abortion (Chung et al. 1963) or still birth (Coghlan and Bain 1969; Faine et al. 1984).

1.2 Transmission

Portals of entry include cuts and abrasions or mucous membranes such as the conjunctival, oral, or genital surfaces. Exposure may occur through either direct contact with an infected animal or through indirect contact via soil or water contaminated with urine from an infected animal. Individuals with occupations at risk for direct contact with potentially infected animals include veterinarians, abattoir workers, farm workers (particularly in dairy milking situations), hunters and trappers, animal shelter workers, scientists, and technologists handling animals in laboratories or during fieldwork. The magnitude of the risk depends on the local prevalence of leptospiral carriage and the degree and frequency of exposure. Most of these infections are preventable by the use of appropriate personal protective equipment such as rubber boots, gloves, and protective eyewear. Since many of these infections are covered by occupational health and safety regulations, local risk assessments and training are essential (Steneroden et al. 2011).

Indirect contact with water or soil contaminated with leptospires is much more common, and can be associated with occupational, recreational, or avocational activities. In addition to the risks associated with outdoor work listed above, sewer work, military exercises, and farming in high rainfall tropical regions are recognized; the latter is by far the most important numerically. Agricultural workers at risk for leptospirosis include rice field workers, taro farmers, banana farmers, and sugar cane and pineapple field harvesters (Levett 2001). These occupations involve activities likely to result in exposure of cuts and abrasions to soil and water contaminated with the urine of rodents and other animals attracted to food sources. For example, banana workers accounted for two-thirds of the reported leptospirosis cases in a tropical region of Queensland, Australia (Smythe et al. 1997).

Recreational exposures include all freshwater water sports including caving (Self et al. 1987), canoeing (Waitkins 1986), kayaking (Jevon et al. 1986; Shaw 1992), rafting (Wilkins et al. 1988), and triathlons (Morgan et al. 2002; Sejvar et al. 2003). The importance of this type of exposure has increased over the past 20 years as the popularity of adventure sports and races has increased, and also because the relative cost of travel to exotic destinations has decreased (Lau et al. 2010a). Competitive events create the potential for large outbreaks; 80 and 98 leptospirosis cases occurred as part of the 2000 Eco-challenge competition (Fig. 2a) (Sejvar et al. 2003) and 1998 Springfield triathlon (Morgan et al. 2002), respectively. Participants in international events may become ill after having returned home, often to multiple destination

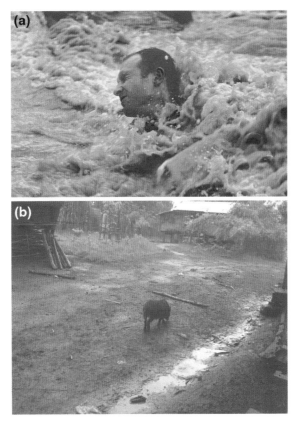

Fig. 2 Epidemiologic settings for leptospirosis. **a** A high proportion of contestants in the 2000 Eco-Challenge multisport race held in Malaysian Borneo developed leptospirosis. Of 189 participants contacted by the Centers for Disease Control, 80 (42 %) met the case definition for leptospirosis. Risk factors included exposure for extended periods of time to the rain-swollen Segama river (*photograph credit* Reed Hoffmann). **b** This rural village in Laos is a typical epidemiologic setting for leptospirosis. Residents of tropical regions of the world with high levels of rainfall are at increased risk of leptospirosis, particularly when standing water is contaminated by urine from wild or domesticated animals, which may serve as reservoir hosts for pathogenic *Leptospira* species (*photograph credit* Ben Adler)

countries, which complicates recognition and investigation of outbreaks. In many series, the incidence of leptospirosis is much higher in males than females (Everard et al. 1992; Guerra-Silveira and Abad-Franch 2013; Katz et al. 2011). However, it seems likely that gender differences in leptospirosis incidence are due entirely to exposure-related bias, as reports of leptospirosis outbreaks related to athletic events where males and females have similar levels of exposure have found no significant effects of gender on development of illness (Morgan et al. 2002; Sejvar et al. 2003).

Avocational exposures are by far the most important exposures, affecting millions of people living in tropical regions. As illustrated in Fig. 2b, lack of adequate sanitation and poor housing combine to exacerbate the risk of exposure to leptospires in both rural and urban slum communities (Bharti et al. 2003; Felzemburgh et al. 2014; Hotez et al. 2008; Reis et al. 2008). The role of poor housing is also suggested by the study of Maciel et al. (2008), which showed a greatly increased risk (odds ratio 5.29) of leptospirosis exposure among individuals who live in the same household as a leptospirosis patient. These factors are most likely surrogates for rat exposure, as proximity to uncollected trash and sighting of rats increased the risk of leptospirosis among residents of urban slums (Reis et al. 2008). The recognition of large outbreaks following excess rainfall events (Ahern et al. 2005; Dechet et al. 2012; Ko et al. 1999; Zaki and Shieh 1996) led to the labeling of leptospirosis as an emerging infectious disease two decades ago (Levett 1999). More recently, the interaction of urbanization and climate change has been identified as a significant risk for both increased incidence and increasing frequency of outbreaks of leptospirosis (Lau et al. 2010b). The need for interdisciplinary research to understand the effects of anthropogenic change and its effect on the epidemiology of leptospirosis has been proposed (Vinetz et al. 2005).

1.3 Global Burden of Disease

Early studies of leptospirosis incidence concentrated on occupational disease, primarily in developed countries related to leptospirosis in livestock animals (Alston and Broom 1958; Faine et al. 1999). As the importance of the disease in tropical countries became better recognized, guidelines were developed for the diagnosis and control of leptospirosis (Faine 1982). As diagnostic methods became more widely available, numerous epidemiologic studies were reported from many countries. An initial attempt to gather global data on the incidence of leptospirosis was published over 15 years ago (WHO 1999). Based on global data collected by International Leptospirosis Society surveys, the incidence was estimated to be 350,000–500,000 severe leptospirosis cases annually (Ahmed et al. 2012). Despite these efforts, the global burden of leptospirosis was felt to be largely underestimated for a number of reasons, including the fact that the vast majority of countries either lack a notification system or notification is not mandatory (Ahmed et al. 2012). To address these shortcomings, the WHO established the Leptospirosis Burden Epidemiology Reference Group (LERG) (Abela-Ridder et al. 2010). The LERG met for the first time in

2009 and for a second time in 2010. The specific objectives of the second LERG meeting were: (1) To review and appraise the revised systematic review of mortality, morbidity, and disability from human leptospirosis; (2) To review a draft disease transmission model for leptospirosis and provide technical input for the further development and refinement of the model; (3) To assemble preliminary estimates of the disease burden; (4) To identify gaps in knowledge and research; and (5) To advise WHO on the next steps for estimation of the burden of human leptospirosis and the implications for policy. The resulting LERG report included a systematic literature review that estimated the overall global annual incidence of endemic and epidemic human leptospirosis at 5 and 14 cases per 100,000 population, respectively (WHO 2011). Endemic human leptospirosis rates varied by region from 0.5/100,000 population in Europe to 95/100,000 population in Africa.

2 Pathology

The first step in the pathogenesis of leptospirosis is penetration of tissue barriers to gain entrance to the body. Potential portals of entry include the skin via a cut or abrasion and the mucous membranes of the conjunctivae or oral cavity. The importance of the oral mucosa as a portal of entry is indicated by a number of studies that found that swallowing while swimming in contaminated water is a risk factor for infection (Corwin et al. 1990; Lingappa et al. 2004; Stern et al. 2010).

The second step in pathogenesis is hematogenous dissemination. Unlike other pathogenic spirochetes such as *B. burgdorferi* and *T. pallidum*, which cause skin lesions indicating establishment of infection in the skin, pathogenic leptospires make their way into the bloodstream and persist there during the leptospiremic phase of the illness. Results from inoculation of blood into leptospiral medium and detection of leptospiremia by quantitative PCR are more likely to be positive during the first 8 days of fever (Agampodi et al. 2012) prior to antibody formation and clearance of organisms from the bloodstream. Quantitative PCR has documented leptospiremia levels as high as 10^6/ml of blood (Agampodi et al. 2012), which is similar to the burden of spirochetes seen in the blood of patients with relapsing fever (Stoenner et al. 1982). Levels of $>10^4$ leptospires/ml in the bloodstream have been associated with severe outcomes (Segura et al. 2005; Truccolo et al. 2001), although a more recent larger study suggests that leptospires with lower virulence may be able to achieve even higher leptospiral bloodstream burdens without causing severe complications (Agampodi et al. 2012).

The levels of bacteremia that occur during leptospirosis are similar to those found in infections caused by the relapsing fever *Borreliae* (Stoenner et al. 1982), and very different from those found in bacteremia caused by *E. coli* and other *Enterobacteriaceae*, in which concentrations are typically <1 cfu/ml (Yagupsky and Nolte 1990). Part of the explanation for these differences is the human innate immune response. Human TLR4 is able to detect *E. coli* lipopolysaccharide (LPS) at extremely low concentrations, but is unable to recognize leptospiral LPS (Werts et al. 2001). A likely explanation for this difference in reactivity of human TLR4 is structural differences between the lipid A component of *E. coli* and leptospiral LPS; leptospiral LPS has a unique methylated phosphate residue not found in any other form of lipid A (Que-Gewirth et al. 2004). In contrast to human TLR4, mouse TLR4 is able to recognize leptospiral LPS (Nahori et al. 2005), suggesting that the murine innate immune response is adapted to leptospiral infection. This notion is consistent with differences in the pathogenesis of leptospirosis between humans and mice; humans are accidental hosts that experience potentially fatal outcomes and rarely transmit infection, while mice are resistant to fatal infection and serve as natural reservoirs.

The importance of TLR4 in determining the outcome of infection was demon-strated in studies showing that young (but not adult) C3H/HeJ mice lacking TLR4 are susceptible to lethal infection with *L. interrogans* (Viriyakosol et al. 2006). However, TLR4 is only one component of the innate immune response to lepto-spirosis. Both human and mouse TLR2 are able to recognize the polysaccharide or 2-keto-3-deoxyoctonoic acid (KDO) component of leptospiral LPS (Nahori et al. 2005; Werts 2010). Only when both TLR4 and TLR2 are mutated do adult C57BL/ 6 J mice experience lethal leptospirosis infections (Nahori et al. 2005). Presumably, TLR2 and other innate immune response mechanisms are responsible for the host response to leptospiral infection that leads to symptoms of disease. TLR2, TLR4, and TLR5 have been shown to be required for virulent leptospires to induce expression of the cytokines IL-6 and TNF-alpha in whole blood (Goris et al. 2011a).

When high levels of leptospiremia occur during infection, innate immune mechanisms eventually trigger tissue-based and systemic responses to infection that lead to severe outcomes such as a sepsis-like syndrome or organ failure. Patients with severe leptospirosis have evidence of a "cytokine storm" with higher levels of IL-6, TNF-alpha, and a number of other cytokines than patients with mild disease (Reis et al. 2013). In particular, IL-6 and IL-10 levels were independent predictors of death, suggesting that overproduction of IL-10 may inhibit a protective Th1 immune response. Superantigen stimulation of nonspecific T cell activation may also play a role in human leptospirosis. A study of athletes participating in the Springfield triathalon found that the human leukocyte antigen (HLA) DQ6 was an independent risk factor for development of leptospirosis after exposure to lake water contaminated with virulent leptospires (Lingappa et al. 2004). The structural location of HLA-DQ6 polymorphisms associated with disease suggested a super-antigen mechanism for this HLA-dependent susceptibility (Lingappa et al. 2004), although the identity of any such antigen(s) remains unknown.

The liver is a major target organ in leptospirosis. Pathology reports from autopsy specimens from fatal cases of leptospirosis have reported congested sinusoids and distention of the space of Disse, located between the sinusoids and hepatocytes (Arean 1962). Immunohistochemistry studies have documented large numbers of leptospires between hepatocytes in animal models. A recent, elegant study has documented leptospiral infiltration of Disse's space and preferential leptospiral attachment to and invasion of the perijunctional region between hepatocytes (Miyahara et al. 2014). Additionally, hepatocyte apoptosis has been documented in

Fig. 3 Histopathology of leptospirosis. **a** Histology of the liver typically shows lack of the normal adhesion between hepatocytes, a hallmark of the disease (*photograph credit* Thales De Brito). **b** Typical renal histopathology showing acute tubular necrosis and interstitial nephritis. The glomerulus is essentially unremarkable. Reproduced from Abdulkader and Silva, The kidney in leptospirosis. Pediatr Nephrol 2008; 23:2111–2120, with permission of the publisher, Springer

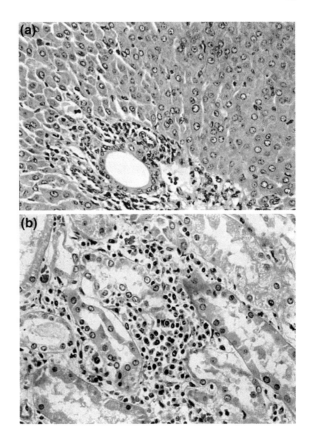

leptospirosis (Merien et al. 1998). Together, hepatocellular damage and disruption of hepatocyte intercellular junctions (Fig. 3a) leads to leakage of bile from bile canaliculi into sinusoidal blood vessels, which accounts for the elevated levels of direct bilirubin seen in icteric forms of leptospirosis. Occasionally, elevation of indirect bilirubin levels may also occur in the setting of leptospirosis-induced hemolysis (Avdeeva et al. 2002).

Pathological changes in the lung are extremely common in leptospirosis. In the 1962 study of fatal leptospirosis cases by Arean, all 33 cases were found to have pulmonary petechiae on the pleural surfaces and 60 % of patients had gross hemorrhage on the cut surfaces of the lungs (Arean 1962). Histologically, hemorrhage was found to occur in both the alveolar septa and intra-alveolar spaces (Arean 1962). A recent Brazilian study of patients with severe pulmonary hemorrhage syndrome (SPHS) performed immunohistochemistry on pulmonary tissue and found finely granular material representing leptospiral antigen within macrophages in septa and alveoli (Silva et al. 2002b). The guinea pig model of leptospirosis replicates the pulmonary hemorrhage seen in humans and studies of this animal model also revealed extensive deposition of immunoglobulin and complement along the alveolar basement membrane (Nally et al. 2004). Petechiae and hemorrhage are noted in a number of different organs beside the lungs and may be related, at least in part, to the coagulation abnormalities associated that frequently occur in severe leptospirosis (Wagenaar et al. 2010). The concept that SPHS is a manifestation of severe systemic disease rather than a strictly pulmonary problem is consistent with the finding that risk factors for SPHS include not only the respiratory rate but also hypokalemia, elevated serum creatinine, shock, and the Glasgow Coma Scale Score (Marotto et al. 2010).

Renal involvement varies in severity from mild nonoliguric renal dysfunction to complete renal failure, a hallmark of Weil's syndrome. The polyuria observed in mild leptospirosis appears to be due to reduced expression of the sodium–hydrogen exchanger 3, resulting in decreased reabsorption of sodium and fluid by the proximal tubule (Araujo et al. 2010). The histologic changes vary in intensity and typically involve tubular changes and interstitial nephritis (Fig. 3b). Tubular damage includes thinning and/or necrosis of the tubular epithelium and distention of the tubular lumen with hyaline casts and cellular debris (Arean 1962). In the reservoir host, the tubular lumen is a key site of colonization in the leptospiral life cycle and immunohistochemistry can show large numbers of organisms attached to the brush border of proximal tubular epithelium. In humans, an inflammatory response is triggered by recognition of leptospiral lipoproteins such as LipL32 by TLR2 on renal tubular epithelial cells, resulting in induction of nitric oxide synthase (iNOS) and monocyte chemoattractant protein-1 (Yang et al. 2006). Tubular inflammation results in interstitial nephritis characterized by edema and infiltration with lymphocytes, monocytes, and plasma cells, and occasionally neutrophils (Arean 1962; Sitprija and Evans 1970). This interstitial nephritis increases in extent and intensity during the first 2 weeks of illness. Most patients with acute renal failure due to leptospirosis who survive regain normal renal function. However, some patients have persistent renal dysfunction associated with tubular atrophy and interstitial fibrosis on kidney biopsy (Herath et al. 2014).

3 Clinical Features

Leptospirosis ranges in severity from a mild, self-limited febrile illness to a fulminant life-threatening illness. When illness occurs, a broad array of organ systems may be involved, reflecting the systemic nature of the infection. As a result, the signs and symptoms of leptospirosis are protean and frequently mistaken for other causes of acute febrile syndrome.

3.1 Incubation Phase

The incubation phase from exposure to onset of symptoms averages from 7 to 12 days, though it can be as short as 3 days or as long as a month. The remarkable variability in the duration of the incubation phase is evident in the 6–29 day lag between exposure and onset of symptoms among 52 athletes who developed laboratory-confirmed leptospirosis after participating (all on the same day) in the Springfield Triathalon (Morgan et al. 2002).

3.2 Presentation

Patients typically present with sudden onset of fever, chills, and headache. These signs and symptoms are nonspecific and also occur with other causes of acute febrile syndrome that, depending on the setting, could also be caused by influenza, dengue fever, or malaria. The headache is often severe and has been described as a bitemporal, frontal throbbing headache accompanied by retro-orbital pain and photophobia.

Muscle pain and tenderness is common and characteristically involves the calves and lower back. A tip-off to identification of leptospirosis is conjunctival suffusion (dilatation of conjunctival vessels without purulent exudate), which occurs frequently in leptospirosis, but is uncommon in other infectious diseases. Additional ocular findings typically include subconjunctival hemorrhages and icterus (Fig. 4a). Rash is uncommon in leptospirosis and when it occurs in the setting of an acute febrile illness, may suggest an alternative diagnosis such as dengue or chikungunya fever (Burt et al. 2012; Zaki and Shanbag 2010). An erythematous rash limited to the pretibial areas of both legs appearing on about the fourth day of illness was a feature of an outbreak of "Fort Bragg Fever" which also included headache, malaise, and splenomegaly among soldiers in North Carolina, the etiology of which was later determined to be *L. interrogans* serovar Autumnalis (Gochenour et al. 1952).

A nonproductive cough has been noted in 20–57 % of leptospirosis patients and can potentially lead clinicians to incorrectly diagnose the patient with influenza or another respiratory illness. Gastrointestinal symptoms are frequently observed, and may include nausea, vomiting, diarrhea, and abdominal pain. Nausea and other gastrointestinal symptoms may contribute to dehydration in patients with high-output nonoliguric renal failure caused by leptospirosis. The abdominal pain may be due to acalculous cholecystitis and/or pancreatitis. In patients admitted to the hospital for leptospirosis, abdominal pain associated with abnormal serum amylase and/or lipase levels is relatively common (O'Brien et al. 1998). It should be kept in mind that impaired renal function alone can elevate pancreatic enzyme levels when the creatinine clearance is less than 50 ml/min (Collen et al. 1990). While most cases of pancreatitis due to leptospirosis are self-limited, some cases are more severe and associated with fatal outcomes (Spichler et al. 2007).

Severe leptospirosis is characterized by dysfunction of multiple organs including the liver, kidneys, lungs, and brain. The combination of jaundice and renal failure, known as Weil's disease, was first described in 1886 (Weil 1886) and remains one

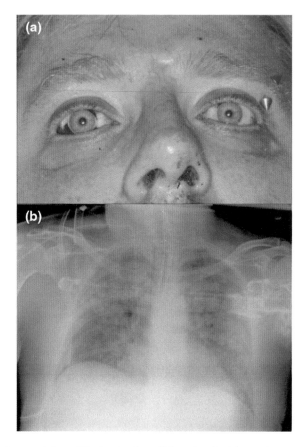

Fig. 4 Clinical presentation of leptospirosis. **a** Subconjunctival hemorrhages and icterus in a 37-year-old man who kept pet rats presented with sudden onset of fever, myalgia, and severe headache. On admission he had abnormal liver and kidney function. Serological tests for leptospiral antibodies converted from negative to positive 1 week after presentation. He was treated with intravenous penicillin and recovered completely. Reproduced from Jansen and Schneider, Weil's disease in a rat owner. Lancet Infect Dis 2011; 11:152, with permission of the publisher, Elsevier Ltd. **b** Severe pulmonary hemorrhage in a 50-year-old man who had recently returned from vacation in Malaysia where he had waded through mangrove forests. Respiratory deterioration occurred on day 2 of hospitalization requiring mechanical ventilation complicated by severe hemoptysis requiring blood transfusion. He was treated initially with doxycycline followed by amoxicillin and made a slow but complete recovery. Blood culture in leptospiral growth medium became positive 4 months after inoculation. Reproduced from Wagenaar et al. Leptospirosis with pulmonary hemorrhage, caused by a new strain of serovar Lai: Langkawi. J Travel Med 2004; 11:379–382. With permission of the publisher, John Wiley and sons. No portion of this figure may be reproduced without permission of the publisher

of the most clinically recognizable forms of leptospirosis (see the chapter by B. Adler, this volume). Evidence of organ dysfunction indicates a more advanced stage of infection, yet may develop suddenly and be present in a large percentage of patients at the time of presentation.

Leptospirosis patients are typically found to have mild to moderate elevations in levels of liver transaminases and direct (conjugated) bilirubin. The frequency of jaundice varies widely among case series, perhaps due in part to the virulence of the causative organism. Katz et al. (2001) found a strong association between infection with the Icterohaemorrhagiae serogroup and jaundice and elevated bilirubin levels. Acute hemolytic anemia can contribute to jaundice which, not surprisingly, is more common in leptospirosis patients with glucose-6-phosphate dehydrogenase deficiency (Avdeeva et al. 2002). Such patients have a higher percentage of unconjugated (i.e., indirect) bilirubin. Many patients have leukocytosis and thrombocytopenia, though usually not to the extent that would cause spontaneous hemorrhage. Leukopenia in the setting of thrombocytopenia and anemia can suggest bone marrow suppression.

Clinical signs of bleeding are common and occur in the majority of patients with severe leptospirosis. Most bleeding manifestations are mild, including petechiae, ecchymoses, and epistaxis. However, some patients have severe gastrointestinal (melena or hematemesis) or pulmonary hemorrhage. Thrombocytopenia frequently occurs, although usually not to the extent that would cause spontaneous hemorrhage. In a study of severe leptospirosis performed in the Netherlands, all patients had coagulation disorders, including prolongation of the prothrombin time (PT) and the length of the PT was associated with severe bleeding manifestations (Wagenaar et al. 2010).

The kidney is a major target organ in leptospirosis, perhaps due to the intrinsic renal-tropic homing ability of leptospires in their reservoir hosts. The kidneys are commonly involved, as manifested by elevations in serum blood urea nitrogen and creatinine levels and findings on urinalysis of pyuria, hematuria, and elevated urine protein levels (Katz et al. 2001). Leptospirosis causes a unique nonoliguric potassium wasting nephropathy characterized by impaired sodium reabsorption and potassium wasting (Seguro et al. 1990). When poor oral intake due to nausea and high-output renal failure combine to cause dehydration, patients are at risk of oliguria and renal failure, a frequent cause of death in areas where peritoneal or hemodialysis is not available.

Progression to severe leptospirosis and circulatory collapse may be accompanied by acute respiratory distress syndrome (ARDS). As in other causes of ARDS, leptospirosis causes diffuse lung injury characterized by impaired gas exchange and the need for mechanical ventilation. Massive hemoptysis, representing extensive alveolar hemorrhage, is an ominous complication of leptospirosis associated with fatality rates >50 % (Gouveia et al. 2008). Pulmonary hemorrhage associated with leptospirosis was first reported in Switzerland in 1943 (Moeschlin 1943), and since then has been reported with increasing frequency from a variety of locations (Park et al. 1989). Leptospirosis-associated severe pulmonary hemorrhage syndrome (SHPS) can occur sporadically or in outbreaks that can be confused clinically with viral pneumonitis (Sehgal et al. 1995; Trevejo et al. 1998). For example, a 1995 outbreak of SPHS that occurred after heavy rainfall and flooding in Nicaragua was initially thought to be due to hantavirus pulmonary syndrome until silver staining and immunohistochemistry of postmortem lung tissue revealed leptospires (Trevejo et al. 1998). SPHS can present as hemoptysis associated with cough or may be discovered after patients undergo pulmonary intubation (Yersin et al. 2000). Chest radiographs show diffuse alveolar infiltrates (Fig. 4b). Epidemiologic evidence suggests that SPHS may be a relatively new problem, suggesting emergence of a new clone of *L. interrogans* with enhanced virulence. However, it is also possible that SPHS is an old problem that is finally being recognized and documented.

As noted above, headache is frequently severe and when accompanied by meningismus may prompt performance of lumbar puncture. Typical findings on CSF examination include a lymphocytic predominance with total cell counts of up to 500/mm^3, protein levels between 50 and 100 mg/mL, and normal glucose levels, consistent with aseptic meningitis (Berman et al. 1973). Depending on the epidemiologic setting, leptospirosis may be a predominant cause of aseptic meningitis in some areas (Silva et al. 2002a). Patients with aseptic meningitis due to leptospirosis may be anicteric, making the diagnosis more challenging (Berman et al. 1973; Karande et al. 2005). In severe leptospirosis, altered mental status may be an indicator of meningoencephalitis. A variety of other neurologic complications may also occur including hemiplegia, transverse myelitis, and Guillain–Barré syndrome (Levett 2001).

3.3 Risk Factors for Morbidity and Mortality

In an active surveillance study of 326 cases of leptospirosis in Salvador, Brazil, the strongest independent predictor of a fatal outcome was altered mental status (odds ratio 9.12), which typically began with confusion and obtundation without focal neurologic signs (Ko et al. 1999). Other independent risk factors for death identified in the Salvador study included oliguria (odds ratio 5.28), age over 36 years (odds ratio 4.38), and respiratory insufficiency (2. 56) (Ko et al. 1999). The risk of a fatal outcome increases with increased age; compared to individuals aged 19–29, the increased risk of death rose from 3.7-fold for 40–49 year olds to 7.3-fold among those 60 or older (Lopes et al. 2004). Lung involvement, as indicated by dyspnea (odds ratio 11.7) or alveolar infiltrates on chest X-ray (odds ratio 7.3), was found to be associated with mortality in a retrospective study of 68 leptospirosis cases at Pointe-à-Pître Hospital in the French West Indies, along with oliguria (odds ratio 9), repolarization abnormalities on electrocardiogram (odds ratio 5.95), and a white blood count >12,900/mm^3 (odds ratio 2.54) (Dupont et al. 1997). A retrospective review of leptospirosis cases associated with an outbreak of leptospirosis in India identified pulmonary involvement and altered mental status as independent predictors of death (Pappachan et al. 2004). Additional poor prognostic signs identified in other studies include acute renal failure, hypotension, and arrhythmias (Daher et al. 1999; Panaphut et al. 2002).

3.4 Recovery Phase

With proper supportive care (see Management below), most leptospirosis patients recover completely (Spichler et al. 2011). Patients with acute renal failure who require dialysis typically regain most of their renal function, although there may be evidence of persistent mild renal impairment (Covic et al. 2003). In addition, there is growing recognition that many patients suffer from chronic postleptospirosis symptoms. In a recent study of laboratory-confirmed leptospirosis patients in the Netherlands, 30 % of patients experienced persistent complaints after acute leptospirosis (PCAC) characterized by fatigue, myalgia, malaise, headache, and weakness (Goris et al. 2013a). Of patients with PCAC, 21 % reported that their complaints lasted for more than 24 months.

Ocular involvement in the form of uveitis is well-known to occur during the convalescent phase of leptospirosis. Eye involvement ranges in severity from insidious onset of mild anterior uveitis to acute, severe panuveitis involving the anterior, middle, and posterior segments of the eye (Rathinam 2005). Leptospiral uveitis may occur either as a single, self-limited event or as a series of recurrent episodes, which appears to occur more frequently in patients with severe uveitis. In one study, 80 % of patients had leptospiral DNA in the aqueous humor, detected by PCR (Chu et al. 1998). However, the relative contributions of infection and autoimmunity are uncertain. There are parallels between recurrent uveitis in humans and equine recurrent uveitis (ERU) and autoimmunity to lens proteins has been suggested to play a role in ERU (Verma et al. 2010).

4 Diagnosis

Diagnosis of leptospirosis may be accomplished by direct detection of the organism or its components in body fluid or tissues, by isolation of leptospires in cultures, or by detection of specific antibodies (Hartskeerl et al. 2011; Schreier et al. 2013). The collection of appropriate specimens and selection of tests for diagnosis depend upon the timing of collection and the duration of symptoms (Fig. 5). For detailed descriptions of historical methods see the following publications (Faine et al. 1999; Galton 1962; Levett 2001; Sulzer and Jones 1978; Turner 1968, 1970; Wolff 1954).

4.1 Molecular Diagnosis

Leptospiral DNA has been amplified from serum, urine, aqueous humor, CSF, and a number of organs post mortem (Levett 2004). Conventional PCR and other assays such as LAMP and NASBA were reviewed recently (Ahmed et al. 2012) and will not be discussed further. Many quantitative PCR assays have been described, which target a number of different genes (Ahmed et al. 2009; Merien et al. 2005;

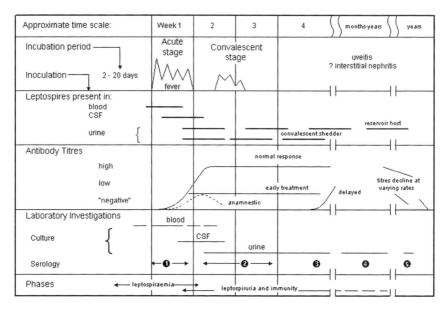

Fig. 5 Biphasic nature of leptospirosis and relevant investigations at different stages of disease. Specimens *1* and *2* for serology are acute-phase specimens, *3* is a convalescent-phase sample which may facilitate detection of a delayed immune response, and *4* and *5* are follow-up samples which can provide epidemiological information, such as the presumptive infecting serogroup. Adapted from Turner LH (1969). Leptospirosis. Br Med J i:231–235, with permission of the publisher. Copyright © American Society for Microbiology, (Clin Microbiol Rev 2001, 14 (2):296–326. doi:10.1128/CMR.14.2.296-326.2001)

Palaniappan et al. 2005; Smythe et al. 2002; Stoddard et al. 2009). Assays developed for diagnostic use can be considered in two broad categories, targeting either housekeeping genes, such as *rrs*, *gyrB*, or *secY*, or pathogen-specific genes such as *lipL32*, *lig*, or *lfb1* (Ahmed et al. 2012). Examples of these two types of quantitative assay were evaluated in a large case-control study in a high-prevalence population in Thailand (Thaipadunpanit et al. 2011), that confirmed earlier reports that PCR detection in blood samples collected at admission to hospital was more sensitive than culture, but serology using the microscopic agglutination test (MAT) ultimately detected more cases (Brown et al. 1995). Real-time PCR assays have been used to quantify the bacterial load in leptospirosis (Agampodi et al. 2012; Segura et al. 2005; Tubiana et al. 2013).

A limitation of PCR-based diagnosis of leptospirosis is the current inability of PCR assays to identify the infecting serovar. While this is not significant for individual patient management, the identity of the serovar has both epidemiological and public health value. Serovar identification requires isolation of the infecting strain from patients or carrier animals. However, whole genome sequencing has recently been applied to the diagnosis of neurological leptospirosis (Wilson et al. 2014) and it is probable that direct serovar identification will be possible in the near future, limited only by the quality of sequences obtained from specimens.

4.2 Isolation and Identification of Leptospires

Culture of leptospires requires specialized media (see the chapter by C.E. Cameron, this volume). Leptospires can be recovered from humans during the acute phase of the illness and during the so-called immune phase. Leptospiremia occurs during the first stage of the disease, beginning before the onset of symptoms and has usually declined by the end of the first week of the acute illness. Timing of culture of different specimens depends upon an accurate date of onset of symptoms, so a careful history is essential. Blood cultures should be taken as soon as possible after the patient's presentation. One or two drops of blood are inoculated into 5–10 ml semisolid or liquid medium at the bedside (Turner 1970). Multiple cultures yield higher recovery rates, but this is rarely possible. Inoculation of media with dilutions of blood samples may increase recovery (Sulzer and Jones 1978). Leptospires have been shown to survive in commercially available conventional blood culture media for periods of time ranging from 48 h to 4 weeks (Palmer and Zochowski 2000). Blood cultures with no growth can be used to inoculate leptospiral culture medium (Turner 1970).

Other samples that may be cultured during the first week of illness include CSF and peritoneal dialysate. Urine should be cultured from the beginning of the second week of symptomatic illness. The duration of urinary excretion varies, but may be several weeks (Bal et al. 1994). Survival of leptospires in voided human urine is limited, so urine should be collected into sterile phosphate buffered saline (Turner 1970). Contamination of urine cultures is a major problem and the use of selective media containing 5-fluorouracil or other antimicrobial agents (see the chapter by C.E. Cameron, this volume) is strongly recommended. Cultures are incubated at 28–30 °C and examined weekly by dark field microscopy, for up to 13 weeks.

Isolated leptospires are identified either by serological methods, or more recently, by molecular techniques. Traditional methods relied on cross-agglutinin absorption (Dikken and Kmety 1978). The number of laboratories which can perform these identification methods is small. Monoclonal antibodies are available for identification of many, but not all, serovars (Korver et al. 1988). The limitations of these approaches are discussed by Hartskeerl and Smythe (see the chapter by R.A. Hartskeerl and L.D. Smythe, this volume).

Molecular methods for identification and subtyping have been studied extensively. Increasingly, sequence-based identification of *Leptospira* is becoming the standard (Ahmed et al. 2012) and this can be performed on the products of diagnostic PCR (Ganoza et al. 2010; Perez and Goarant 2010). Pulsed-field gel electrophoresis (PFGE) has been shown to identify most serovars (Galloway and Levett 2010; Herrmann et al. 1992), but complements, rather than replaces, serological identification (Ahmed et al. 2012). Identification of serovars by whole genome sequencing will likely become standardized in the near future (Ahmed et al. 2012).

Strain subtyping for epidemiological purposes can be accomplished by simple methods using restriction enzymes or variations of PCR conditions that can generate banding patterns that allow strains to be differentiated (Ahmed et al. 2012).

However, reproducibility is poor, particularly between laboratories. More recently, sequence-based methods such as MLVA (Pavan et al. 2008; Salaun et al. 2006; Slack et al. 2005) and MLST (Ahmed et al. 2006, 2011; Boonsilp et al. 2013; Leon et al. 2009; Thaipadungpanit et al. 2007) have been applied. These methods are reproducible and can yield significant information at a subserovar level (Boonsilp et al. 2013). MLST data can be analyzed online (http://leptospira.mlst.net).

4.3 Serological Diagnosis

Most cases of leptospirosis are diagnosed by serology, because capacity for culture and PCR is limited. IgM antibodies are detectable in the blood 5–7 days after the onset of symptoms. Serological methods can be divided into those which are genus-specific and those which are serogroup-specific. The use of agglutination tests was described soon after the first isolation of the organism and the microscopic agglutination test remains the definitive serological investigation in both human and animals.

4.3.1 Microscopic Agglutination Test

In the microscopic agglutination test (MAT), patients' sera are reacted with live antigen suspensions of leptospiral serovars. After incubation, the serum/antigen mixtures are examined microscopically for agglutination and the titers are determined. The MAT can be a complex test to control, perform, and interpret (Turner 1968). Live cultures must be maintained of all the serovars required for use as antigens. The range of antigens used should include serovars representative of all serogroups (Faine 1982; Turner 1968) and locally common serovars (Torten 1979). A wide range of antigens is used in order to detect infections with uncommon, or previously undetected, serovars (Katz et al. 1991). The MAT is a serogroup-specific assay and cannot be relied upon to detect the infecting serovar (Levett 2003; Murray et al. 2011; Smythe et al. 2009).

The MAT is read by dark field microscopy. The endpoint is the highest dilution of serum in which 50 % agglutination occurs. Because of the difficulty in detecting when 50 % of the leptospires are agglutinated, the endpoint is determined by the presence of approximately 50 % free, unagglutinated leptospires, by comparison with the control suspension (Faine 1982). Considerable effort is required to reduce the subjective effect of observer variation, even within laboratories.

Interpretation of the MAT is complicated by the high degree of cross-reaction that occurs between different serogroups, especially in acute-phase samples. Patients often have similar titers to all serovars of an individual serogroup, but "paradoxical" reactions, in which the highest titers are detected to a serogroup unrelated to the infecting one, may also occur (Alston and Broom 1958; Levett 2001). The broad cross-reactivity in the acute phase, followed by relative serogroup specificity in convalescent samples, results from the detection in the MAT of both IgM and IgG antibodies (Adler and Faine 1978).

Paired sera are required to confirm a diagnosis with certainty. A fourfold or greater rise in titre between paired sera confirms the diagnosis, regardless of the interval between samples. The interval between first and second samples depends very much on the delay between onset of symptoms and presentation of the patient. If symptoms typical of leptospirosis are present, then an interval of 3–5 days may be adequate to detect rising titers. However, if the patient presents earlier in the course of the disease, or if the date of onset is not known precisely, then an interval of 10–14 days between samples is more appropriate. Less often, seroconversion does not occur with such rapidity, and a longer interval between samples (or repeated sampling) is necessary. MAT serology is insensitive in early acute-phase specimens (Appassakij et al. 1995; Brandão et al. 1998; Cumberland et al. 1999). Moreover, patients with fulminant leptospirosis may die before seroconversion occurs (Brown et al. 1995; Cumberland et al. 1999; Ribeiro et al. 1994).

Acute infection is suggested by a single elevated titer detected in association with an acute febrile illness. The magnitude of such a titer is dependent upon the background level of exposure in the population, and hence the seroprevalence. The application of single titers for presumptive diagnosis has been reviewed (Levett 2001) and will not be discussed further. Titers following acute infection may be extremely high ($\geq 25,600$) and may take months, or even years, to fall to low levels (Alston and Broom 1958; Blackmore et al. 1984; Cumberland et al. 2001; Lupidi et al. 1991; Romero et al. 1998). Rarely, seroconversion may be delayed for many weeks after recovery, and longer serological follow-up will be necessary to confirm the diagnosis.

The MAT is the most appropriate test to employ in epidemiological sero-surveys, since it can be applied to sera from any animal species, and because the range of antigens utilized can be expanded or decreased as required. It is usual to use a titer ≥ 100 as evidence of past exposure (Faine 1982). However, conclusions about infecting serovars cannot be drawn without isolates; MAT data can give only a general impression about which serogroups are present within a population (Everard and Everard 1993).

4.3.2 Other Serological Tests

Because of the complexity of the MAT, rapid screening tests for leptospiral antibodies in acute infection have been developed. IgM antibodies become detectable during the first week of illness, allowing the diagnosis to be confirmed and treatment to be initiated while it is likely to be most effective. IgM detection has repeatedly been shown to be more sensitive than MAT when the first specimen is taken early in the acute phase of the illness (Cumberland et al. 1999; Goris et al. 2011b; Ribeiro et al. 1994; Winslow et al. 1997).

Detection of IgM using ELISA has been employed widely, most often using antigen prepared from cultures of *L. biflexa*, although pathogenic species have also been used. Several products are available commercially. Recombinant antigens have also been employed, but none has been evaluated widely (Signorini et al. 2013). Specificity of IgM detection by ELISA is affected by the antigen used in the assay, by the presence of antibodies due to previous exposure (in endemic regions), and by the presence of other diseases (Bajani et al. 2003).

More recently, IgM detection assays have been developed in several rapid test formats intended for use in laboratories without extensive instrumentation, or potentially in field settings. These have included two dipstick formats (Smits et al. 2000a; Levett and Branch 2002), latex agglutination (Smits et al. 2000b, 2001a), lateral flow (Smits et al. 2001b) and dual path platform (Nabity et al. 2012).

However, there are significant limitations to early diagnosis using any serological test (Goris et al. 2011b; Signorini et al. 2013) and testing of a second sample should be considered mandatory. Moreover, confirmation of rapid diagnostic test results by a reference test has been recommended (Goris et al. 2013b).

4.3.3 Evaluation of Serological Tests

Evaluation of serological tests for leptospirosis has been problematic because there are few laboratories equipped to perform the definitive serological test (MAT), and there are fewer laboratories with the capacity to isolate and identify leptospires from patients. A large body of the literature consists of reports on studies that have been ill-designed and which use less than perfect case definitions, leading to misleading estimates of sensitivity and specificity. Ideally, new serological assays should be evaluated in clinical trials of consecutive patients investigated using a case definition which includes both MAT and culture results, and which are conducted in multiple regions, where different leptospiral serovars are prevalent and where the differential diagnoses may vary widely (Smits et al. 2000a, b). Assays may perform differently in different populations (Desakorn et al. 2012; Levett and Branch 2002). Alternatively, well-designed studies conducted in individual centers may be compared, providing the limitations of this approach are recognized (Levett 2001). Evaluations performed using collections of sera in reference laboratories may be useful for determining sensitivity of assays, but specificity is dependent upon the selection of noncase sera representative both of other diseases and the normal population. Parallel studies in clinical and reference settings may yield quite different results (Bajani et al. 2003; Hull-Jackson et al. 2006).

5 Management

Most leptospirosis cases are mild and resolve spontaneously. Early initiation of antimicrobial therapy may prevent some patients from progressing to more severe disease. Identification of leptospirosis in its early stages is largely a clinical diagnosis and relies on a high index of suspicion based on the patient's risk factors, exposure history, and presenting signs and symptoms. Rapid diagnostic tests for leptospirosis are improving, but a negative result should not be relied on to rule out early infection. For these reasons, empirical therapy should be initiated as soon as the diagnosis of leptospirosis is suspected.

Therapy for patients with leptospirosis severe enough to merit hospitalization usually involves intravenous penicillin (1.5 million units IV every 6 h), ampicillin (0.5–1 g IV every 6 h), ceftriaxone (1 g IV every 24 h), or cefotaxime (1 g IV every 6 h). Ceftriaxone has been shown to be noninferior to penicillin for serious leptospirosis (Panaphut et al. 2003) and in addition to once daily dosing has the added benefit of intramuscular administration as an alternative to intravenous therapy in settings where hospitalization is not possible. Adult outpatients with early disease should receive either doxycycline 100 mg orally twice per day or azithromycin 500 mg orally once per day. When the dosage is adjusted for weight, either azithromycin or amoxicillin can also be given to pregnant women and children. These recommendations are based on in vitro susceptibility data (Hospenthal and Murray 2003; Ressner et al. 2008), animal studies (Alexander and Rule 1986; Truccolo et al. 2002), and clinical experience including a randomized, placebo-controlled, double-blinded study which found that doxycycline therapy shortened the duration of illness due to leptospirosis by 2 days and improved fever, malaise, headache, and myalgias (McClain et al. 1984). Doxycycline treatment also prevented shedding of organisms in the urine.

There are strong grounds for administering antibiotics as soon as possible to patients with risk factors and clinical features of severe leptospirosis. A placebo-controlled trial of intravenous penicillin for leptospirosis conducted in the Philippines found that penicillin shortened the duration of fever, abnormal renal function, and hospitalization and prevented leptospiral shedding in the urine (Watt et al. 1988). A flaw in this study was that a number of patients in both groups had received antibiotics prior to entry into the study. A second placebo-controlled study of intravenous penicillin for leptospirosis patients was conducted in Barbados, most of whom were icteric. Although the Barbados study failed to show significant differences between the penicillin and placebo groups, patients receiving penicillin had a lower mortality rate than patients receiving placebo (2.6 vs. 7.3 %, respectively) (Edwards et al. 1988). It can be difficult to demonstrate a beneficial effect of antibiotics in patients who have already begun to experience some degree of organ dysfunction, which of course cannot be reversed with antibiotics. As imperfect as these studies are, they are likely to be the only placebo-controlled studies that will ever be conducted, given the ethical barriers to placebo-controlled studies involving life-threatening illnesses caused by antibiotic-susceptible bacteria.

Severe leptospirosis is a medical emergency requiring both antibiotics and proper supportive therapy to improve mortality rates. Patients with severe leptospirosis are frequently found to have a unique form of potassium wasting high-output renal dysfunction (Abdulkader et al. 1996; Seguro et al. 1990). For this reason, patients should receive intravenous hydration to correct dehydration and prevent oliguric renal failure. Potassium supplementation should be included for patients with hypokalemia. When oliguric renal failure occurs, early initiation of peritoneal or hemodialysis can be lifesaving and is usually needed only on a short-term basis (Andrade et al. 2008). In a comparative study, prompt initiation of daily dialysis in critically ill leptospirosis patients reduced mortality from 67 to 17 % (Andrade et al. 2007). Patients with respiratory failure who require intubation typically have poor pulmonary compliance (i.e., "stiff lungs") and have been found to benefit from ventilation with low tidal volumes (<6 mL/kg) to reduce ventilation pressures, protect patients from alveolar injury, and improve survival rates (Amato et al. 1998).

5.1 Antimicrobial Susceptibilities

Leptospires are susceptible to β-lactams, macrolides, tetracyclines, fluoroquinolones, and streptomycin (Alexander and Rule 1986; Faine et al. 1999). Problems in the determination of susceptibility include the long incubation time required, the use of media containing serum, and the difficulty in quantifying growth accurately. These constraints have limited the development of rapid, standardized methods for susceptibility testing. Most studies have used a limited range of laboratory strains and/or a small number of antimicrobial agents. However, microdilution methods have been described recently (Murray et al. 2004; Ressner et al. 2008), which will facilitate the study of large numbers of isolates against a wide range of antimicrobial agents, with the potential of identifying new agents for prophylaxis or treatment of leptospirosis.

6 Prevention

Strategies for prevention of leptospirosis are based on awareness of leptospirosis epidemiology and transmission mechanisms, as presented earlier in this chapter. Once the local epidemiology and transmission risks have been defined, it is possible to greatly mitigate risk by taking steps to reduce exposure and implement protective measures, immunization, and pre- or postexposure chemoprophylaxis.

From a global perspective, human leptospirosis is strongly linked to poverty wherever poor housing standards and local infrastructure result in exposure to rodent reservoirs. Rodent abatement efforts may have short-term benefit but rodenticides create risks for children and wildlife and are not good long-term solutions. Housing construction that prevents rodents from invading residential living spaces greatly reduces risk. Flood control projects that prevent inundation of residential areas would greatly reduce the potential for leptospirosis outbreaks. These measures are difficult to implement, but should be recognized as an important part of an overall prevention strategy.

Occupational activities that put workers at risk through exposure to contaminated water or infected animals should be identified. Personal protective equipment such as gloves, boots, goggles, and overalls for workers in high-risk occupations are important to prevent exposure of mucous membranes and skin, but can be difficult to implement in hot and humid environments. Abrasions, cuts, and damaged skin are particularly important as portals of entry. Walking barefoot and water sports in endemic areas are notoriously high-risk activities. The 2001 Eco-challenge multi-sport competition in Borneo involving jungle trekking and leach bites followed by prolonged emersion in the rain-swollen Segama River resulted in an astounding 42 % attack rate and illustrates how endemic factors and susceptible hosts combine to create high-risk exposures (Sejvar et al. 2003).

Source reduction through immunization of agricultural and companion animals with killed whole-cell vaccines is an extremely important strategy for reducing the risk of human leptospirosis. Humans may also become infected through exposure to acutely or chronically infected animals that are shedding leptospires in their urine. Diagnosis and treatment of infected animals, and immunization of uninfected companion and agricultural animals is another cornerstone of leptospirosis prevention and is covered in chapter by W.A. Ellis, this volume.

6.1 Human Leptospirosis Vaccines

Immunization of humans with killed, whole-cell vaccines has generally been restricted to individuals in high-risk occupations and in response to floods and epidemics. One of the first reports of human leptospirosis immunization involved the vaccination of thousands of miners in Japan using a culture-derived *L. interrogans* serovar Icterohaemorrhagiae vaccine (Wani 1933). Although local and generalized reactions were common, a significant decrease in the incidence of leptospirosis among the miners was observed. Immunization of large populations at risk of leptospirosis due to extensive flooding has been performed in China (Chen 1985). A Cuban leptospirosis vaccine trial involving >100,000 persons reported that local pain and "general discomfort" were significantly greater than in a control group given a recombinant hepatitis B vaccine (Martinez et al. 2004). The vaccine showed an efficacy of >97 % against the prevalent local serovars. Concern over reactions to host proteins led to the development of a leptospiral vaccine derived from leptospires grown in a chemically defined medium (Shenberg and Torten 1973); however, growth in protein media is generally poorer and such media have not gained widespread use.

Some of the most detailed safety and efficacy studies involved a leptospirosis vaccination program for Parisian sewer workers. In response to a request by the City of Paris, the Pasteur Institute developed a killed, whole-cell vaccine derived from *L. interrogans* serovar Icterohaemorrhagiae strain Verdun. Mailloux et al. (1983) examined the safety of this vaccine and reported three systemic (nausea) reactions and seven local reactions among 1,157 immunizations of 454 vaccines. Importantly, after the vaccine was introduced in 1979, the incidence of leptospirosis dropped from 1.3 cases per year (29 cases from 1951 to 1979) to zero (no cases reported from 1981 to 1988) during a 7 year follow-up period. The recommended vaccination protocol involves two booster doses after the initial immunization followed by reimmunization every 2 years. More recent reports of safety and efficacy have been published since the vaccine was marketed as Spirolept™ (Benbrick et al. 2001; Laurichesse et al. 2007; Pouliquen and Catilina 2000).

As described in chapter by B. Adler, this volume, the active component of killed, whole-cell vaccines is leptospiral LPS, a serovar-specific antigen (Chapman et al. 1990). LPS-based immunity is generally considered to provide protection against homologous or closely related, but not heterologous, serovars. For example, Fukumura (1984) reported that individuals immunized with a serovar Pyrogenes vaccine were protected from infection by that serovar but not from serovars Autumnalis and Hebdomadis with antigenically unrelated LPS, leading to development of a trivalent vaccine consisting of all three serovars. Research on development of leptospirosis vaccines with a low side-effect profile that induce long-lasting, cross-protective immunity is focused on an improved understanding of the leptospiral outer membrane (see the chapters by D.A. Haake and W.R. Zückert and by B. Adler, this volume).

6.2 Chemoprophylaxis

Unavoidable short-term exposure can be mitigated by chemoprophylaxis. Pre-exposure prophylaxis with doxycycline (200 mg orally once per week) was effective for military personnel undergoing high-risk jungle training exercises (Takafuji et al. 1984). Doxycycline has also been studied for postexposure prophylaxis of local populations after heavy rainfall in endemic areas (Gonsalcz ct al. 1998; Sehgal et al. 2000). One of these two studies found that postexposure doxycycline prophylaxis reduced the incidence of symptomatic disease (Sehgal et al. 2000). Alternatives to doxycycline, such as azithromycin or amoxicillin, have not been studied, but may be considered in pregnant women and children and individuals at risk of photosensitivity.

Acknowledgments Current work in Prof. Haake's laboratory is supported by NIH Grant R01 AI034431 and a VA Merit Award.

References

Abdulkader RC, Seguro AC, Malheiro PS, Burdmann EA, Marcondes M (1996) Peculiar electrolytic and hormonal abnormalities in acute renal failure due to leptospirosis. Am J Trop Med Hyg 54:1–6
Abela-Ridder B, Sikkema R, Hartskeerl RA (2010) Estimating the burden of human leptospirosis. Int J Antimicrob Agents 36(Suppl 1):S5–S7
Adler B, Faine S (1978) The antibodies involved in the human immune response to leptospiral infection. J Med Microbiol 11:387–400

Adler B, de la Peña-Moctezuma A (2010) *Leptospira* and leptospirosis. Vet Microbiol 140:287–296

Agampodi SB, Matthias MA, Moreno AC, Vinetz JM (2012) Utility of quantitative polymerase chain reaction in leptospirosis diagnosis: association of level of leptospiremia and clinical manifestations in Sri Lanka. Clin Infect Dis 54:1249–1255

Ahern M, Kovats RS, Wilkinson P, Few R, Matthies F (2005) Global health impacts of floods: epidemiologic evidence. Epidemiol Rev 27:36–46

Ahmed A, Engelberts MF, Boer KR, Ahmed N, Hartskeerl RA (2009) Development and validation of a real-time PCR for detection of pathogenic *Leptospira* species in clinical materials. PLoS ONE 4:e7093

Ahmed A, Grobusch MP, Klatser PR, Hartskeerl RA (2012) Molecular approaches in the detection and characterization of *Leptospira*. J Bacteriol Parasitol 3:1000133

Ahmed A, Thaipadungpanit J, Boonsilp S, Wuthiekanun V, Nalam K, Spratt BG, Aanensen DM, Smythe LD, Ahmed N, Feil EJ, Hartskeerl RA, Peacock SJ (2011) Comparison of two multilocus sequence based genotyping schemes for *Leptospira* species. PLoS Negl Trop Dis 5: e1374

Ahmed N, Devi SM, Valverde Mde L, Vijayachari P, Machang'u RS, Ellis WA, Hartskeerl RA (2006) Multilocus sequence typing method for identification and genotypic classification of pathogenic *Leptospira* species. Ann Clin Microbiol Antimicrob 5:28

Alexander AD, Rule PL (1986) Penicillins, cephalosporins, and tetracyclines in treatment of hamsters with fatal leptospirosis. Antimicrob Agents Chemother 30:835–839

Alston JM, Broom JC (1958) Leptospirosis in man and animals. E. & S. Livingstone, Edinburgh

Amato MB, Barbas CS, Medeiros DM, Magaldi RB, Schettino GP, Lorenzi-Filho G, Kairalla RA, Deheinzelin D, Munoz C, Oliveira R, Takagaki TY, Carvalho CR (1998) Effect of a protective-ventilation strategy on mortality in the acute respiratory distress syndrome. N Engl J Med 338:347–354

Andrade L, Cleto S, Seguro AC (2007) Door-to-dialysis time and daily hemodialysis in patients with leptospirosis: impact on mortality. Clin J Am Soc Nephrol 2:739–744

Andrade L, de Francesco Daher E, Seguro AC (2008) *Leptospiral* nephropathy. Semin Nephrol 28:383–394

Appassakij H, Silpapojakul K, Wansit R, Woodtayakorn J (1995) Evaluation of the immuno-fluorescent antibody test for the diagnosis of human leptospirosis. Am J Trop Med Hyg 52:340–343

Araujo ER, Seguro AC, Spichler A, Magaldi AJ, Volpini RA, De Brito T (2010) Acute kidney injury in human leptospirosis: an immunohistochemical study with pathophysiological correlation. Virchows Arch 456:367–375

Arean VM (1962) The pathologic anatomy and pathogenesis of fatal human leptospirosis (Weil's disease). Am J Pathol 40:393–423

Avdeeva MG, Moisova DL, Gorodin VN, Kostomarov AM, Zotov SV, Cherniavskaia OV (2002) The role glucose-6-phosphate dehydrogenase in pathogenesis of anemia in leptospirosis. Klin Med (Mosk) 80:42–44

Babudieri B, Carlos ER, Carlos ET Jr (1973) Pathogenic *Leptospira* isolated from toad kidneys. Trop Geogr Med 25:297–299

Bajani MD, Ashford DA, Bragg SL, Woods CW, Aye T, Spiegel RA, Plikaytis BD, Perkins BA, Phelan M, Levett PN, Weyant RS (2003) Evaluation of four commercially available rapid serologic tests for diagnosis of leptospirosis. J Clin Microbiol 41:803–809

Bal AE, Gravekamp C, Hartskeerl RA, de Meza-Brewster J, Korver H, Terpstra WJ (1994) Detection of leptospires in urine by PCR for early diagnosis of leptospirosis. J Clin Microbiol 32:1894–1898

Benbrick E, Pouliquen P, Domont A (2001) Evaluation de la tolerance de la vaccination contre *Leptospira icterohaemorrhagiae* chez 50 employe´s de canaux. Arch Mal Prof 62:35–40

Berman SJ, Tsai C, Holms K, Fresh JW, Walten RH (1973) Sporadic anicteric leptospirosis in South Vietnam. A study of 150 patients. Ann Intern Med 79:167–173

Bharti AR, Nally JE, Ricaldi JN, Matthias MA, Diaz MM, Lovett MA, Levett PN, Gilman RH, Willig MR, Gotuzzo E, Vinetz JM (2003) Leptospirosis: a zoonotic disease of global importance. Lancet Infect Dis 3:757–771

Blackmore DK, Schollum LM, Moriarty KM (1984) The magnitude and duration of titres of leptospiral agglutinins in human sera. NZ Med J 97:83–86

Bolin CA, Koellner P (1988) Human-to-human transmission of *Leptospira interrogans* by milk. J Infect Dis 158:246–247

Boonsilp S, Thaipadungpanit J, Amornchai P, Wuthiekanun V, Bailey MS, Holden MT, Zhang C, Jiang X, Koizumi N, Taylor K, Galloway R, Hoffmaster AR, Craig S, Smythe LD, Hartskeerl RA, Day NP, Chantratita N, Feil EJ, Aanensen DM, Spratt BG, Peacock SJ (2013) A single multilocus sequence typing (MLST) scheme for seven pathogenic *Leptospira* species. PLoS Negl Trop Dis 7:e1954

Brandão AP, Camargo ED, da Silva ED, Silva MV, Abrão RV (1998) Macroscopic agglutination test for rapid diagnosis of human leptospirosis. J Clin Microbiol 36:3138–3142

Brown PD, Gravekamp C, Carrington DG, Van de Kemp H, Hartskeerl RA, Edwards CN, Everard COR, Terpstra WJ, Levett PN (1995) Evaluation of the polymerase chain reaction for early diagnosis of leptospirosis. J Med Microbiol 43:110–114

Burt FJ, Rolph MS, Rulli NE, Mahalingam S, Heise MT (2012) Chikungunya: a re-emerging virus. Lancet 379:662–671

Chapman AJ, Faine S, Adler B (1990) Antigens recognized by the human immune response to vaccination with a bivalent hardjo/pomona leptospiral vaccine. FEMS Microbiol Immunol 2:111–118

Chen T (1985) Development and present status of leptospiral vaccine and technology of production of the vaccine in China. Nihon Saikingaku Zasshi 40:755–762

Chu KM, Rathinam R, Namperumalsamy P, Dean D (1998) Identification of *Leptospira* species in the pathogenesis of uveitis and determination of clinical ocular characteristics in South India. J Infect Dis 177:1314–1321

Chung HL, Ts'ao WC, Mo PS, Yen C (1963) Transplacental or congenital infection of leptospirosis. Clinical and experimental observations. Chin Med J 82:777–782

Coghlan JD, Bain AD (1969) Leptospirosis in human pregnancy followed by death of the foetus. Brit Med J 1:228–230

Collen MJ, Ansher AF, Chapman AB, Mackow RC, Lewis JH (1990) Serum amylase in patients with renal insufficiency and renal failure. Am J Gastroenterol 85:1377–1380

Corwin A, Ryan A, Bloys W, Thomas R, Deniega B, Watts D (1990) A waterborne outbreak of leptospirosis among United States military personnel in Okinawa, Japan. Int J Epidemiol 19:743–748

Covic A, Goldsmith DJ, Gusbeth-Tatomir P, Seica A, Covic M (2003) A retrospective 5-year study in Moldova of acute renal failure due to leptospirosis: 58 cases and a review of the literature. Nephrol Dial Transplant 18:1128–1134

Cumberland PC, Everard COR, Levett PN (1999) Assessment of the efficacy of the IgM enzyme-linked immunosorbent assay (ELISA) and microscopic agglutination test (MAT) in the diagnosis of acute leptospirosis. Am J Trop Med Hyg 61:731–734

Cumberland PC, Everard COR, Wheeler JG, Levett PN (2001) Persistence of anti-leptospiral IgM, IgG and agglutinating antibodies in patients presenting with acute febrile illness in Barbados 1979–1989. Eur J Epidemiol 17:601–608

Daher E, Zanetta DM, Cavalcante MB, Abdulkader RC (1999) Risk factors for death and changing patterns in leptospirosis acute renal failure. Am J Trop Med Hyg 61:630–634

Dechet AM, Parsons M, Rambaran M, Mohamed-Rambaran P, Florendo-Cumbermack A, Persaud S, Baboolal S, Ari MD, Shadomy SV, Zaki SR, Paddock CD, Clark TA, Harris L, Lyon D, Mintz ED (2012) Leptospirosis outbreak following severe flooding: a rapid assessment and mass prophylaxis campaign; Guyana, January–February 2005. PLoS ONE 7:e39672

Desakorn V, Wuthiekanun V, Thanachartwet V, Sahassananda D, Chierakul W, Apiwattanaporn A, Day NP, Limmathurotsakul D, Peacock SJ (2012) Accuracy of a commercial IgM ELISA for the diagnosis of human leptospirosis in Thailand. Am J Trop Med Hyg 86:524–527

Dikken H, Kmety E (1978) Serological typing methods of leptospires. In: Bergan T, Norris JR (eds) Methods in microbiology. Academic Press, London, pp 259–307

Doeleman FPJ (1932) Ziekte van Weil, rechstreeks overgebracht van mensch op mensch. Ned Tijdschr Geneeskd 76:5057

Dupont H, Dupont-Perdrizet D, Perie JL, Zehner-Hansen S, Jarrige B, Daijardin JB (1997) Leptospirosis: prognostic factors associated with mortality. Clin Infect Dis 25:720–724

Edwards CN, Nicholson GD, Hassell TA, Everard CO, Callender J (1988) Penicillin therapy in icteric leptospirosis. Am J Trop Med Hyg 39:388–390

Everard CO, Carrington D, Korver H, Everard JD (1988) Leptospires in the marine toad (*Bufo marinus*) on Barbados. J Wildl Dis 24:334–338

Everard COR, Bennett S, Edwards CN, Nicholson GD, Hassell TA, Carrington DG, Everard JD (1992) An investigation of some risk factors for severe leptospirosis on Barbados. J Trop Med Hyg 95:13–32

Everard JD, Everard COR (1993) Leptospirosis in the Caribbean. Rev Med Microbiol 4:114–122

Faine S (1982) Guidelines for the control of leptospirosis. World Health Organization, Geneva

Faine S, Adler B, Christopher W, Valentine R (1984) Fatal congenital human leptospirosis. Zentralbl Bakteriol Mikrobiol Hyg [A] 257:548

Faine S, Adler B, Bolin C, Perolat P (1999) *Leptospira* and leptospirosis, 2nd edn. MediSci, Melbourne

Felzemburgh RD, Ribeiro GS, Costa F, Reis RB, Hagan JE, Melendez AX, Fraga D, Santana FS, Mohr S, Dos Santos BL, Silva AQ, Santos AC, Ravines RR, Tassinari WS, Carvalho MS, Reis MG, Ko AI (2014) Prospective study of leptospirosis transmission in an urban slum community: role of poor environment in repeated exposures to the *Leptospira* agent. PLoS Negl Trop Dis 8:e2927

Fukumura K (1984) Epidemiological studies on leptospirosis in Okinawa. Part 1. Prevalence of leptospirosis in Izena Island and the prevention by vaccination. Yamaguchi Med J 33:257–268

Galloway RL, Levett PN (2010) Application and validation of PFGE for serovar identification of *Leptospira* clinical isolates. PLoS Negl Trop Dis 4:e824

Galton MM (1962) Methods in the laboratory diagnosis of leptospirosis. Ann NY Acad Sci 98:675–684

Ganoza CA, Matthias MA, Saito M, Cespedes M, Gotuzzo E, Vinetz JM (2010) Asymptomatic renal colonization of humans in the peruvian Amazon by *Leptospira*. PLoS Negl Trop Dis 4: e612

Gochenour WS, Smadel JE, Jackson EB, Evans LB, Yager RH (1952) Leptospiral etiology of Fort Bragg fever. Publ Hlth Rep 67:811–813

Gonsalez CR, Casseb J, Monteiro FG, Paula-Neto JB, Fernandez RB, Silva MV, Camargo ED, Mairinque JM, Tavares LC (1998) Use of doxycycline for leptospirosis after high-risk exposure in Sao Paulo, Brazil. Rev Inst Med Trop Sao Paulo 40:59–61

Goris MG, Wagenaar JF, Hartskeerl RA, van Gorp EC, Schuller S, Monahan AM, Nally JE, van der Poll T, van't Veer C (2011a) Potent innate immune response to pathogenic *Leptospira* in human whole blood. PLoS ONE 6:e18279

Goris MGA, Leeflang MMG, Boer KR, Goeijenbier M, van Gorp ECM, Wagenaar JFP, Hartskeerl RA (2011b) Establishment of valid laboratory case definition for human leptospirosis. J Bacteriol Parasitol S5-001:1–8

Goris MG, Kikken V, Straetemans M, Alba S, Goeijenbier M, van Gorp EC, Boer KR, Wagenaar JF, Hartskeerl RA (2013a) Towards the burden of human leptospirosis: duration of acute illness and occurrence of post-leptospirosis symptoms of patients in the Netherlands. PLoS ONE 8:e76549

Goris MGA, Leeflang MMG, Loden M, Wagenaar JFP, Klatser PR, Hartskeerl RA, Boer KR (2013b) Prospective evaluation of three rapid diagnostic tests for diagnosis of human leptospirosis. PLoS Negl Trop Dis 7:e2290

Gouveia EL, Metcalfe J, de Carvalho ALF, Aires TSF, Villalobos-Bisneto JC, Queiroz A, Santos AC, Salgado K, Reis MG, Ko AI (2008) Leptospirosis-associated severe pulmonary hemorrhage syndrome, Salvador, Brazil. Emerg Infect Dis 14:505–508

Gravekamp C, Korver H, Montgomery J, Everard COR, Carrington D, Ellis WA, Terpstra WJ (1991) Leptospires isolated from toads and frogs on the island of Barbados. Zentralbl Bakteriol 275:403–411

Guerra-Silveira F, Abad-Franch F (2013) Sex bias in infectious disease epidemiology: patterns and processes. PLoS ONE 8:e62390

Harrison NA, Fitzgerald WR (1988) Leptospirosis—can it be a sexually transmitted disease? Postgrad Med J 64:163–164

Hartskeerl RA, Collares-Pereira M, Ellis WA (2011) Emergence, control and re-emerging leptospirosis: dynamics of infection in the changing world. Clin Microbiol Infect 17:494–501

Herath NJ, Kularatne SA, Weerakoon KG, Wazil A, Subasinghe N, Ratnatunga NV (2014) Long term outcome of acute kidney injury due to leptospirosis? A longitudinal study in Sri Lanka. BMC Res Notes 7:398

Herrmann JL, Bellenger E, Perolat P, Baranton G, Saint Girons I (1992) Pulsed-field gel electrophoresis of *Not*I digests of leptospiral DNA: a new rapid method of serovar identification. J Clin Microbiol 30:1696–1702

Hospenthal DR, Murray CK (2003) In vitro susceptibilities of seven *Leptospira* species to traditional and newer antibiotics. Antimicrob Agents Chemother 47:2646–2648

Hotez PJ, Bottazzi ME, Franco-Paredes C, Ault SK, Periago MR (2008) The neglected tropical diseases of Latin America and the Caribbean: a review of disease burden and distribution and a roadmap for control and elimination. PLoS Negl Trop Dis 2:e300

Hull-Jackson C, Glass MB, Ari MD, Bragg SL, Branch SL, Whittington CU, Edwards CN, Levett PN (2006) Evaluation of a commercial latex agglutination assay for serological diagnosis of leptospirosis. J Clin Microbiol 44:1853–1855

Jevon TR, Knudson MP, Smith PA, Whitecar PS, Blake RL (1986) A point-source epidemic of leptospirosis. Postgrad Med 80:121–129

Karande S, Patil S, Kulkarni M, Joshi A, Bharadwaj R (2005) Acute aseptic meningitis as the only presenting feature of leptospirosis. Pediatr Infect Dis J 24:390–391

Katz AR, Manea SJ, Sasaki DM (1991) Leptospirosis on Kauai: investigation of a common source waterborne outbreak. Am J Public Health 81:1310–1312

Katz AR, Ansdell VE, Effler PV, Middleton CR, Sasaki DM (2001) Assessment of the clinical presentation and treatment of 353 cases of laboratory-confirmed leptospirosis in hawaii, 1974–1998. Clin Infect Dis 33:1834–1841

Katz AR, Buchholz AE, Hinson K, Park SY, Effler PV (2011) Leptospirosis in Hawaii, USA, 1999–2008. Emerg Infect Dis 17:221–226

Ko AI, Galvao Reis M, Ribeiro Dourado CM, Johnson WD Jr, Riley LW, The Salvador Leptospirosis Study Group (1999) Urban epidemic of severe leptospirosis in Braz Lancet 354:820–825

Ko AI, Goarant C, Picardeau M (2009) *Leptospira*: the dawn of the molecular genetics era for an emerging zoonotic pathogen. Nat Rev Microbiol 7:736–747

Korver H, Kolk AHJ, Vingerhoed J, van Leeuwen J, Terpstra WJ (1988) Classification of serovars of the Icterohaemorrhagiae serogroup by monoclonal antibodies. Israel J Vet Med 44:15–18

Lau C, Smythe L, Weinstein P (2010a) Leptospirosis: an emerging disease in travellers. Travel Med Infect Dis 8:33–39

Lau CL, Smythe LD, Craig SB, Weinstein P (2010b) Climate change, flooding, urbanisation and leptospirosis: fuelling the fire? Trans R Soc Trop Med Hyg 104:631–638

Laurichesse H, Gourdon F, Smits HL, Abdoe TH, Estavoyer JM, Rebika H, Pouliquen P, Catalina P, Dubray C, Beytout J (2007) Safety and immunogenicity of subcutaneous or intramuscular administration of a monovalent inactivated vaccine against *Leptospira interrogans* serogroup Icterohaemorrhagiae in healthy volunteers. Clin Microbiol Infect 13:395–403

Leon A, Pronost S, Fortier G, Andre-Fontaine G, Leclercq R (2009) Multilocus sequence analysis for typing *Leptospira interrogans* and *Leptospira kirschneri*. J Clin Microbiol 48:581–585

Levett PN (1999) Leptospirosis: re-emerging or re-discovered disease? J Med Microbiol 48:417–418

Levett PN (2001) Leptospirosis. Clin Microbiol Rev 14:296–326

Levett PN, Branch SL (2002) Evaluation of two enzyme-linked immunosorbent assay methods for detection of immunoglobulin M antibodies in acute leptospirosis. Am J Trop Med Hyg 66:745–748

Levett PN (2003) Usefulness of serologic analysis as a predictor of the infecting serovar in patients with severe leptospirosis. Clin Infect Dis 36:447–452

Levett PN (2004) Leptospirosis: a forgotten zoonosis? Clin Appl Immunol Rev 4:435–448

Lingappa J, Kuffner T, Tappero J, Whitworth W, Mize A, Kaiser R, McNicholl J (2004) HLA-DQ6 and ingestion of contaminated water: possible gene-environment interaction in an outbreak of leptospirosis. Genes Immun 5:197–202

Lopes AA, Costa E, Costa YA, Sacramento E, De Oliveira Junior AR, Lopes MB, Lopes GB (2004) Comparative study of the in-hospital case-fatality rate of leptospirosis between pediatric and adult patients of different age groups. Rev Inst Med Trop Sao Paulo 46:19–24

Lupidi R, Cinco M, Balanzin D, Delprete E, Varaldo PE (1991) Serological follow-up of patients in a localized outbreak of leptospirosis. J Clin Microbiol 29:805–809

Maciel EA, de Carvalho AL, Nascimento SF, de Matos RB, Gouveia EL, Reis MG, Ko AI (2008) Household transmission of *Leptospira* infection in urban slum communities. PLoS Negl Trop Dis 2:e154

Mailloux M, Lambert R, Chenu M (1983) Human vaccination against leptospirosis icterohaemorrhagiae. Med Hyg (Geneve) 41:1025–1030

Marotto PC, Ko AI, Murta-Nascimento C, Seguro AC, Prado RR, Barbosa MC, Cleto SA, Eluf-Neto J (2010) Early identification of leptospirosis-associated pulmonary hemorrhage syndrome by use of a validated prediction model. J Infect 60:218–223

Martinez R, Perez A, Quinones Mdel C, Cruz R, Alvarez A, Armesto M, Fernandez C, Menendez J, Rodriguez I, Baro M, Diaz M, Rodriguez J, Sierra G, Obregon AM, Toledo ME, Fernandez N (2004) Efficacy and safety of a vaccine against human leptospirosis in Cuba. Rev Panam Salud Publica 15:249–255

McBride AJ, Athanazio DA, Reis MG, Ko AI (2005) Leptospirosis. Curr Opin Infect Dis 18:376–386

McClain JBL, Ballou WR, Harrison SM, Steinweg DL (1984) Doxycycline therapy for leptospirosis. Ann Intern Med 100:696–698

Merien F, Truccolo J, Rougier Y, Baranton G, Perolat P (1998) In vivo apoptosis of hepatocytes in guinea pigs infected with *Leptospira interrogans* serovar icterohaemorrhagiae. FEMS Microbiol Lett 169:95–102

Merien F, Portnoi D, Bourhy P, Charavay F, Berlioz-Arthaud A, Baranton G (2005) A rapid and quantitative method for the detection of *Leptospira* species in human leptospirosis. FEMS Microbiol Lett 249:139–147

Miyahara S, Saito M, Kanemaru T, Villanueva SY, Gloriani NG, Yoshida SI (2014) Destruction of the hepatocyte junction by intercellular invasion of *Leptospira* causes jaundice in a hamster model of Weil's disease. Int J Exp Pathol 95:271–281

Moeschlin S (1943) Lungeninfiltrate beim Ikterus infeciosus Weil. Schweitz Med Wochenschr 73:1227–1230

Morgan J, Bornstein SL, Karpati AM, Bruce M, Bolin CA, Austin CC, Woods CW, Lingappa J, Langkop C, Davis B, Graham DR, Proctor M, Ashford DA, Bajani M, Bragg SL, Shutt K, Perkins BA, Tappero JW (2002) Outbreak of leptospirosis among triathlon participants and community residents in Springfield, Illinois, 1998. Clin Infect Dis 34:1593–1599

Murray CK, Ellis MW, Hospenthal DR (2004) Susceptibility of *Leptospira* serovars to antimalarial agents. Am J Trop Med Hyg 71:685–686

Murray CK, Gray MR, Mende K, Parker TM, Samir A, Rahman BA, Habashy EE, Hospenthal DR, Pimentel G (2011) Use of patient-specific *Leptospira* isolates in the diagnosis of leptospirosis employing microscopic agglutination testing (MAT). Trans R Soc Trop Med Hyg 105:209–213

Nabity SA, Ribeiro GS, Lessa Aquino C, Takahashi D, Damião AO, Gonçalves AH, Miranda-Filho DB, Greenwald R, Esfandiari J, Lyashchenko KP, Reis MG, Medeiros MA, Ko AI (2012) Accuracy of a dual path platform (DPP) assay for the rapid point-of-care diagnosis of human leptospirosis. PLoS Negl Trop Dis 6:e1878

Nahori MA, Fournie-Amazouz E, Que-Gewirth NS, Balloy V, Chignard M, Raetz CR, Saint Girons I, Werts C (2005) Differential TLR recognition of leptospiral lipid A and lipopolysaccharide in murine and human cells. J Immunol 175:6022–6031

Nally JE, Chantranuwat C, Wu XY, Fishbein MC, Pereira MM, Da Silva JJ, Blanco DR, Lovett MA (2004) Alveolar septal deposition of immunoglobulin and complement parallels pulmonary hemorrhage in a guinea pig model of severe pulmonary leptospirosis. Am J Pathol 164:1115–1127

O'Brien MM, Vincent JM, Person DA, Cook BA (1998) Leptospirosis and pancreatitis: a report of ten cases. Pediatr Infect Dis J 17:436–438

Palaniappan RU, Chang YF, Chang CF, Pan MJ, Yang CW, Harpending P, McDonough SP, Dubovi E, Divers T, Qu J, Roe B (2005) Evaluation of lig-based conventional and real time PCR for the detection of pathogenic leptospires. Mol Cell Probes 19:111–117

Palmer MF, Zochowski WJ (2000) Survival of leptospires in commercial blood culture systems revisited. J Clin Pathol 53:713–714

Panaphut T, Domrongkitchaiporn S, Thinkamrop B (2002) Prognostic factors of death in leptospirosis: a prospective cohort study in Khon Kaen, Thailand. Int J Infect Dis 6:52–59

Panaphut T, Domrongkitchaiporn S, Vibhagool A, Thinkamrop B, Susaengrat W (2003) Ceftriaxone compared with sodium penicillin G for treatment of severe leptospirosis. Clin Infect Dis 36:1507–1513

Pappachan MJ, Mathew S, Aravindan KP, Khader A, Bharghavan PV, Kareem MM, Tuteja U, Shukla J, Batra HV (2004) Risk factors for mortality in patients with leptospirosis during an epidemic in northern Kerala. Natl Med J India 17:240–242

Park SK, Lee SH, Rhee YK, Kang SK, Kim KJ, Kim MC, Kim KW, Chang WH (1989) Leptospirosis in Chonbuk Province of Korea in 1987: a study of 93 patients. Am J Trop Med Hyg 41:345–351

Pavan ME, Cairó F, Brihuega B, Samartino L (2008) Multiple-locus variable-number tandem repeat analysis (MLVA) of Leptospira interrogans serovar Pomona from Argentina reveals four new genotypes. Comp Immunol Microbiol Infect Dis 31:37–45

Perez J, Goarant C (2010) Rapid Leptospira identification by direct sequencing of the diagnostic PCR products in New Caledonia. BMC Microbiol 10:325

Pouliquen P, Catilina P (2000) Enquete de pharmacosurveillance aupres des medecins vaccinateurs. Rev Med Trav 27:83–88

Que-Gewirth NS, Riberio AA, Kalb SR, Cotter RJ, Bulach DM, Adler B, Saint Girons I, Werts C, Raetz CRH (2004) A methylated phosphate group and four amide-linked acyl chains in Leptospira interrogans lipid A. J Biol Chem 279:25420–25429

Rathinam SR (2005) Ocular manifestations of leptospirosis. J Postgrad Med 51:189–194

Reis EA, Hagan JE, Ribeiro GS, Teixeira-Carvalho A, Martins-Filho OA, Montgomery RR, Shaw AC, Ko AI, Reis MG (2013) Cytokine response signatures in disease progression and development of severe clinical outcomes for leptospirosis. PLoS Negl Trop Dis 7:e2457

Reis RB, Ribeiro GS, Felzemburgh RD, Santana FS, Mohr S, Melendez AX, Queiroz A, Santos AC, Ravines RR, Tassinari WS, Carvalho MS, Reis MG, Ko AI (2008) Impact of environment and social gradient on Leptospira infection in urban slums. PLoS Negl Trop Dis 2:e228

Ressner RA, Griffith ME, Beckius ML, Pimentel G, Miller RS, Mende K, Fraser SL, Galloway RL, Hospenthal DR, Murray CK (2008) Antimicrobial susceptibilities of geographically diverse clinical human isolates of Leptospira. Antimicrob Agents Chemother 52:2750–2754

Ribeiro MA, Assis CSN, Romero EC (1994) Serodiagnosis of human leptospirosis employing immunodominant antigen. Serodiagn Immunother Infect Dis 6:140–144

Romero EC, Caly CR, Yasuda PH (1998) The persistence of leptospiral agglutinins titers in human sera diagnosed by the microscopic agglutination test. Rev Inst Med Trop São Paulo 40:183–184

Salaun L, Merien F, Gurianova S, Baranton G, Picardeau M (2006) Application of multilocus variable-number tandem-repeat analysis for molecular typing of the agent of leptospirosis. J Clin Microbiol 44:3954–3962

Schreier S, Doungchawee G, Chadsuthi S, Triampo D, Triampo W (2013) Leptospirosis: current situation and trends of specific laboratory tests. Expert Rev Clin Immunol 9:263–280

Segura ER, Ganoza CA, Campos K, Ricaldi JN, Torres S, Silva H, Cespedes MJ, Matthias MA, Swancutt MA, Lopez Linan R, Gotuzzo E, Guerra H, Gilman RH, Vinetz JM (2005) Clinical spectrum of pulmonary involvement in leptospirosis in a region of endemicity, with quantification of leptospiral burden. Clin Infect Dis 40:343–351

Seguro AC, Lomar AV, Rocha AS (1990) Acute renal failure of leptospirosis: nonoliguric and hypokalemic forms. Nephron 55:146–151

Sehgal SC, Murhekar MV, Sugunan AP (1995) Outbreak of leptospirosis with pulmonary involvement in North Andaman. Indian J Med Res 102:9–12

Sehgal SC, Sugunan AP, Murhekar MV, Sharma S, Vijayachari P (2000) Randomized controlled trial of doxycycline prophylaxis against leptospirosis in an endemic area. Int J Antimicrob Agents 13:249–255

Sejvar J, Bancroft E, Winthrop K, Bettinger J, Bajani M, Bragg S, Shutt K, Kaiser R, Marano N, Popovic T, Tappero J, Ashford D, Mascola L, Vugia D, Perkins B, Rosenstein N (2003) Leptospirosis in "eco-challenge" athletes, Malaysian Borneo, 2000. Emerg Infect Dis 9:702–707

Self CA, Iskrzynska WI, Waitkins SA, Whicher JW, Whicher JT (1987) Leptospirosis among British cavers. Cave Sci 14:131–134

Shaw RD (1992) Kayaking as a risk factor for leptospirosis. Mo Med 89:354–357

Shenberg E, Torten M (1973) A new leptospiral vaccine for use in man. I. Development of a vaccine from *Leptospira* grown on a chemically defined medium. J Infect Dis 128:642–646

Signorini ML, Lottersberger J, Tarabla HD, Vanasco NB (2013) Enzyme-linked immunosorbent assay to diagnose human leptospirosis: a meta-analysis of the published literature. Epidemiol Infect 141:22–32

Silva HR, Tanajura GM, Tavares-Neto J, Gomes Md Mde L, Linhares Ad Ada C, Vasconcelos PF, Ko AI (2002a) Aseptic meningitis syndrome due to enterovirus and *Leptospira* sp in children of Salvador, Bahia. Rev Soc Bras Med Trop 35:159–165

Silva JJ, Dalston MO, Carvalho JE, Setubal S, Oliveira JM, Pereira MM (2002b) Clinicopathological and immunohistochemical features of the severe pulmonary form of leptospirosis. Rev Soc Bras Med Trop 35:395–399

Sitprija V, Evans H (1970) The kidney in human leptospirosis. Am J Med 49:780–788

Slack AT, Dohnt MF, Symonds ML, Smythe LD (2005) Development of a multiple-locus variable number of tandem repeat analysis (MLVA) for *Leptospira interrogans* and its application to *Leptospira interrogans* serovar Australis isolates from far North Queensland. Australia. Ann Clin Microbiol Antimicrob 4:10

Smits HL, Hartskeerl RA, Terpstra WJ (2000a) International multi-centre evaluation of a dipstick assay for human leptospirosis. Trop Med Int Health 5:124–128

Smits HL, van Der Hoorn MA, Goris MG, Gussenhoven GC, Yersin C, Sasaki DM, Terpstra WJ, Hartskeerl RA (2000b) Simple latex agglutination assay for rapid serodiagnosis of human leptospirosis. J Clin Microbiol 38:1272–1275

Smits HL, Chee HD, Eapen CK, Kuriakose M, Sugathan S, Gasem MH, Yersin C, Sakasi D, Lai AFRF, Hartskeerl RA, Liesdek B, Abdoel TH, Goris MG, Gussenhoven GC (2001a) Latex based, rapid and easy assay for human leptospirosis in a single test format. Trop Med Int Health 6:114–118

Smits HL, Eapen CK, Sugathan S, Kuriakose M, Gasem MH, Yersin C, Sasaki D, Pujianto B, Vestering M, Abdoel TH, Gussenhoven GC (2001b) Lateral-flow assay for rapid serodiagnosis of human leptospirosis. Clin Diagn Lab Immunol 8:166–169

Smythe L, Dohnt M, Norris M, Symonds M, Scott J (1997) Review of leptospirosis notifications in Queensland 1985 to 1996. Commun Dis Intell 21:17–20

Smythe LD, Smith IL, Smith GA, Dohnt MF, Symonds ML, Barnett LJ, McKay DB (2002) A
    quantitative PCR (TaqMan) assay for pathogenic *Leptospira* spp. BMC Infect Dis 2:13
Smythe LD, Wuthiekanun V, Chierakul W, Suputtamongkol Y, Tiengrim S, Dohnt MF, Symonds
    ML, Slack AT, Apiwattanaporn A, Chueasuwanchai S, Day NP, Peacock SJ (2009) The
    microscopic agglutination test (MAT) is an unreliable predictor of infecting *Leptospira* serovar
    in Thailand. Am J Trop Med Hyg 81:695–697
Spichler A, Spichler E, Moock M, Vinetz JM, Leake JA (2007) Acute pancreatitis in fatal anicteric
    leptospirosis. Am J Trop Med Hyg 76:886–887
Spichler A, Athanazio D, Seguro AC, Vinetz JM (2011) Outpatient follow-up of patients
    hospitalized for acute leptospirosis. Int J Infect Dis 15:e486–e490
Steneroden KK, Hill AE, Salman MD (2011) Zoonotic disease awareness in animal shelter
    workers and volunteers and the effect of training. Zoonoses Public Health 58:449–453
Stern EJ, Galloway R, Shadomy SV, Wannemuehler K, Atrubin D, Blackmore C, Wofford T,
    Wilkins PP, Ari MD, Harris L, Clark TA (2010) Outbreak of leptospirosis among adventure
    race participants in Florida, 2005. Clin Infect Dis 50:843–849
Stoddard RA, Gee JE, Wilkins PP, McCaustland K, Hoffmaster AR (2009) Detection of
    pathogenic *Leptospira* spp. through TaqMan polymerase chain reaction targeting the LipL32
    gene. Diagn Microbiol Infect Dis 64:247–255
Stoenner HG, Dodd T, Larsen C (1982) Antigenic variation of *Borrelia hermsii*. J Exp Med
    156:1297–1311
Sulzer CR, Jones WL (1978) Leptospirosis: methods in laboratory diagnosis. U.S. Department of
    Health, Education and Welfare, Atlanta
Takafuji ET, Kirkpatrick JW, Miller RN, Karwacki JJ, Kelley PW, Gray MR, McNeill KM,
    Timboe HL, Kane RE, Sanchez JL (1984) An efficacy trial of doxycycline chemoprophylaxis
    against leptospirosis. N Engl J Med 310:497–500
Thaipadungpanit J, Wuthiekanun V, Chierakul W, Smythe LD, Petkanchanapong W, Limpaiboon
    R, Apiwatanaporn A, Slack AT, Suputtamongkol Y, White NJ, Feil EJ, Day NP, Peacock SJ
    (2007) A dominant clone of *Leptospira interrogans* associated with an outbreak of human
    leptospirosis in Thailand. PLoS Negl Trop Dis 1:e56
Thaipadunpanit J, Chierakul W, Wuthiekanun V, Limmathurotsakul D, Amornchai P, Boonslip S,
    Smythe LD, Limpaiboon R, Hoffmaster AR, Day NP, Peacock SJ (2011) Diagnostic accuracy
    of real-time PCR assays targeting 16S rRNA and LipL32 genes for human leptospirosis in
    Thailand: a case-control study. PLoS ONE 6:e16236
Torten M (1979) Leptospirosis. In: Stoenner HE, Torten M, Kaplan W (eds) CRC handbook series
    in zoonoses section a: bacterial, rickettsial and mycotic diseases, pp 363–420. CRC press, Boca
    Raton
Trevejo RT, Rigau-Perez JG, Ashford DA, McClure EM, Jarquin-Gonzalez C, Amador JJ, de los
    Reyes JO, Gonzalez A, Zaki SR, Shieh WJ, McLean RG, Nasci RS, Weyant RS, Bolin CA,
    Bragg SL, Perkins BA, Spiegel RA (1998) Epidemic leptospirosis associated with pulmonary
    hemorrhage-Nicaragua, 1995. J Infect Dis 178:1457–1463
Truccolo J, Serais O, Merien F, Perolat P (2001) Following the course of human leptospirosis:
    evidence of a critical threshold for the vital prognosis using a quantitative PCR assay. FEMS
    Microbiol Lett 204:317–321
Truccolo J, Charavay F, Merien F, Perolat P (2002) Quantitative PCR assay to evaluate ampicillin,
    ofloxacin, and doxycycline for treatment of experimental leptospirosis. Antimicrob Agents
    Chemother 46:848–853
Tubiana S, Mikulski M, Becam J, Lacassin F, Lefevre P, Gourinat AC, Goarant C, D'Ortenzio E
    (2013) Risk factors and predictors of severe leptospirosis in New Caledonia. PLoS Negl Trop
    Dis 7:e1991
Turner LH (1968) Leptospirosis II. Serology. Trans R Soc Trop Med Hyg 62:880–889
Turner LH (1970) Leptospirosis III. Maintenance, isolation and demonstration of leptospires.
    Trans R Soc Trop Med Hyg 64:623–646

Verma A, Kumar P, Babb K, Timoney JF, Stevenson B (2010) Cross-reactivity of antibodies against leptospiral recurrent uveitis-associated proteins A and B (LruA and LruB) with eye proteins. PLoS Negl Trop Dis 4:e778

Vinetz JM, Wilcox BA, Aguirre A, Gollin LX, Katz AR, Fujioka RS, Maly K, Horwitz P, Chang H (2005) Beyond disciplinary boundaries: leptospirosis as a model of incorporating transdisciplinary approaches to understand infectious disease emergence. EcoHealth 2:1–16

Viriyakosol S, Matthias MA, Swancutt MA, Kirkland TN, Vinetz JM (2006) Toll-like receptor 4 protects against lethal *Leptospira interrogans* serovar Icterohaemorrhagiae infection and contributes to in vivo control of leptospiral burden. Infect Immun 74:887–895

Wagenaar JF, Goris MG, Partiningrum DL, Isbandrio B, Hartskeerl RA, Brandjes DP, Meijers JC, Gasem MH, van Gorp EC (2010) Coagulation disorders in patients with severe leptospirosis are associated with severe bleeding and mortality. Trop Med Int Health 15:152–159

Waitkins S (1986) Leptospirosis in man, British Isles: 1984. Brit Med J 292:1324

Wani H (1933) Über die prophylaxe der pirochaetosis icterohaemorrhagica Inada (Weilschen Krankheit) durch Schutzimpfung. Zeitschr Immunforsch Exp Therap 79:1–26

Watt G, Padre LP, Tuazon ML, Calubaquib C, Santiago E, Ranoa CP, Laughlin LW (1988) Placebo-controlled trial of intravenous penicillin for severe and late leptospirosis. Lancet 1:433–435

Weil A (1886) Ueber eine eigenthümliche, mit Milztumor, Icterus und Nephritis einhergehende, acute Infectionskrankheit. Dtsch Arch Klin Med 39:209

Werts C, Tapping RI, Mathison JC, Chuang T-H, Kravchenko V, Saint Girons I, Haake D, Godowski PJ, Hayashi F, Ozinsky A, Underhill D, Aderem A, Tobias PS, Ulevitch RJ (2001) Leptospiral endotoxin activates cells via a TLR2-dependent mechanism. Nat Immunol 2:346–352

Werts C (2010) Leptospirosis: a Toll road from B lymphocytes. Chang Gung Med J 33:591–601

WHO (1999) Leptospirosis worldwide, 1999. Wkly Epidemiol Rec 74:237–242

WHO (2011) Report of the second meeting of the leptospirosis burden epidemiology reference group

Wilkins E, Cope A, Waitkins S (1988) Rapids, rafts, and rats. Lancet 2:283–284

Wilson MR, Naccache SN, Samayoa E, Biagtan M, Bashir H, Yu G, Salamat SM, Somasekar S, Federman S, Miller S, Sokolic R, Garabedian E, Candotti F, Buckley RH, Reed KD, Meyer TL, Seroogy CM, Galloway R, Henderson SL, Gern JE, DeRisi JL, Chiu CY (2014) Actionable diagnosis of neuroleptospirosis by next-generation sequencing. N Engl J Med 370:2408–2417

Winslow WE, Merry DJ, Pirc ML, Devine PL (1997) Evaluation of a commercial enzyme-linked immunosorbent assay for detection of immunoglobulin M antibody in diagnosis of human leptospiral infection. J Clin Microbiol 35:1938–1942

Wolff JW (1954) The laboratory diagnosis of leptospirosis. C.C.Thomas, Springfield, Illinois

Yagupsky P, Nolte FS (1990) Quantitative aspects of septicemia. Clin Microbiol Rev 3:269–279

Yang CW, Hung CC, Wu MS, Tian YC, Chang CT, Pan MJ, Vandewalle A (2006) Toll-like receptor 2 mediates early inflammation by leptospiral outer membrane proteins in proximal tubule cells. Kidney Int 69:815–822

Yersin C, Bovet P, Merien F, Clement J, Laille M, Van Ranst M, Perolat P (2000) Pulmonary haemorrhage as a predominant cause of death in leptospirosis in Seychelles. Trans R Soc Trop Med Hyg 94:71–76

Zaki SA, Shanbag P (2010) Clinical manifestations of dengue and leptospirosis in children in Mumbai: an observational study. Infection 38:285–291

Zaki SR, Shieh WJ (1996) Leptospirosis associated with outbreak of acute febrile illness and pulmonary haemorrhage, Nicaragua, 1995. Lancet 347:535–536

Animal Leptospirosis

William A. Ellis

Abstract Leptospirosis is a global disease of animals, which can have a major economic impact on livestock industries and is an important zoonosis. The current knowledge base is heavily biased towards the developed agricultural economies. The disease situation in the developing economies presents a major challenge as humans and animals frequently live in close association. The severity of disease varies with the infecting serovar and the affected species, but there are many common aspects across the species; for example, the acute phase of infection is mostly sub-clinical and the greatest economic losses arise from chronic infection causing reproductive wastage. The principles of, and tests for, diagnosis, treatment, control and surveillance are applicable across the species.

Contents

W.A. Ellis (✉)
OIE Leptospira Reference Laboratory, AFBI Veterinary Sciences Division,
Belfast, Northern Ireland
e-mail: billellisellktj@hotmail.com

© Springer-Verlag Berlin Heidelberg 2015
B. Adler (ed.), *Leptospira and Leptospirosis*, Current Topics in Microbiology
and Immunology 387, DOI 10.1007/978-3-662-45059-8_6

1   Introduction

Animal leptospirosis is fundamentally different from human leptospirosis in important aspects of epidemiology, pathogenesis, clinical features, requirements of diagnostic methods used and the control measures applied. It is characterised by the acute clinical features seen in human disease, but also chronic infection which can result in important economic losses due to reproductive wastage.

2   Epidemiology: General Considerations

Leptospirosis in animals is ubiquitous. It has been found in almost all regions, with the exception of the polar regions, and in virtually every animal species examined by experienced investigators. Within the domestic species there appears to be a range of susceptibility to infection, with horses being susceptible to a wide range of leptospires while infection in cats is rare. The central point in the epidemiology of leptospirosis is the renal carrier excreting leptospires into the environment. Sexual transmission is also important in within species transmission.

In theory any parasitic *Leptospira* may infect any animal species. Fortunately, only a small number of serovars is endemic in any particular region or country. Furthermore, leptospirosis is a disease that shows a natural nidality, and each serovar tends to be maintained in specific maintenance hosts (Hathaway 1981). Therefore, in any region, an animal species will be infected by serovars maintained by that species or by serovars maintained by other animal species present in the area. The relative importance of these incidental infections is determined by the opportunity that prevailing social, management, and environmental factors provide for contact and transmission of leptospires from other species. As with humans, incidental infections are most common in warm, moist climates, with poor sanitation, poor rodent control and mixed domestic animal management systems leading to conditions which provide for environmental contamination by a diverse range of *Leptospira* strains and for the maximum survival of those strains in the environment.

Incidental infections are more likely to be associated with acute clinical disease and renal excretion is usually of limited duration. Limited host ranges for the major host maintained infections allows for the development of control/eradication schemes.

The major host maintained infections of global importance are Ict-erohaemorrhagiae infection in the brown rat, *Rattus norvegicus*, Hardjo in cattle and sheep and Canicola and possibly Bratislava in pigs and possibly dogs. Other host maintained infections have a more limited geographical spread either due to limitations in host distribution or to unrecognized factors, e.g., serovars Kenniwicki or Tarassovi infection in pigs. Whether a population maintains an infection may also depend on population density and environmental conditions. For example, in a New Zealand study the brown rat did not maintain Ballum infection under most conditions, but it did so when present in high density populations found on rubbish dumps (Hathaway and Blackmore 1981).

Host maintained leptospires are excellent parasites and have little clinical effect on, and cause minimal pathological damage to, their hosts, except under certain circumstances e.g., immune-compromised animals, such as females in late pregnancy and the neonate or where there is concurrent infection such as bovine virus diarrhea in cattle or circavirus infection in pigs. Renal persistence and urinary excretion may last for years even and leptospires may have a major tropism for tissues other than kidney, for example the genital tract (Ellis et al. 1986a, b).

3 Pathogenesis

Infection most frequently occurs through the mucous membranes of the eye, mouth, nose or genital tract. Oral infection has also been shown in predators. Vertical transmission can also occur. A period of bacteremia, which may last for a week, begins 1 or 2 days after infection. During this period, leptospires can be isolated from blood and most organs of the body and also from the cerebrospinal fluid. This primary bacteremic phase ends with the appearance of circulating antibodies, which are detectable usually after 10–14 days. A secondary bacteremic period (after 15–26 days) has rarely been reported (Hathaway et al. 1983).

Acute clinical disease coincides with the bacteremic phase of the disease. It is seen mainly in young animals. It is usually associated with incidental infections, particularly hemolysin-producing strains such as Pomona or Icterohaemorrhagiae serogroup strains, which cause hemolytic disease, hemoglobinuria, jaundice and death. Renal damage can be an important feature, particularly in Canicola infection in dogs. Agalactia may occur in cattle, sheep and buffalo. Acute disease can be important in individual herds/flocks, but not on a national basis.

Antileptospiral agglutinins appear at detectable levels in the blood at approximately 10–14 days after infection and reach maximum levels at around 3–6 weeks. Peak titers vary considerably (1,000 to 100,000 in the MAT), and these may be maintained for up to 6 weeks, depending on the species, after which a subsequent gradual decline occurs. Low titers may be detectable for several years in many animals.

Following the period of leptospiremia, leptospires localize in the proximal renal tubules where they multiply and are voided in the urine. The duration and intensity of urinary shedding varies from species to species, animal to animal and with the infecting serovar. In the case of Pomona infection in pigs, the intensity of excretion is highest during the first month of shedding (Bolt and Marshall 1995a, b); urine shedding is very constant during this period. A variable period of intermittent, low-intensity leptospiruria then ensues, and this may last for up to 2 or more years in some cases.

Leptospires may also localize in the uterus of pregnant females; abortion,abortion, stillbirth, and neonatal disease may result from intrauterine infections occurring in late gestation. If immune competence has developed, antibodies to the infecting leptospire may be found in pig, cattle and horse fetuses. The pathogenesis of reproductive disease is poorly understood, but some authors believe that transplacental infection, occurring during the very limited period of maternal leptospiremia, is the sole cause. The low antibody titers detected in dogs and sows aborting Bratislava-infected fetuses has led to the hypothesis that infection may occur as a result of waning uterine immunity being unable to prevent transplacental infection by leptospires present in the genital tract. In multiparous species there may be sequential infection in the uterus with offspring being born/aborted at various stages of infection, i.e., some uninfected, some septicemic and some dead and starting to autolyse. Limited post abortion excretion in uterine discharges may occur.

An additional feature, seen in host-maintained infection, is persistence of leptospires in the oviduct and uterus of non-pregnant females and in the genital tracts of males (Ellis et al. 1986a, b, c, d; Oliveira et al. 2007). In vitro studies have also shown that leptospires have the ability to adhere to and penetrate the zona pellucida and enter embryonic cells (Bielanski and Surujballi 1998). Chronic persistence in the mammary gland and its drainage lymph nodes has also been reported (Thiermann 1982). Leptospires localize and persist in the eye of some species, most notably the horse, leading to uveitis and blindness (Hartskeerl et al. 2004). Symptomless infection is thought to be very common as evidenced by the wide disparity between seroprevalence and apparent disease prevalence.

The cellular and molecular basis of pathogenesis is described in detail in chapter by G.L. Murray.

4 Disease in Animals

4.1 Large Ruminants

4.1.1 Cattle

Bovine leptospirosis occurs world-wide and results from infection by a wide variety of serovars. Cattle maintain serovar Hardjo, which has an almost global distribution, although there are some cattle rearing areas where it is absent or only present at a very low levels, most notably the Scandinavian countries. *Leptospira borgpetersenii* serovar Hardjo (Hardjobovis, HB) is the common strain of this serovar maintained by cattle, but *Leptospira interrogans* serovar Hardjo (Hardjoprajitno, HP) also occurs in cattle in some parts of the world. Both strains have the ability to colonise and persist in the genital tract of infected cows and bulls suggesting that venereal spread may be a factor in transmission.

The host-parasite relationship between HP and cattle has been a conundrum. It was first isolated from cattle in Scotland (Michna and Campbell 1969) and subsequently in Northern Ireland where it was common in the 1970s and early 1980s (Ellis et al. 1988), often in mixed infection with HB, but has not been isolated there for than 20 years. Isolation has been reported from cattle from a number of countries from around the world, including such diverse locations as Nigeria (Ezeh et al. 1989), Brazil (Moreira 1994; Chiareli et al. 2012) and Mexico (Carmona-Gasca et al. 2011). Whether it has been superseded by a more successful parasite, such as HB which may have been introduced in the late 1960s by imported cattle, or whether some other factor such as vaccinal pressure has contributed to its demise is a matter of speculation. It has never been isolated from cattle in the USA (Alt et al. 2001), where it has been isolated from a horse (Kinde et al. 1996), and where HP vaccination has been practiced since the 1960s. Its apparent demise in the UK coincided with the introduction of HP vaccination for cattle in the mid-1980s.

The major risk factors that have been identified for Hardjo infection in cattle are open herds, co-grazing with sheep, access to contaminated water courses, use of natural service, and herd-size (Bennett 1994; Ryan et al. 2012; Van Schaik et al. 2002; Oliveira et al. 2010). Infection rates in zero-grazed dairy cattle are very low or absent, while there is little evidence of spread of infection in dairy animals which are housed for the winter, leading to speculation that diets which give rise to acid pH urine may also be a factor in reducing transmission (Leonard et al. 1992). Alternatively, it may be that artificial insemination, the norm in such circumstances, rather than natural service is the key factor in reducing transmission.

Serovar Kennewicki is the other common serovar in cattle, but its distribution is largely limited to north and south America, Australia, and New Zealand. It can persist in cattle and propagating epidemics can occur under certain circumstances, but it is also dependent on external environmental factors and the presence of other host species (Elder et al. 1986; Kingscote 1988), such as pigs or skunks, whereas the maintenance of serovar Hardjo is based solely on host factors. Other members of the Pomona serogroup can infect cattle, but they are strictly incidental infections, e.g., serovars Mozdok and Pomona.

A wide variety of other serovars belonging to the Icterohaemorrhagiae, Canicola, Hebdomadis, Sejroe, Pyrogenes, Autumnalis, Australis, Javanica, Tarassovi, and Grippotyphosa serogroups have been reported as causing incidental infections in cattle in some parts of the world.

Severe disease is uncommon and is usually associated with infection by strains belonging to the Pomona, Icterohaemorrhagiae, and Grippotyphosa serogroups in young animals. Clinical signs include pyrexia, hemolytic anemia, hemoglobinuria, jaundice, occasionally meningitis, and death. In lactating cows, incidental infections are often associated with small quantities of blood-tinged milk. The acute phase of clinical disease in serovar Hardjo (both subtypes) infection is usually subclinical, with the exception of lactating cows, where agalactia may occur. The characteristics of this acute "milk drop syndrome" are: (1) a sudden drop in milk production; (2) a soft flabby udder with all four quarters affected; (3) pyrexia may or may not be present; (4) the milk has a yellow colostrum-like appearance, contains clots, has a high somatic cell count and appears free of common mastitis causing organisms; (5) most animals return to almost full milk production in 10–14 days with or without treatment, the exception being animals in late gestation which may dry off; (6) the number of animals affected can vary from 1 to 50 %, depending on herd immunity and herd management practices. Large outbreaks, while very dramatic, are rare and individual cases (even herd outbreaks) can go unobserved unless milk production is recorded (Higgins et al. 1980).

Abortion, stillbirth, premature birth, the birth of weakly calves and reduced birth weight are the most important economic aspects of chronic leptospirosis in cattle. In incidental infections it occurs 4–6 weeks after acute disease, but with Hardjo infection the interval is longer at 6–12 weeks. Abortion is not a consistent feature after agalactia and vice versa (Ellis et al. 1985a). Placental infection may also affect the weight of calves; stillborn or weak calves with Hardjo infected placentas were significantly lighter than uninfected controls (Smyth et al. 1999). There has also been an association with retention of fetal membranes (Ellis et al. 1985a). Leptospires have been detected for up to 8 days in post abortion/calving vaginal discharges (Ellis et al. 1985b). Infertility, which responds to antibiotic and/or vaccination, is described in Hardjo infection (Dhaliwal et al. 1996a, b).

The pattern of Hardjo infection in a herd varies with the husbandry conditions and the strains of Hardjo present. In endemically infected herds, where young stock are exposed to infection before breeding, levels of associated reproductive wastage are very low. Management systems, found particularly in intensive dairy farming, can contribute to clinical disease prevalence, most notably the practice of separating calves at birth and only exposing them to the adult infected herd after sexual maturity, thus ensuring a regular supply of fully susceptible animals. Strains of Hardjo in some parts of the world are associated with reproductive failure, while in others, most notably Australia and New Zealand they are not; however, new evidence suggests that the situation there is changing (Sanhueza et al. 2013).

There are large parts of the world where cattle are important, but where very little is known about the role of leptospirosis in disease. This is particularly true in Africa where studies in Nigeria (Jagun et al. 2011) and Zimbabwe (Feresu 1992) have shown high prevalences of renal carriage.

4.1.2 Buffalo

The limited information available indicates a picture in domestic buffalo resembling that in cattle. High seroprevalences have been found in virtually all investigations. Acute disease has been associated with jaundice, fatal hemorrhagic syndrome and agalactia (Upadhye et al. 1983; Pande et al. 1961; Khalacheva and Sherkov 1981; Ahmed 1990) with abortion as a sequel (Marianelli et al. 2007; Dehkordi and Taghizadeh 2012).

4.1.3 Cervidae

Reports of leptospirosis in deer species have been dominated by seroprevalence investigations, with very few isolation studies or clinical reports. These studies have shown that all species of wild deer examined have shown evidence of seroconversion and renal carrier rates of up to 19 % have been recorded (Koizumi et al. 2008).

Most of the detailed information available results from the investigation of farmed red deer in New Zealand, where serovar Hardjo is endemic, but largely subclinical, with losses between birth and weaning and poorer live weight gain being the only possible clinical effects identified (Subharat et al. 2011, 2012a). Infection has been identified in a fetus from a hind with a Hardjo titer (Subharat et al. 2010). Pomona infection is less common, but more likely to cause clinical disease, while Copenhageni infection is uncommon, but has been associated with clinical disease (Ayanegui-Alcerreca et al. 2007).

Hardjo has also been recovered from rusa deer (Perez and Gorant 2010) while mixed Hardjo and Copenhageni infections have been observed in some animals (Flint et al. 1986). Experimental infection of pronghorns has shown that Hardjo may persist in that species for more 381 days (Thorne 1985).

Pomona strains have been the most common isolates from deer, having been recovered from red deer, white-tailed deer (Abdulla et al. 1962; Roth et al. 1964) and rusa deer (Perez and Gorant 2010). Pomona infection has been implicated in acute hemolytic disease of red deer (Ayanegui-Alcerreca et al. 2007), mule deer (Rapley et al. 1981) and white-tailed deer (Ferris et al. 1960).

4.1.4 Camelids

Information about leptospirosis in camelids is sparse. In south America high seroprevalences have been reported in alpacas (Rosadio et al. 2012), vicunas (Rosadio et al. 2012; Llorente et al. 2002) and llamas (Marin et al. 2008; Llorente et al. 2002) and lower seroprevalences in guanacos (Llorente et al. 2002).

Seroprevalence rates have been low (0–12 %) in dromedaries from north Africa and the Arabian peninsula (Shigidi 1974; Burgmeister et al. 1975, Afzal and Sakkir 1994; Wernery et al. 2008), but a 50 % seroprevalence has been reported in Rajasthan (Mathur et al. 1984). Information on clinical leptospirosis in camels is lacking. As with other animal species, abortion (Dehkordi and Taghizadeh 2012) is a feature; leptospires were demonstrated in 8/49 aborted fetuses (7 by PCR and culture and 1 by PCR only). An interesting observation has been the finding that 19/130 camel bloods were PCR positive (Doosti et al. 2012).

4.2 Small Ruminants

4.2.1 Sheep

Relative to cattle and pigs, sheep have been considered resistant to leptospiral infection, with historical low seroprevalences and only a small number of sero-groups being implicated in clinical disease, namely Pomona (Vermunt et al. 1994), Grippotyphosa (Trap and Garin 1988), Icterohaemorrhagiae (Leon et al. 1987), Australis, and Sejroe (Ellis et al. 1983a; McKeown and Ellis 1986). Infections by the first four serogroups are incidentally acquired and have resulted in sporadic outbreaks of acute disease characterised by hematuria, hemoglobinuria, jaundice, and death, usually in lambs and occasional abortions (Ellis et al. 1983a, b, c; Leon et al. 1987). Serological studies would indicate high levels of exposure to some incidental infections, Icterohaemorrhagiae infection in Brazil (da Silva et al. 2012) and Tunisia (Khbou et al. 2010), Canicola in Iran (Hassanpour et al. 2011), Pomona in India (Balakrishnan et al. 2011) and Nigeria (Agunloye 2002). PCR studies would suggest that abortion may be more common than previously thought (Moshkelani et al. 2011). Lilenbaum et al. (2008) have detected leptospiral DNA in the semen of infected rams and vaginal fluids of ewes. Noguchi, Javanica, and Bratislava have been isolated from sheep (Silva et al. 2007; Natarajaseenivasan and Ratnam 1999; Little et al. 1981), in Brazil, India, and the UK respectively. Leon et al. (1987) isolated Pomona and Icterohaemorrhagiae from aborted fetuses in Spain.

In contrast, sheep have emerged as an alternative maintenance host for serovar Hardjo. This is based on (1) significant serological prevalences to serovar Hardjo (Egan and Yearsley 1987; Cerri et al. 2003; Ridler et al. 2005; Herrmann et al. 2004; Martins et al. 2012) in some sheep populations; (2) abattoir studies (Bahaman et al. 1980; Dorjcc et al. 2008); (3) experimental studies (Cousins et al. 1989; Farina et al. 1996; Gerritsen et al. 1994); (4) the apparent independence of sheep infections from cattle (Pekelder et al. 1993), and (5) sheep have been identified as a risk factor for Hardjo infection in cattle and deer (Bennett 1994; Subharat et al. 2012a, b). The organism can persist for long periods of time in the kidney of infected animals (Cousins et al. 1989; Farina et al. 1996; Gerritsen et al. 1994) and a recent study has shown that it can also persist in the genital tract of ewes (Arent et al. 2013) PCR studies would indicate that excretion in semen also occurs (Lilenbaum et al. 2008).

Most infections are subclinical and clinical Hardjo infection is rarely seen in extensively managed flocks. In intensively managed flocks, Hardjo has been reported as causing clinical infection in the peri-parturient ewe and the neonate, with abortion, stillbirth, the birth of weak lambs and agalactia being reported (Ellis et al. 1983a, b, c; McKeown and Ellis 1986; McTague 1997). It has also been implicated in infertility (Lilenbaum et al. 2009).

4.2.2 Goats

The literature on leptospirosis in goats is considerably smaller than that for cattle, pigs, and even sheep, which is probably a reflection of the fact that goat production and losses have not been seen as economic priorities in the animal production systems of the developed economies. Various serovars have been isolated from goats in many parts of the world (Anonymous 1966, 1974). These serovars belong to the Australis, Grippotyphosa, Hebdomadis, Sejroe, Pomona serogroups (Torten 1979; Schollum and Blackmore 1981; Lilenbaum et al. 2007). Goats are susceptible to experimental infection with Icterohaemorrhagiae (Michna 1970), Pomona (Morse and Langham 1958) and Hardjo (Tripathy et al. 1985) and severe disease with high mortality, associated Grippotyphosa infection, has been reported (Torten 1979). As with other leptospiral infections, abortion may be the most important clinical consequence (Leon et al. 1987; Dehkordi and Taghizadeh 2012).

4.3 Swine

Leptospirosis is a common disease of swine throughout the world and can be a significant cause of reproductive loss. Knowledge of the incidence and economic impact of the disease is biased towards the intensive pig industries of the northern hemisphere, Australia, New Zealand, Argentina, and Brazil. The serogroups most commonly associated with infection of pigs are the Pomona, Australis, and Tarassovi groups, and include strains maintained by pigs, but all of which have alternative wildlife maintenance hosts. Significant incidental infections include strains belonging to the Grippotyphosa, Icterohaemorrhagiae, and Canicola serogroups.

The three host-maintained infections differ in terms of available information, geographical distribution, clinical impact, disease patterns and how they have been affected by industry moves to modern, total confinement systems.

4.3.1 Pomona Infection

Serovar Pomona and the closely related serovar Kennewicki have been the most common serovars isolated from pigs worldwide. Many strains of serovars Pomona and Kennewicki, especially those found in the United States and Canada, are adapted to swine. In the past, they have been the cause of widespread clinical disease in swine in north and south America, Australia, New Zealand, and eastern and central Europe, and were thought to be endemic in many of these regions (Ellis 2012). The situation appears to have changed, although this should be caveated by the lack of recent surveillance data. Widespread vaccination has been practiced in eastern Europe and north America and there has been a move to indoor housing. No carriers were detected in a 1989 meat-plant survey carried out in Iowa (Bolin and Cassells 1992), while no evidence of Pomona infection was found in Quebec (Ribotta et al. 1999). A move to indoor housing systems would also have prevented contact with the known wildlife host, the skunk (Mitchell et al. 1966). Studies in Europe suggest a similar decline, although there is still evidence of infection in Sardinia where there is close contact between domestic pigs and wild boar (Pintore et al. 2012). Such strains are apparently absent from the more westerly parts of Europe where rodent maintained strains of serovar Mozdok and serovar Pomona may cause occasional small outbreaks of clinical disease (Barlow 2004; Rocha 1990; Zieris 1991). There is now evidence of high levels of Pomona infection in parts of Africa (Agunloye 2001) and Southeast Asia (Al-Khleif et al. 2009).

Serovar Kennewicki infection can cause an acute febrile illness in young pigs, characterised by hemorrhage, hematuria, jaundice, signs of renal failure; infection may be fatal. This is also a feature of some incidental infections, including infections by other members of the Pomona serogroup (serovars Mozdok and Pomona). Adult non-pregnant animals are usually asymptomatic carriers, with infected pigs shedding enormous numbers of leptospires in their urine for as long as a year after infection. Abortion, stillbirth or the birth of weak or ill piglets are often the only signs of leptospirosis in a breeding herd. During the initial herd infection, clinical disease may occur in all ages of sows, while in herds with endemic infection, clinical disease is usually restricted to gilts that have either been reared in isolation since weaning and reintroduced into the herd, or more commonly brought in from an uninfected herd (Ellis 2012). Following abortions due to Pomona, there does not appear to be any subsequent limitation on reproductive performance, even in pigs that remain infected for long periods (Ferguson and Powers 1956; Kemenes and Suveges 1976; Mitchell et al. 1966).

4.3.2 Australis Infection

Serovar Bratislava has a global distribution but it remains poorly understood due to difficulties in culturing these strains. In contrast to the high seroprevalences reported worldwide, serovar Bratislava or closely related strains have only been recovered from pigs in a few countries, namely The Netherlands (Hartman et al. 1975), United Kingdom (Ellis et al. 1986e, 1991), the United States (Ellis and Thiermann 1986; Bolin and Cassells 1990, 1992), Germany (Schonberg et al. 1992), and Vietnam (Boqvist et al. 2003).

The epidemiology of these strains is poorly understood. There are specific pig-adapted strains, strains that are maintained by pigs, dogs, horses, and hedgehogs, and strains that are found only in wildlife. Within the pig isolates, there are genotypes that are more likely to be associated with disease (Ellis et al. 1991; Ellis, W.A., unpublished data).

Two very distinct serological profiles may be seen in endemically infected herds. In indoor sow units infected with pig-adapted strains of Bratislava, the prevalence of sows with antibody titers of greater than 100 in the MAT is usually very low, although many sows will have titers of less than 100. This is thought to result from infection being primarily due to venereal transmission. In contrast, in units where the sows are kept outside, the seroprevalence (≥100) may be greater than 50 %. This is thought to be due to the sows being infected systemically as a result of exposure to infected rodent urine. Seropositivity in outdoor reared pigs is directly related to rainfall (Boquist et al. 2012).

Although the renal-carrier state does become established, urinary excretion is poor compared with Pomona excretion, and transmission within the fattening house is inefficient. Important additional carrier sites have been identified, namely, the upper genital tracts of sows and boars (Ellis et al. 1986b, d; Bolin and Cassells 1992; Power 1991). Venereal transmission is thought to play an important role in the spread of Bratislava infection. Infertility is also a feature (Hathaway and Little 1981; Frantz et al. 1989).

4.3.3 Tarassovi Infection

Information on the epidemiology of Tarassovi infection in pigs is limited. It would appear that pigs could have acted as a maintenance host for some strains of Tarassovi found in Eastern Europe. Tarrasovi does not spread as rapidly in a pig population as does Pomona, but endemic infection is readily maintained (Kemenes and Suveges 1976). While it was common in eastern and southern Europe, it would appear to have almost disappeared in most regions. The reasons for this are unclear. In Spain and Portugal, it has apparently disappeared without any specific control measures (Pumarola et al. 1987; Perea et al. 1994), whereas in the east of Europe vaccination was practiced.

4.3.4 Incidental Infections

Incidental infections can cause both acute and chronic infections in pigs, but clinical cases are focal with limited in-contact spread. The serovars involved and the prevalence of these infections vary around the world depending on the sophistication of the management systems in those regions. They are very rare in housed populations, but may be more important in outdoor-rearing systems. Treatment of clinical disease is by a combination of systemic and oral antibiotics and, where available, vaccination.

4.4 Horses and Donkeys

Apart from seroprevalence studies, leptospirosis in horses has largely been ignored until relatively recently (Verma et al. 2013). The recognition that leptospiral infections can have major economic consequences, through the loss of very expensive foals or recurrent uveitis ending the career of valuable horses, has brought about a change in attitudes. Seroprevalence and isolation studies indicate that the horse is susceptible to a wide range of incidental infections, in particular serovars belonging to the Pomona (serovar Kennewicki) and Grippotyphosa serogroups, but also the Icterohaemorrhagiae, Autumnalis, Sejroe, Canicola, and Ballum serogroups (Wood and Townsend 1999). Serovar Kennewicki is the major serovar associated with disease in horses in the USA and one particular genotype has been associated with abortion. That genotype has also been recovered from skunk, racoon, and red fox (Timoney et al. 2011). Small rodents are the source of Grippotyphosa infection in mainland Europe.

Serovar Bratislava antibodies are the most common antibodies detected in horses globally, but the nature of the host pathogen relationship is a matter of debate (Ellis 1999) and it has been postulated that both horse-maintained and incidental infections may occur.

The majority of infections are sub-clinical, but where acute infection in horses occurs, it resembles that seen in severe disease in other species with hemoglobin-uria, jaundice, depression, and impaired renal function (Wood and Townsend 1999). Abortion, stillbirth, and the birth of infected foals which may show severe clinical signs are common sequels to infection (Ellis et al. 1983c: Pooncha et al. 1993). Two to 8 months after initial infection, some horses may develop periodic opthalmia (recurrent uveitis or ERU). It is accompanied by the presence of specific antibodies in the aqueous and vitreous humor, and the persistence of leptospires in the eye. An auto-immune response to persistent infection results in periodic opthalmia and blindness. This appears to be an organ-specific autoimmune cross reaction involving two leptospiral proteins LruA and LruB which are expressed in the eyes of uveitis cases (Verma et al. 2010).

Certain serovars appear to be more commonly associated with ERU, in particular serovar Kennewicki in the USA and serovar Grippotyphosa in Europe (Harskeerl et al. 2004). The distribution of these serovars appears to dictate the frequency of uveitis in the horse population. The incidence of recurrent uveitis is particularly high in Germany, where it has been estimated that about 10 % of horses suffer from ERU, with more than half of the cases being associated with leptospiral infection (Borstel et al. 2010; Kulbock et al. 2013).

Fatigue (Baverud et al. 2009; Twigg et al. 1971) and pulmonary hemorrhage following exercise have also been reported as features of equine leptospirosis. The limited data available suggest that renal carriage rates may be high in some horse populations (Ellis et al. 1983b; Hamond et al. 2012a, b, 2013a). Whether there is chronic persistence in the non-pregnant female genital tract or the genital tract of stallions as in other species has yet to be determined, but PCR-positive material has been found in semen (Genovez et al. 2004; Hamond et al. 2013b).

The study of leptospirosis in donkeys and mules has been neglected, but seroprevalence studies indicate that the situation is likely to be similar to that in horses (Ali and Saeid 2012; Hajikolaei et al. 2005).

4.5 Dogs and Cats

4.5.1 Dogs

Because of human's close affection for pets, there has been more detailed investigation of clinical infection in individual dogs than in other animal species. Dogs are top predators for many rodent species and because of their close association with humans in many societies they provide a unique conduit of transmission from rodents to human.

Serovar Canicola is maintained by dogs worldwide and has no other known maintenance host, but seroprevalence has been falling in many countries (Claus et al. 2008; Ellis 2010). This has been attributed to the use of vaccine for more than 50 years and possible mutations in the prevalent strains (Ellis 2010). Serovars belonging to the Icterohaemorrhagiae serogroup remain important incidental infections of dogs globally (Ellis 2010). Seroprevalence studies would suggest that serovar Bratislava is maintained by dogs in many parts of the world. Grippotyphosa and Pomona have emerged as important incidental causes of clinical disease in dogs in the USA (Anonymous 1998; Bolin 2002; Moore et al. 2006; Gautam et al. 2010). Serological data suggest that Autumnalis infection could also occur there, but in the absence of isolates the belief is that these are cross reactions to Pomona infection. In Europe, Grippotyphosa, and Bratislava have emerged as major causes of canine leptospirosis (Ellis 2010; Mayer-Scholl et al. 2013; Renaud et al. 2013).

Differences in the predominant incidental infections differ elsewhere; e.g., in Japan, Hebdomadis infection has emerged as the major infection in dogs (Koizumi et al. 2013), while in Brazil, Canicola, and Icterohaemorrhagiae infections remain important (Oliveira et al. 2012).

The symptoms and treatment of canine leptospirosis have been documented in detail (Greene et al. 2007; Tangeman and Littman 2013). As with other species, many infections are subclinical. The spectrum of clinical disease in dogs is very similar to that in man. The main forms of the disease are an acute anicteric illness (usually with biphasic pyrexia) and an icteric form. Anicteric leptospirosis is a febrile illness of sudden onset. The fever is often bi-phasic. The initial phase coincides with the bacteremic phase of infection and may last for up to a week. Sometimes a secondary phase may occur after a remission of 3–4 days and coincides with the immune response to infection. The febrile phases are accompanied by a variety of symptoms, which may include combinations of dullness, photophobia, severe myalgia, conjuctival suffusion, anorexia, nausea, vomiting, and prostration. They may be accompanied by leucocytopenia, increased liver transaminases and decreased glomerular filtration rates.

In contrast, icteric leptospirosis is usually more severe and is characterised by liver, kidney and vascular symptoms in addition to the spectrum of symptoms associated with anicteric leptospirosis. Jaundice usually occurs early in the illness and with increasing severity of jaundice the risks of renal failure, hemorrhage, and cardiovascular collapse increase.

While any serovar can produce severe disease, serovars of the Icterohaemorrhagiae and Pomona serogroups tend to be more commonly associated with jaundice. In contrast, other serovars, are usually associated with anicteric disease.

The severe pulmonary form of leptospirosis is a less well known, but increasingly recognized, entity (Tochetto et al. 2012), and is characterised by intra-pulmonary hemorrhage which can lead to acute respiratory failure and death. A variety of chronic sequelae have been described, including chronic interstitial nephritis, and occasionally uveitis (Gallagher 2011).

4.5.2 Cats

Cats are regarded as being very resistant to leptospirosis and attempts at experimental infection have failed (Larsson et al. 1985). Significant seroprevalences have been detected in various cat populations (Mylonakis et al. 2005; Alves et al. 2003; Modric and Knezevic 1997; Batza and Weiss 1987; Dickeson and Love 1993; Agunloye and Nash 1996; Jamshidi et al. 2009), but there are very few reports of clinical disease (Arbour et al. 2012, Bryson and Ellis 1976; Reilly et al. 1994; Borku et al. 2000). Until recently there has been no evidence of renal carriage in cat populations, but urine studies conducted in strays in Reunion Island and Taiwan have found 29 and 67 % PCR positive rates respectively (Desvars et al. 2013; Chan et al. 2014).

The situation is similar in wild felidae, with only the Iberian lynx being associated with significant clinical disease (Jimenez et al. 2013).

4.6 Non-human Primates

There are very little published data about leptospirosis in non-human primates. High seroprevalences have been found in a various species in captivity, principally in new world monkeys (Romero et al. 2012; Pinna et al. 2012; Lilenbaum et al. 2005), but also in macaques (Bain et al. 1988; Ibanez et al. 2010; Jaffe et al. 2007). Seroprevalences of up to 42 % were found in captured vervet monkeys (Baulu et al. 1987). Antibodies to Icterohaemorrhagiae, Pomona and Grippotyphosa strains have predominated in captive primates (Stasilevich et al. 2000), but Ballum was the predominant serovar detected in free-living vervet monkeys following capture (Balulu et al. 1987). Severe, sometimes fatal, disease has been observed in capuchins (Scarcelli et al. 2003; Szonyi et al. 2011), squirrel monkeys (Perolat et al. 1992), marmosets (Baitchman et al. 2006), tamarins (Reid et al. 1993) and macaques (Shive et al. 1969). The disease spectrum resembles that seen in humans, with severe icteric, anicteric, and pulmonary forms observed (Pereira et al. 2005). Meningo-encephalitis has also been reported, as has abortion (Perolat et al. 1992).

4.7 Rodents and Other Wild Animals

There is an extensive literature on leptospirosis in wild rodent as carriers of leptospirosis, but given the large number of species and diverse habitats there remains much that is not known. In contrast, there is a dearth of information on clinical disease in wild rodents.

There are reports of clinical disease in a diverse range of zoo animals, black rhinosceros (Neiffer et al. 2001), a giant anteater (Monteiro et al. 2003), a polar bear (Kohm 1988), black tailed deer (Rapley et al. 1981) and a wild dog (Vijayarani et al. 2010). Given the potential for human infection, zoos need to be aware of this possibility.

Leptospirosis is one of the most common causes of stranding and mortality in the Californian sea lion, where infection is characterised by liver and kidney infection leading to acute renal failure and death (Mancia et al. 2012). Other pinnipeds are also affected, including northern fur seals, northern elephant seals and harbor seals (Cameron et al. 2008).

Some bat populations are carriers of leptospires (Mueldorfer 2013), but there is little characterisation of the organisms other than several molecular studies which show that they are pathogens (Cox et al. 2005; Mathias et al. 2005) and while there is some evidence of fruit bats transmitting infection to rodents (Tulsiani et al. 2011), there is no evidence of significant spread to domestic animals.

4.8 Laboratory Animals

Young, susceptible laboratory animals, most notably guinea pigs, hamsters and to a lesser extent gerbils, have been widely used as experimental models for studying the disease processes in acute leptospirosis. They have also been used in the indirect isolation of leptospires, as a means of recovering leptospires from contaminated environments, passaging leptospires to enhance virulence and in vaccine potency testing. Welfare legislation and ethical review processes in many countries discourage these uses and alternative methods of vaccine potency testing are being developed (Klaasen et al. 2013; Stokes et al. 2012; Romberg et al. 2012).

Models utilizing the Wistar strain of *R. norvegicus* have been developed to provide valuable information on the proteomics, pathology and immunology of chronic renal infection in a maintenance host (Tucunduva de Faria et al. 2007; Athanazio et al. 2008; Monahan et al. 2008; Nally et al. 2011). Balb/c mice are also susceptible to renal colonisation with some serovars (Faine 1963; Masuzawa et al. 1991).

4.9 Reptiles and Other Poikilothermic Vertebrates

The role of reptiles and other poikilothermic vertebrates has been historically neglected, which is unfortunate given that many have a close association with water, an important risk factor for leptospirosis in higher vertebrates. Seroprevalence studies have been the primary surveillance tool used in higher vertebrates, but natural serum factors which cause agglutination in lower vertebrate sera have raised doubts about the value of seroprevalence studies in those species (Charon et al. 1975).

Infection has been demonstrated by culture and PCR in a range of frogs and toads (Diesch et al. 1966; Babudieri et al. 1973; Gravekamp et al. 1991; Jiang et al. 2011). Similarly, infection has been demonstrated in snakes and turtles (Ferris et al. 1961; Glosser et al. 1974; Hyakutake et al. 1980; Biscola et al. 2011). Long term persistence of Pomona in hibernating snakes suggested an overwintering mechanism for leptospires.

5 Pathology

The main pathological changes are essentially the same for all infections, with the primary lesion being damage to the endothelial cells of small blood vessels (Fig. 1). The consequences of this vary considerably with the infecting serovar, the animal species, its age, and the stage of infection. The findings in acute disease, particularly in dogs, are similar to those found in humans.

In acute fatal leptospirosis, there are no pathognomonic gross changes; however, there are changes which would indicate the inclusion of acute leptospirosis in a differential diagnosis. These include icterus and the presence of ecchymotic and petechial hemorrhages on the serosal surface of major organs including the lungs, kidney (Fig. 2), abomasum and the peritoneum and pleura and blood in the bladder.

Fig. 1 Vasculitis in a horse which died of acute leptospirosis

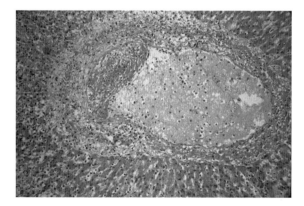

Fig. 2 Acute Canicola
infection in a pig showing the
surface of the kidney covered
in hemorrhages

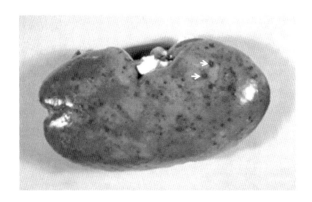

Liver may be enlarged with accentuation of the hepatic lobes. Hepatocellular dissociation, intracanicular cholestasis, hepatocellular necrosis and Kupffer cell hypertrophy may be found on histological examination. The kidneys may be swollen and when cut exhibit a marked pale infiltrate, particularly at the cortico-medullary junction, particularly in dogs (Fig. 3). Acute interstitial nephritis, with tubular and glomerular degeneration, and the infiltration of mononuclear cells, lymphocytes, plasma cells and macrophages, may be seen on histological examination.

Myocarditis and meningitis may also be present. The clinical pathological features of acute leptospirosis in dogs have been reviewed recently by Tangeman and Littman (2013).

In chronic leptospirosis, lesions are confined to the kidneys and consist of scattered small gray foci, often surrounded by a ring of hyperemia (Fig. 4). Microscopic examination shows these lesions to be a progressive focal interstitial nephritis. The interstitial leukocytic infiltrations, which consist mainly of lymphocytes, macrophages, and plasma cells, may be extensive in some areas, particularly in dogs. Focal damage may also involve the glomeruli and renal tubules. Older lesions mainly consist of fibrosis and interstitial infiltration. In the host-maintained infections, lesions are usually very small and focal in nature (Fig. 5) and may even be visible only on microscopic examination.

Fig. 3 Acute Canicola
infection in a dog showing
gross infiltration (*arrowed*) of
the renal cortex by monocytes

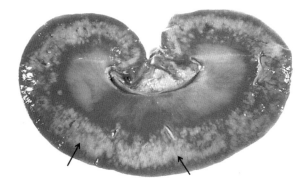

Fig. 4 Focal pale lesion
surrounded by hyperaemia on
a serovar Hardjo infected
Bovine kidney

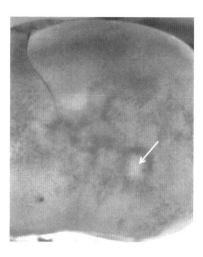

Fig. 5 Mild focal interstitial
nephritis in serovar Hardjo
infected Bovine kidney

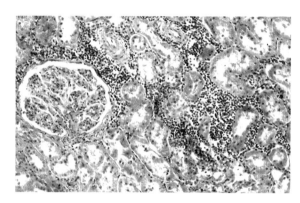

Fetal pathology varies considerably and depends on the species, the stage of gestation at which infection occurred and the infecting serovar. In cattle, sheep, and swine, pathological examination of fetuses usually reveals only nonspecific findings either as a result of autolysis or which cannot be differentiated satisfactorily from autolytic changes. Jaundice may occasionally be seen in subcutaneous tissues of late term abortions, while stillborn fetuses frequently exhibit lesions similar to those produced by anoxia—i.e., petechial hemorrhages on the surface of the thymus, thyroid, lungs, and heart and in the parietal pleura, peritoneum, and mesentery. Vascultis and perivascular hemorrhage, particularly in the liver and to a lesser extent the lung and meninges plus mild tubular necrosis and interstitial nephritis have been features of experimental fetal disease (Ellis 1994, 2012). In contrast, Pooncha et al. (1993) reported gross and histopathological changes in 80 and 96 % respectively of aborted equine fetuses (largely due to Kenniwicki infection). These were consistent with what is seen in acute leptospirosis in young animals. Placentitis was also a feature. Funisitis has also been horses (Sebastian et al. 2005).

Aspects of the pathology of ocular lesions in horses has been reviewed by several authors (Kalsow and Dwyer 1998; Matthews 1999). The clinical pathology of canine leptospirosis has been reviewed recently (Tangeman and Littman 2013).

6 Diagnosis

A diagnosis of leptospirosis may be required not only for the confirmation of leptospirosis as a cause of clinical disease, but also for other reasons, such as (1) the assessment of the infection and/or the immune status of a herd for the purposes of a control or eradication program on either a herd or national basis; (2) epidemiological studies; and (3) an assessment of the infectivity status of an individual animal to assess its suitability for international trade or for introduction into an uninfected herd.

Leptospirosis should be differentiated from other diseases where (1) acute milk drop may occur, such as acute viral infections and sudden withdrawal of drinking water: (2) diseases with liver and kidney failure; (3) diseases characterized by abortion, stillbirth, birth of weakly offspring or infertility, such as brucellosis, Neospora infection, Q-fever and bovine viral diarrhea virus infection in cattle, chlamydiosis and toxoplasmosis in sheep, equine herpes virus in horses etc.

The mild, often inapparent, clinical signs of acute leptospirosis make clinical diagnosis difficult; therefore, diagnosis is usually dependent on laboratory procedures. Laboratory diagnostic procedures for leptospirosis fall into two groups. The first group consists of tests for the demonstration of leptospires in tissues; the second contains the tests for antibody detection. The selection of tests to be carried out depends on the purpose for which a diagnosis is to be made and the resources available.

The appropriateness of the two groups of tests at the various stages of infection is outlined in Fig. 6.

6.1 Demonstration of Leptospires in Animals

The use of organism detection methods has a role in: (1) the initial bacteremic phase of infection when organisms may be detected in blood and milk; (2) untreated fatal cases and aborted or stillborn fetuses, where there may be multiple organ infection; and (3) the localization phase where following the onset of the immune response, leptospires localize in immunologically protected sites such as the proximal renal tubules, genital tract, and eye, and may be demonstrated in urine, products of abortion, etc. and the aqueous humor (horse and fetus—all species). The methods available fall into the following categories: direct visualization of organisms by dark-field microscopy, culture, DNA detection methods and staining (silver and immunochemical).

Appropriateness of diagnostic procedure to stage of infection

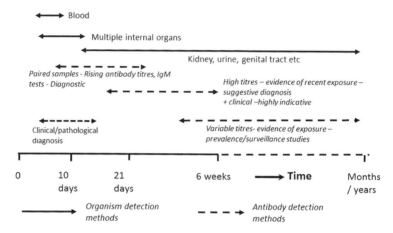

Fig. 6 The appropriateness of serological and organism based tests at various stages of infection

The demonstration of leptospires in blood and milk of animals showing clinical signs suggestive of acute leptospirosis is considered to be diagnostic. However, isolation of leptospires from blood and milk is often unsuccessful because of their transient nature and frequent lack of accompanying clinical signs. Animals may have been treated with antibiotics before samples were collected for testing for *Leptospira,* which further decreases the likelihood of identifying the agent. The demonstration of generalised leptospiral infection in a range of organs taken at post mortem examination is also considered to be diagnostic. However, if the animal lives long enough or has been treated with antibiotics, it may be difficult to detect intact organisms. Demonstration of leptospires in the genital tract, kidneys, or urine only, must be interpreted with caution as these findings may merely indicate that the animal was a carrier.

Failure to demonstrate leptospires in the urine of an animal does not rule out the possibility that the animal is a chronic renal carrier; it merely indicates that the animal was not excreting detectable numbers of leptospires at the time of testing. Collection of urine following treatment of the animals with a diuretic enhances the chances of detecting the organism (Nervig and Garrett 1979). Urine samples should be mixed immediately with an equal volume of phosphate buffered saline containing 1 % bovine serum albumin on collection (Ellinghausen 1973).

The demonstration of leptospires in body fluids or internal organs (usually kidney, liver, lung, brain, adrenal gland, mesenteric lymph nodes or stomach contents) of aborted or stillborn fetuses is considered to be diagnostic of chronic leptospirosis of the mother, and is evidence of active infection of the fetus. Infection of only placental tissue should not be taken as evidence of fetal infection.

Dark-field microscopy is a rapid method for demonstrating leptospires in body fluids, but the method is insensitive and lacks specificity (Levett 2001; Vijayachari et al. 2001) with artefacts in blood and urine giving rise to false positives (Frerichs and Maley 1980). It is most successful in the examination of urine from those species which may produce high concentrations of leptospires in their urine such as rats, but its use should be avoided if possible.

PCR is increasingly used for diagnosis because of its perceived sensitivity, its not requiring the presence of viable organisms and its ability to give an early diagnosis. There is now a considerable literature on its use in the diagnosis of animal leptospirosis. Real-time PCR (SYBR Green or Taqman technology) is faster than regular PCR and less sensitive to contamination (Picardeau 2013). Assays fall into two categories based on the detection of genes which are universally present in bacteria, for example, *gryB*, *rrs* (16S rRNA gene) and *secY*, or the detection of genes restricted to pathogenic *Leptospira*, for example, *lipL21*, *lipL32*, *lipL41*, *ligA* and *ligB* (Thaipadunpanit et al. 2011). There remain problems with the validation of reported PCRs, as comparisons with culture, which has 100 % specificity, have usually been carried out in seeded material and not in naturally infected material, or comparisons have been made with the microscopic agglutination test, a procedure which can have a sensitivity of less than 50 %. Where it has been compared with culture of naturally infected material the quality of the culture component has usually been questionable. A positive PCR demonstrates the presence of pathogenic leptospires, but does not currently allow direct identification of the serovar. Analyzing the melting curves of the amplification products or sequencing may allow identification of the species and in some cases the genotype (Perez and Goarant 2010; Cerqueira et al. 2010). There have been particular problems with the use of PCR in aborted fetal material due to the presence of inhibitors resulting from tissue autolysis, but recent reports are more positive (Artiushin et al. 2012), with some of the problems being circumvented by testing stomach contents (Dosti and Tamimian 2011; Hamond et al. 2012a), a fluid commonly used in the diagnosis of other abortifacient bacterial infections.

Culture, if successful, is far too slow to provide treatment guidance; however, it can provide retrospective information which is useful in epidemiological studies and advising control measures. It is difficult and resource-demanding, with successful isolation taking up to 6 months and no single medium supporting the primary isolation of all pathogenic leptospires. While culture has 100 % specificity, sensitivity is often very poor. In the majority of publications the quality of the culture technique used is poor and lacks an understanding of the requirements for isolating, what may be small numbers of viable leptospires, from contaminated and/or autolytic material. Permutations of liquid and semi-solid (0.1–0.2 % agar) EMJH (Johnson and Seiter 1976) and supplemented Tween 80/40 media (Ellis et al. 1985a, b, c) with various levels of rabbit serum (0.4–5 %), with and without selective agents (5-fluorouracil, nalidixic acid, fosfomycin, and a cocktail of rifamycin, polymyxin, neomycin, 5-fluorouracil, bacitracin, and actidione), are required. When combined with a dilution technique, these media offer the optimum chance of successful isolation. Culture media containing 5-fluorouracil at levels between 200 and 500 µg/mL should be used as transport media for the submission of samples. Cultures should be incubated at 28–30 °C for up 26 weeks and examined by dark-field microscopy every 7–10 days. The time required for detection of a positive culture varies with the leptospiral serovar and the number of viable organisms present in the sample. Less fastidious serovars such as Icterohaemorrhagiae may result in positive cultures in less than 2 weeks, but other serovars such as pig and dog Bratislava strains may take considerably longer and require topping up with fresh medium during the incubation period.

In the event of death, staining methods such as immunofluorescence and immunochemical staining are appropriate additional methods (Ross et al. 2011). Immunofluorescence is particularly useful in the diagnosis of fetal infection (Ellis et al. 1982a, b).

6.2 Serological Tests

Serological testing is the most widely used method for diagnosing leptospirosis, and the MAT is the standard serological test. The minimum antigen requirements are that the test should employ representative strains of all the serogroups known to exist in the particular country or region, plus those known to be maintained elsewhere by the species under examination. It is labor and resource demanding and its sensitivity depends on the stage of infection in an individual animal.

As an individual animal test, the MAT is most sensitive when used in diagnosing acute infection; rising antibody titers in paired acute and convalescent serum samples are diagnostic. High titres (≥1,000) in animals showing recent clinical signs are highly suggestive of leptospirosis. As with human sera, paradoxical reactions can present a problem in interpreting the initial MAT response to acute infection; antibody titers to heterologous strains may give equal or higher titers than the infecting serovar. This is particularly the case with dog sera, but it can occur in all species. The presence of antibody in fetal serum is diagnostic of fetal infection.

The MAT has severe limitations in the diagnosis of chronic infection in individual animals, both in the diagnosis of abortion and in the identification of renal or genital carriers where titers are falling or static. Infected animals may have MAT titers below the widely accepted minimum significant titer of 100 (Ellis et al. 1982b, 1986b; Otaka et al. 2012; Hamond et al. 2012b).

The MAT is used primarily as a herd test. To obtain useful information, at least 10 animals or 10 % of the herd, whichever is greater, should be tested (Hathaway et al. 1986). A retrospective diagnosis of both acute leptospirosis and abortion may be inferred when the majority of affected animals have titers of 1,000 or greater (Ellis et al. 1982b); however, the converse is not true. Increasing the sample size and sampling a number of different cohorts markedly improves epidemiological information, investigations of clinical disease, assessments of vaccination needs, and public health tracebacks.

ELISA tests for detection of anti-leptospiral antibodies have been developed using a number of different antigen preparations, assay protocols and assay platforms, including plate tests and dipstick tests. The antigen preparations have mainly been either whole cell preparations or outer membrane protein (OMP) preparations, with recent emphasis on developing tests using recombinant OMPs. The antigen used dictates the specificity of the ELISA. Recombinant OMP-based ELISAs are broadly reactive to antibodies to all pathogenic leptospires and so their value will be mainly in the diagnosis of acute infection in those species, such as the dog, where such a diagnosis is required (Dey et al. 2004; La-ard et al. 2011; Subathra et al. 2013), but will have limited value in epidemiological investigations (possibly as a screening test) or retrospective diagnosis of chronic disease where the emphasis is in determining the infecting serovar for assessing the practicalities of vaccine use. They have no value in control programs for host maintained infections, such as serovar Hardjo, where naturally infected cattle produce a weak or no response to OMPs, but where the major serological response is to outer envelope lipopolysaccharide antigens (Ellis et al. 2000). In contrast, lipopolysaccharide antigen based ELISAs are serogroup specific and have value in epidemiological investigations and control schemes. IgM ELISAs have been shown to be useful in the diagnosis of acute infection in dogs (Hartman 1984). A total-Ig ELISA is useful in the identification of fully susceptible animals suitable for experimental challenge work (Ellis et al. 1989). ELISAs have also been developed for use in milk from individual cows or in bulk tank milk for the detection of serovar Hardjo antibodies. These tests have been helpful in identifying Hardjo-infected herds and in serovar Hardjo control/eradication programs (Pritchard 1999). However, herds that are vaccinated against serovar Hardjo will also be positive in these various ELISAs, decreasing their usefulness in regions where is a routine practice.

Problems with validation have been major constraints in assessing ELISA tests. Almost all have been validated against the MAT (using MAT titres of 100 or greater), which is an imperfect test, having very low a sensitivities in chronic infections.

7 Treatment and Control

7.1 Treatment

The treatment of acute leptospirosis in individual animals or in herds is dependent on the use of antibiotics plus supportive symptomatic treatment. In the case of valuable companion animals, intensive supportive therapy may be required; fluid therapy is almost always indicated and blood transfusions and dialysis may be deemed appropriate. When treating herd problems in pigs, cattle and sheep, vaccination may be combined with antibiotic treatment to obviate chronic reproductive wastage. The principles are the same for all species, but the antibiotics used may vary according to their safety in a particular species, their availability in a particular country, the cost and the route of administration.

A combination of penicillin and streptomycin has been the antibiotic therapy of choice for the treatment of acute leptospirosis, but ampicillin, amoxycillin, tetracyclines, tulathromycin and third generation cephalosporins have also been used (Alt and Bolin 1996; Alt et al. 2001; Cortese et al. 2007; Smith et al. 1997). In food-producing animals, withdrawal times are an important consideration. In the face of an outbreak of Hardjo agalactia in cattle, the cost of withdrawing milk has to be balanced against the risk of subsequent abortions. The usual decision is not to treat, but only vaccinate; however, the owner must be cautioned that vaccination alone may not stop abortion if genital infection has already taken place.

Antibiotics also have a role in chronic disease. Systemic treatment with penicillin and streptomycin should be considered in the face of an abortion storm in pigs, while in cattle in the same situation, streptomycin may be given to dairy animals in late gestation which have already dried-off or are about to. Vaccination should also be given to all at risk animals.

Treatment with a third generation cephalosporin has proved useful in the treatment of equine recurrent uveitis (ERU) (Dixon and Coppack 2002; Speiss 2008). Pars plana vitrectomy is commonly used in treatment of ERU in horses (Tomordy et al. 2010; Borstel et al. 2005).

Antibiotics are used for the treatment of chronic renal and genital leptospirosis, an important component of control programs. Streptomycin at 25 mg/kg has been the most widely used antibiotic for the treatment of renal carrier animals, but in some experiments it has not been effective (Hodges et al. 1979; Ellis et al. 1985c).

The use of tetracyclines as a feed supplement has been widely used for the control of clinical leptospirosis in pigs. While it suppresses clinical signs, it does not give a microbiological cure (Ellis 2012). A combination of penicillin and streptomycin in semen diluent is effective in killing leptospires (Rodrigues et al. 2003).

7.2 Control

The principles of control are the same for most animal species and are based on the interruption of direct and indirect transmission of infection. Variations occur in the particular methods used, depending on ease of access to the animals, the numbers involved, the tools available and the economic viability of control. Control may be needed not only to control infection in a particular species but also to reduce the zoonotic risk.

Control strategies must take into consideration the location, number of animals, infecting serovars, maintenance hosts, means of transmission,risk factors, and the control options available. Good surveillance information is required. This can come from disease surveillance through diagnostic services, sero-epidemiological surveys, or culture-based data on prevalence rates in wild and/or domestic animal populations, or from combinations of these methodologies. Surveillance should prioritize species where economic losses have been identified, species with a known history of maintaining leptospires and novel species identified in epidemiological studies of human disease. This establishes the relative importance of serovars and host species, leading to the possibilities for reducing/managing risk factors, vaccination programs, rodent control programs and animal health programs.

Control decisions are not always based on the obvious ones of reducing/preventing human infections and preventing clinical disease and economic loss in animals. Other considerations include achieving economic or strategic advantage for either the national or individual herds or the generation of laboratory/practice income.

The type of control program varies depending on the objectives—control of clinical disease, an immune population or eradication which leaves a susceptible population. The tools for control include: vaccination, antibiotic therapy, assessment of herd/population status (profiling), identification, and removal of infected animals, rodent control, reducing risk factors through management systems and permutations of all these methods.

Vaccination is the easiest and often the only practical method of control. It is the method of choice for the dog owner or the commercial farmer who wants an immune animal population rather than a susceptible population. Its use is limited by availability, expense, quality, and appropriateness of the antigens in the vaccine in terms of relevance to the species and country. Efficacy data for some products is poor in terms of microbiological protection data, and often based on inappropriate studies, including unnatural routes of challenge and very short duration of immunity studies. Suggested examples of inappropriate antigens are the inclusion of Canicola and Icterohaemorrhagiae antigens in US cattle and pig vaccines, for which there is little or no supportive evidence.

Vaccines have been most widely used in cattle, pigs, and dogs. They may contain anywhere from one to five or more serovars. Some monovalent or bivalent products, containing the cattle maintained serovar Hardjo and where appropriate serovar Pomona have been shown to provide good microbiological protection for up to a year (Bolin et al. 1991; Dhaliwal et al. 1996a) and modern dog five-way products have produced a similar duration of immunity (Klaasen et al. 2013). Multivalent vaccines for cattle compared very unfavorably with monovalent product in a series of experiments (Bolin et al. 1989a, b, 1991) but they continue to be sold and the debate about their efficacy continues (Rinehart et al. 2012a, b; Alt et al. 2012).

Pig vaccines have not been put under the same critical scrutiny as cattle vaccines, as the pig industry has been prepared to accept shorter periods of immunity, namely one gestation. In dogs, the move has been to evidence-based vaccine requirements with microbiological immunity being seen as important as clinical immunity (Klaasen et al. 2013).

Even the best cattle and pig vaccines may not protect the fetus(es) if placental infection has already occurred before vaccination.

Vaccination in dogs should be given as early as possible after the decline in maternally derived antibody, usually at around 10 weeks. The timing of vaccination in other species is variable, with some products licensed for use in animals as young as 3 months. However it is important that vaccination is completed before mating in cattle and pigs.

Problems arise in countries which do not have surveillance or diagnostic facilities for leptospirosis, and there is reliance on imported multivalent products which may not be appropriate to the particular species or region. The number of species for which vaccines are licensed is often limited and situations arise where vaccines have to be used off license, for example, the use of cattle Hardjo vaccines in sheep, or multivalent product in alpacas.

Antibiotics have a role in control programs. Where active infection has been established in a herd, antibiotics are often used at the start of a program to reduce or eliminate infection from carrier animals before initiating a vaccination or testing and eradication program, or in the case of pigs, before embarking on an oral antibiotic program. Antibiotics may also be used as part of a quarantine process, whereby bought-in animals are quarantined and treated with systemic antibiotics (penicillin and streptomycin) before being released into the herd or country.

Oral antibiotic treatment is widely used in the control of clinical disease in pig herds, e.g., in tetracycline-medicated feed, but its use in eradicating infection has met with variable results (Ellis 2012). It has been very useful in controlling reproductive wastage due to Bratislava infection, but has proved unsuccessful in eliminating infection from a herd (Ellis unpublished data).

Identification and removal of carrier animals is a procedure used in the control of many infectious diseases of animals, but has no value in animal leptospirosis as no single test will reliably identify carrier animals in any of the domestic species.

Rodent (and other wildlife) control is very important in pig and equine leptospirosis. This should involve the use of rodenticides and rodent proof housing.

Livestock management has an important role in preventing the introduction and spread of infection through controlling risk factors other than rodent contact. These are particularly important in dealing with host-maintained infections, where freedom from infection is the objective. A closed herd policy is optimal, but usually impractical. Brought-in animals should be quarantined and treated with antibiotics and artificial insemination should be used in place of natural service. Animals should be purchased from herds of a similar health status. Bull or boar sharing should be avoided as should the use multiple boars in multiple service systems, particularly on gilts. Co-grazing or mixing with other hosts should be avoided, e.g., cattle with sheep. Avoid access to common water sources.

Eradication is an option where it is a component of a wider health scheme e.g., the schemes for cattle farmers in the Netherlands or in the UK (Weber and Verhoeff 2001; Anonymous 2012). It is also an important consideration for farmers who wish to sell bulls into AI stations or be involved in embryo transfer.

The approach to eradication of Hardjo in cattle has been to establish the immune/infection status of herd, through the use of bulk milk ELISA tests and serum ELISAs. If there is no evidence of infection, then control risk factors and maintain free status by regular antibody checks, e.g., bulk milk ELISA. If infected, treat with antibiotics and/or initiate a vaccination program for several years and move to eradication.

8 Challenges

Many challenges remain in animal leptospirosis, for example:

- The impact of leptospirosis on the pastoral economies, particularly in Africa, where the limited available knowledge indicates widespread infection by *Leptospira*, where climate and agricultural practices favor the transmission of infection and where humans and animals live in close contact.
- Goats are a major food source in many developing countries and yet so little is known about the disease in that species.
- In the developed economies, understanding of the role of Bratislava in pigs, dogs and horses remains poorly understood, due to problems in diagnosis which need to be resolved.
- There is a need to balance developments in molecular diagnostics with epidemiological and control requirements, e.g., the validation of novel techniques which identify the infecting strain.
- Maintaining vigilance on the emergence of new host parasite relationships which may be of economic importance, through active surveillance.
- Maintaining a critical mass of expertise. This is in danger in the developed economies where governments have lost interest in endemic disease. In the developing world there is a need to develop expertise.

Acknowledgments My grateful thanks are due to Professor N. Wright for the picture of acute Canicola infection a dog kidney and to the late Dr. S.W. Michna for the photograph of acute Canicola infection in a pig.

References

Abdulla PK, Karstad L, Fish NA (1962) Cultural and serological evidence of leptospirosis in deer in Ontario. Can Vet J 3:71–78
Afzal M, Sakkir M (1994) Survey of antibodies against various infectious disease agents in racing Camels in Abu Dhabi, United Arab Emirates. Revue-Scientifique-et-Technique -Office-International-des-Epizooties 13:787–792
Agunloye CA (2001) Agglutinating antibodies to leptospires in slaughter pigs in Ibadan, Nigeria. Trop Veterinarian 19:188–190
Agunloye CA (2002) Leptospiral agglutinating antibodies in sheep and goats in South-West Nigeria. Israel J Vet Med 57:28–30
Agunloye CA, Nash AS (1996) Investigation of possible leptospiral infection in cats in Scotland. J Small Anim Pract 37:126–129

Ahmed R (1990) Leptospiral infection in lactating buffaloes. Pakistan Vet J 10:98–99
Al-Khleif A, Damriyasa IM, Bauer C, Menge C, Herbst W (2009) A serosurvey for infections with
    Leptospira serovars in pigs from Bali, Indonesia. Dtsch Tierarztl Wochenschr 116:389–391
Ali H, Saeid S (2012) Seroprevalence of leptospiral infection in Horses, Donkeys and Mules in
    East Azerbaijan province. Afr J Microbiol Res 6:4384–4387
Alt DP, Bolin CA (1996) Preliminary evaluation of antimicrobial agents for treatment of
    Leptospira interrogans serovar pomona infection in hamsters and swine. Am J Vet Res 57
    (59–62):24
Alt DP, Zuerner RL, Bolin CA (2001) Evaluation of antibiotics for treatment of cattle infected with
    Leptospira borgpetersenii serovar Hardjo. J Am Vet Med Assoc 219:636–639
Alt DP, Olsen S, Bolin C (2012) Concerns about *Leptospira* vaccine efficacy study. Am J Vet Res
    73:928–929
Alves CJ, Vasconcellos SA, Morais ZM, JSLd A, Clementino IJ, Azevedo SS, Santos FA (2003)
    Valuation the level of antibodies anti-leptospira in cats from the city of Patos, PB. La Clinica
    Veterinaria 8:48–54
Anonymous (1966) C.D.C. Zoonosis surveillance: leptospiral serotypes distribution lists according
    to host and geographical area. U.S. Department of Health Education and Welfare, Atlanta
Anonymous (1974) C.D.C. Zoonosis surveillance: Leptopsiral serotypes distribution lists
    according to host and geographical area. Supplement July 1966 to July 1973. U.S. Department
    of Health, Education and Welfare, Atlanta
Anonymous (1998) Leptospirosis cases rising in United States. J Am Vet Med Assoc 212:472
Anonymous (2012) Cattle health certification standards, incorporating rules for cattle health
    schemes. CHeCS technical document:July 2012, 43pp
Arbour J, Blais MC, Carioto L, Sylvestre D (2012) Clinical leptospirosis in three cats
    (2001–2009). J Am Anim Hosp Assoc 48:256–260
Arent Z, Frizzel C, Gilmore C, Mackie D, Ellis WA (2013) Isolation of leptospires from genital
    tract of sheep. Vet Rec 173:582
Athanazio DA, Silva EF, Santos CS, Rocha GM, Vannier-Santos MA, McBride AJA, Ko AI, Reis
    MG (2008) Rattus norvegicus as a model for persistent renal colonization by pathogenic
    Leptospira interrogans. Acta Trop 105:176–180
Artiushin SC, Timoney JF, Balasuriya UB, Erol E, Sells SF (2012) Real-time PCR for detection of
    Leptospira interrogans serovar Pomona type kennewicki in equine clinical specimens.
    J Equine Vet Sci 32:S53
Ayanegui-Alcerreca MA, Wilson PR, Mackintosh CG, Collins-Emerson JM, Heuer C, Midwinter
    AC, Castillo-Alcala F (2007) Leptospirosis in farmed deer in New Zealand : a review. NZ Vet J
    55:102–108
Babudieri B, Carlos ER, Carlos ET Jr (1973) Pathogenic *Leptospira* isolated from toad kidneys.
    Trop Geogr Med 25:297–299
Bain CB, Cruz NC, Fortugaleza DO, Guzman LE (1988) Prevalence of antibodies to arboviruses
    and *Leptospira interrogans* among captive Phillipine monkeys. Philippine J Vet Med 25:19–22
Balakrishnan G, Govindarajan R, Meenambigai TV, Manohar BM (2011) Seroprevalence of
    leptospirosis among sheep in Tamilnadu. Tamilnadu J Vet Anim Sci 7:285–289
Barlow AM (2004) Reproductive failure in sows associated with *Leptospira* mozdok from a
    wildlife source. Pig J 54:123–131
Batza HJ, Weiss R (1987) Occurrence of *Leptospira* antibodies in cat serum samples.
    Kleintierpraxis 32(171–172):174
Baulu J, Everard COR, Everard JD (1987) Leptospires in vervet monkeys (*Cercopithecus aethiops
    sabaeus*) on Barbados. J Wildl Dis 23:60–66
Baverud V, Gunnarsson A, Engvall EO, Franzen P, Egenvall A, Engvall EO (2009) *Leptospira*
    seroprevalence and associations between seropositivity, clinical disease and host factors in
    horses. Acta Vet Scand 51:15
Bennett RB (1994) A computer-based decision model of leptospirosis control in dairy herds—
    what use for veterinary practice? cattle Practice 2:541–546

Bahaman AR, Marshall RB, Blackmore DK, Hathaway SW (1980) Isolation of *Leptospira interrogans* serovar hardjo from sheep in New Zealand (correspondence). NZ Vet J 28 (171):178

Baitchman EJ, Calle PP, James SB, Linn MJ, Raphael BL (2006) Leptospirosis in Wied's marmosets (*Callithrix kuhlii*). J Zoo Wildl Med 37:182–185

Bielanski A, Surujballi O (1998) Penetration of in vitro fertilized bovine embryos by *Leptospira* after in vitro exposure. Theriogenology 49:250

Biscola NP, Fornazari F, Saad E, Richini-Pereira VB, Campagner MV, Langoni H, Barraviera B, Ferreira Junior RS (2011) Serological investigation and PCR in detection of pathogenic leptospires in snakes. Pesquisa Veterinaria Brasileira 31:806–811

Bolin C (2002). Leptospirosis posing new threat for canine hepatic, renal disease. In Focus:31-34

Bolin CA, Cassells JA (1990) Isolation of *Leptospira interrogans* serovar bratislava from stillborn and weak pigs in Iowa. J Am Vet Med Assoc 196:1601–1604

Bolin CA, Cassells JA (1992) Isolation of *Leptospira interrogans* serovars bratislava and hardjo from swine at slaughter. J Vet Diagn Invest 4:87–89

Bolin CA, Cassells JA, Zuerner RL, Trueba G (1991) Effect of vaccination with a monovalent *Leptospira interrogans* serovar hardjo type hardjo-bovis vaccine on type hardjo-bovis infection of cattle. Am J Vet Res 52:1639–1643

Bolin CA, Thiermann AB, Handsaker A, Foley JW (1989a) Effect of vaccination with a pentovalent leptospiral vaccine on *Leptospira interrogans* serovar hardjo type hardjo-bovis infection of pregnant cattle. Am J Vet Res 50:161–165

Bolin CA, Zuerner RL, Trueba G (1989b) Effect of vaccination with a pentavalent leptospiral vaccine containing *Leptospira interrogans* serovar hardjo type hardjo-bovis on type hardjo-bovis infection in cattle. Am J Vet Res 50:2004–2008

Bolt I, Marshall RB (1995a) The epidemiology of *Leptospira interrogans* serovar pomona in grower pig herds. NZ Vet J 43:10–15

Bolt I, Marshall RB (1995b) The epidemiology of *Leptospira interrogans* serovar pomona in grower pig herds. NZ Vet J 43:204

Boqvist S, Montgomery JM, Hurst M, Thu HTV, Engvall EO, Gunnarsson A, Magnusson U (2003) *Leptospira* in slaughtered fattening pigs in southern Vietnam: presence of the bacteria in the kidneys and association with morphological findings. Vet Microbiol 93:361–368

Boqvist S, Eliasson-Selling L, Bergström K, Magnusson U (2012) The association between rainfall and seropositivity to *Leptospira* in outdoor reared pigs. Vet J 193:135–139

Borku MK, Kurtdede A, Aydin Y, Durgut R, Pekkaya S, Ozkanlar Y (2000) Clinical, laboratory and pathological findings in cats and Dogs exhibiting chronic renal failure signs. Ankara Universitesi Veteriner Fakultesi Dergisi 47:281–289

Borstel MV, Oppen TV, Glitz F, Fruhauf B, Deegen E, Boeve MH, Ohnesorge B (2005) Long-term results of pars-plana (double-port) vitrectomy in equine recurrent uveitis. Pferdeheilkunde 21:13–18

Borstel MV, Oey L, Strutzberg-Minder K, Boeve MH, Ohnesorge B (2010) Direct and indirect detection of leptospires in vitreal samples of horses with ERU. Pferdeheilkunde 26:219–225

Bryson DG, Ellis WA (1976) Leptospirosis in a British domestic cat. J Small Anim Pract 17:459–465

Burgemeister R, Leyk W, Gossler R (1975) Studies on the occurrence of parasites and bacterial and viral infections in southern Tunisian dromedaries. Dtsch Tierarztl Wochenschr 82:352–354

Cameron CE, Zuerner RL, Raverty S, Colegrove KA, Norman SA, Lambourn DM, Jeffiies SJ, Gulland FM (2008) Detection of pathogenic *Leptospira* bacteria in pinniped populations via PCR and identification of a source of transmission for zoonotic leptospirosis in the marine environment. J Clin Microbiol 46:1728–1733

Carmona-Gasca AC, Lara LL, Castillo-Sanchez OL, Ramirez-Ortega MJ, Ko A, Palomera LC, de la Pena-Moctezuma A (2011) Detection of *Leptospira santarosai* and *L. kirschneri* in cattle: new isolates with potential impact in bovine production and public health. Veterinaria Mexico 42:277–288

Cerqueira GM, McBride AJA, Hartskeerl RA et al (2010) Bioinformatics describes novel loci for high resolution discrimination of *Leptospira* isolates. PLoS One 5(10):1533

Cerri D, Ebani VV, Fratini F, Pinzauti P, Andreani E (2003) Epidemiology of leptospirosis: observations on serological data obtained by a "Diagnostic Laboratory for Leptospirosis" from 1995 to 2001. Microbiologica 26:383–389

Charon NW, Johnson RC, Muschel LH (1975) Antileptospiral activity in lower vertebrate sera. Infect Immun 12:1386–1391

Chan K-W, Hsu Y-H, Hu W-L, Pan M-J, Lai J-M, Huang K-C, Chou S-J (2014) Serological and PCR detection of feline *Leptospira* in southern Taiwan. Vector Borne Zoon Dis 14:118–123

Chiareli D, Cosate MRV, Moreira EC, Leite RC, Lobato FCF, da Silva JA, Teixeira JFB, Marcelino AP (2012) Control of leptospirosis in dairy cattle with autogenous vaccine in Santo Antonio do Monte, MG, Brazil. Pesquisa Veterinaria Brasileira 32:633–639

Claus A, de Maele IV, Pasmans F, Gommeren K, Daminet S (2008) Leptospirosis in dogs: a retrospective study of seven clinical cases in Belgium. Vlaams Diergeneeskundig Tijdschrift 77:259–263

Cortese V, Behan S, Galvin J, Penka D, Ramsey D, Bryson W, Lucas M (2007) Evaluation of two antimicrobial therapies in the treatment of *Leptospira borgpetersenii* serovar hardjo infection in experimentally infected cattle. Vet Therap 8:201–208

Cousins DV, Ellis TM, Parkinson J, McClashan CH (1989) Evidence for sheep as a maintenance host for *Leptospira interrogans* serovar hardjo. Vet Rec 124:123–124

Cox TE, Smythe LD, Leung LKP (2005) Flying foxes as carriers of pathogenic *Leptospira* species. J Wildl Dis 41:753–757

da Silva RC, da Costa VM, Shimabukuro FH, Richini-Pereira VB, Menozzi BD, Langoni H (2012) Frequency of *Leptospira* spp. in sheep from Brazilian slaughterhouses and its association with epidemiological variables. Pesquisa Vet Bras 32:194–198

Dehkordi FS, Taghizadeh F (2012) Prevalence and some risk factors associated with brucellosis and leptospirosis in aborted fetuses of ruminant species. Res Opin Anim Vet Sci 2:275–281

Desvars A, Naze F, Benneveau A, Cardinale E, Michault A (2013) Endemicity of leptospirosis in domestic and wild animal species from Reunion Island (Indian Ocean). Epidemiol Infect 141:1154–1165

Dey S, Mohan CM, Kumar T, Ramadass P, Nainar AM, Nachimuthu K (2004) Recombinant Lipl32 antigen-based single serum dilution elisa for detection of canine leptospirosis. Vet Microbiol 103:99–106

Dhaliwal GS, Murray RD, Dobson H, Montgomery J, Ellis WA (1996a) Effect of vaccination against *Leptospira interrogans* serovar hardjo on milk-production and fertility in dairy cattle. Vet Rec 138:334–335

Dhaliwal GS, Murray RD, Dobson H, Montgomery J, Ellis WA (1996b) Reduced conception rates in dairy cattle associated with serological evidence of *Leptospira interrogans* serovar hardjo infection. Vet Rec 139:110–114

Dickeson D, Love DN (1993) A serological survey of dogs, cats and horses in south-eastern Australia for leptospiral antibodies. Aust Vet J 70:389–390

Diesch SL, McCulloch WF, Braun JL, Ellinghausen HC (1966) Leptospires isolated from frog kidneys. Nature 209:939–940

Dixon P, Coppack R (2002) Equine recurrent uveitis. Vet Rec 150:556

Doosti A, Tamimian NH (2011) Diagnosis of leptospiral abortion in bovine by polymerase chain reaction. Global Veterinaria 7:79–82

Doosti A, Ahmadi R, Arshi A (2012) PCR detection of leptospirosis in Iranian Camels. Bulgarian J Vet Med 15:178–183

Dorjee S, Heuer C, Jackson R, West DM, Collins-Emerson JM, Midwinter AC, Ridler AL (2008) Prevalence of pathogenic *Leptospira* spp. in sheep in a sheep-only abattoir in New Zealand. NZ Vet J 56:164–170

Egan J, Yearsley D (1987) Serological survey of leptospiral antibodies in cattle, sheep and pigs in the Republic of Ireland. Irish Vet J 41:213–214

Elder JK, McKeon GM, Duncalfe F, Ward WH, Leutton RD (1986) Epidemiological studies on the ecology of *Leptospira interrogans* serovars pomona and hardjo in Queensland. Prev Vet Med 3:501–521

Ellinghausen HC (1973) Growth teperatures, virulence, survival, and nutrition of leptospires. J Med Microbiol 6:487–497

Ellis WA (1999). Equine leptospirosis. Equine infectious diseases VIII. In: Proceedings of the 8th international conference, Dubai. R&W Publications (Newmarket) Ltd, Newmarket, pp 155–158, 23–26 March 1998

Ellis WA (1994) Leptospirosis as a cause of reproductive failure. Vet Clin Nth Am Food Anim Pract 10:463–478

Ellis WA (2010) Control of canine leptospirosis in Europe: time for a change? Vet Rec 167:602–605

Ellis WA (2012) Leptospirosis. In: Zimmerman JJ, Karriker LA, Ramirez A, Swartz KJ, Stevenson GW (eds) Diseases of swine. Wiley, New York, pp 770–778

Ellis WA, O'Brien JJ, Neill SD, Ferguson HW, Hanna J (1982a) Bovine leptospirosis: microbiological and serological findings in aborted fetuses. Vet Rec 110:147–150

Ellis WA, O'Brien JJ, Neill SD, Hanna J (1982b) Bovine leptospirosis: serological findings in aborting Cows. Vet Rec 110:178–180

Ellis WA, Bryson DG, Neill SD, McParland PJ, Malone FE (1983a) Possible involvement of leptospires in abortion, stillbirths and neonatal deaths in sheep. Vet Rec 112:291–293

Ellis WA, O'Brien JJ, Cassells JA, Montgomery J (1983b) Leptospiral infection in horses in Northern Ireland: serological and microbiological findings. Equine Vet J 15:317–320

Ellis WA, Bryson DG, O'Brien JJ, Neill SD (1983c) Leptospiral infection in aborted equine foetuses. Equine Vet J 15:321–324

Ellis WA, O'Brien JJ, Bryson DG, Mackie DP (1985a) Bovine leptospirosis: some clinical features of serovar hardjo infection. Vet Rec 117:101–104

Ellis WA, O'Brien JJ, Cassells JA, Neill SD, Hanna J (1985b) Excretion of *Leptospira interrogans* serovar hardjo following calving or abortion. Res Vet Sci 39:296–298

Ellis WA, Montgomery J, Cassells JA (1985c) Dihydrostreptomycin treatment of bovine carriers of *Leptospira interrogans* serovar hardjo. Res Vet Sci 39:292–295

Ellis WA, Songer JG, Montgomery J, Cassells JA (1986a) Prevalence of *Leptospira interrogans* serovar Hardjo in the genital and urinary tracts of non pregnant cattle. Vet Rec 118:11–13

Ellis WA, McParland PJ, Bryson DG, Thiermann AB, Montgomery J (1986b) Isolation of leptospires from the genital tract and kidneys of aborted sows. Vet Rec 118:294–295

Ellis WA, Cassells JA, Doyle J (1986c) Genital leptospirosis in bulls. Vet Rec 118:333

Ellis WA, McParland PJ, Bryson DG, Cassells JA (1986d) Boars as carriers of leptospires of the Australis serogroup on farms with an abortion problem. Vet Rec 118:563

Ellis WA, McParland PJ, Bryson DG, Cassells JA (1986e) Prevalence of *Leptospira* infection in aborted pigs in Northern Ireland. Vet Rec 118:63–65

Ellis WA, Thiermann AB (1986) Isolation of *Leptospira interrogans* serovar bratislava from sows in Iowa. Am J Vet Res 47:1458–1460

Ellis WA, Thiermann AB, Montgomery J, Handsaker A, Winter PJ, Marshall RB (1988) Restriction endonuclease analysis of *Leptospira interrogans* serovar hardjo isolates from cattle. Res Vet Sci 44:375–379

Ellis WA, Montgomery JM, McParland PJ (1989) An experimental study with a *Leptospira interrogans* serovar bratislava vaccine. Vet Rec 125:319–321

Ellis WA, Montogomery JM, Thiermann AB (1991) Restriction endonuclease analysis as a taxonomic tool in the study of pig isolated belonging to the australis serogroup of *Leptospira interrogans*. J Clin Microbiol 29:957–961

Ellis WA, Yan KT, McDowell SWJ, Mackie DP, Pollock JM, Taylor MJ (2000) Immunity to bovine leptospirosis. In: Proceedings of the 21st World Buiatrics Congress, pp 10601–10611

Ezeh AO, Kmety E, Ellis WA, Addo PB, Adesiyun AA (1989) Characterisation of leptospires isolated from cattle and man in Plateau State, Nigeria. Revue Scientifique et Technique Office International des Epizooties 8(1009–1020):1026

Faine S (1963) Antibody in the renal tubles and urine of mice. Aust J Exp Biol Med Sic 41:81–91

Farina R, Cerri D, Renzoni G, Andreani E, Mani P, Ebani V, Pedrini A, Nuvoloni R (1996) *Leptospira interrogans* in the genital tract of sheep. Research on ewes and rams experimentally infected with serovar hardjo (Hardjobovis). Microbiologica 19:235–242

Feresu SB (1992) Isolation of *Leptospira interrogans* from kidneys of Zimbabwe beef cattle. Vet Rec 130:446–448

Ferguson LC, Powers TE (1956) Experimental leptospirosis in pregnant swine. Am J Vet Res 17:471–477

Ferris DH, Hanson LE, Hoerlein AB, Beamer PD (1960) Experimental infection of white-tailed deer with *Leptospira pomona*. Corn Vet 50:236–250

Ferris DH, Rhoads WE, Hanson LE, Galton M, Manfield ME (1961) Research into the Nidality of *Leptospira ballum* in campestral host including the hog-nosed snake (*Heterodon platyrhinus*). Cornell Vet 51:406–419

Flint SH, Marshall RB, Winter PJ (1986) Dual infections of red deer (*Cervus elaphus*) by *Leptospira interrogans* serovars copenhageni and hardjo. NZ Vet J 34:70–71

Frantz JC, Hanson LE, Brown AL (1989) Effect of vaccination with a bacterin containing *Leptospira interrogans* serovar bratislava on the breeding performance of swine herds. Am J Vet Res 50:1044–1047

Frerichs GN, Maley AD (1980) Pseudoleptospires in blood culture [letter]. J Clin Pathol 33:905–906

Gallagher A (2011) Leptospirosis in a dog with uveitis and presumed cholecystitis. J Am Anim Hosp Assoc 47:162–167

Gautam R, Wu CC, Guptill LF, Potter A, Moore GE (2010) Detection of antibodies against *Leptospira* serovars via microscopic agglutination tests in dogs in the United States, 2000–2007. J Am Vet Med Assoc 237:293–298

Genovez ME, Scarcelli E, Piatti RM, Girio RJS, Cardoso MV, Miyashiro S, Castro V (2004) *Leptospira* spp. detected by polymerase chain reaction (PCR) in thoroughbred equine semen— case report. Arquivos do Instituto Biologico (Sao Paulo) 71:546–548

Gerritsen MJ, Koopmans MJ, Peterse D, Olyhoek T (1994) Sheep as maintenance host for *Leptospira interrogans* serovar hardjo subtype hardjobovis. Am J Vet Res 55:1232–1237

Glosser JW, Sulzer CR, Eberhardt M, Winkler WG (1974) Cultural and serologic evidence of *Leptospira interrogans* serotype Tarassovi infection in turtles. J Wildl Dis 10:429–435

Gravekamp C, Korver H, Montgomery J, Everard COR, Carrington D, Ellis WA, Terpstra WJ (1991) Leptospires isolated from toads and frogs on the island of Barbados. Int J Med Microbiol 275:403–411

Greene CE, Sykes JE, Brown CA et al (2007) Leptospirosis. In: Greene CE (ed) Infectious diseases of the dog and cat, 3rd edn. Elsevier, St Louis, pp 402–417

Hajikolaei MRH, Gorbanpour M, Haidari M, Abdollapour G (2005) Comparison of leptospiral infection in the horse and Donkey. Bull Vet Inst Pulawy 49:175–178

Hamond C, Martins G, Lilenbaum W, Medeiros MA (2012a) PCR detection of leptospiral carriers among seronegative horses. Vet Rec 171:105

Hamond C, Martins G, Lilenbaum W, Medeiros MA (2012b) Rapid and efficient diagnosis of leptospirosis in an aborted foal by PCR of gastric juice. Vet Microbiol 160:274–275

Hamond C, Martins G, Lawson-Ferreira R, Medeiros MA, Lilenbaum W (2013a) The role of horses in the transmission of leptospirosis in an urban tropical area. Epidemiol Infect 141:33–35

Hamond C, Martins G, Medeiros MA, Lilenbaum W (2013b) Presence of leptospiral DNA in semen suggests venereal transmission in horses. J Equine Sci 33:1157–1159

Hartman EG, Brummelman B, Dikken H (1975) *Leptospirae* of serotype lora of the serogroup Australis isolated for the first time from swine in the Netherlands. Tijdschr Diergeneeskd 100:421–425

Hartman EG (1984) An IgM- and IgG-specific enzyme-linked immunosorbent assay (ELISA) to detect anti-leptospiral immunoglobulins in dogs. Ztlbt Bakteriol Mikrobiol Hyg Series A 257:508–510

Hartskeerl RA, Goris MGA, Brem S, Meyer P, Kopp H, Gerhards H, Wollanke B (2004) Classification of *Leptospira* from the eyes of horses suffering from recurrent uveitis. J Vet Med Series B 51:110–115

Hassanpour A, Imandar M, Abdollahpour GR, Mahsayekhi M (2011) Seroprevalence of leptospiral infection in ewes in Khoy-Iran. Adv Environ Biol 5:2033–2038

Hathaway SC (1981) Leptospirosis in New Zealand: an ecological view. NZ Vet J 29:109–112

Hathaway SC, Little TWA (1981) Prevalence and clinical significance of leptospiral antibodies in pigs in England. Vet Rec 108:224–228

Hathaway SC, Blackmore DK (1981) Ecological aspects of the epidemiology of infection with leptospires of the Ballum serogroup in the black Rat (*Rattus rattus*) and the brown Rat (*Rattus norvegicus*) in New Zealand. J Hyg (Lond) 87:427–436

Hathaway SC, Ellis WA, Little TW, Stevens AE, Ferguson HW (1983) *Leptospira interrogans* serovar hardjo in pigs: a new host-parasite relationship in the United Kingdom. Vet Rec 113:153–154

Hathaway SC, Little TW, Pritchard DG (1986) Problems associated with the serological diagnosis of *Leptospira interrogans* serovar hardjo infection in bovine populations. Vet Rec 119:84–86

Herrmann GP, Lage AP, Moreira EC, Haddad JPA, JRd R, Rodrigues RO, Leite RC (2004) Seroprevalence of agglutinins of anti-*Leptospira* sp in sheep from the Southeast and Southwest Meso-regions of the State of Rio Grande do Sul, Brazil. Ciencia Rural 34:443–448

Higgins RJ, Harbourne JF, Little TW, Stevens AE (1980) Mastitis and abortion in dairy cattle associated with *Leptospira* of the serotype hardjo. Vet Rec 107:307–310

Hodges RT, Thomson J, Townsend KG (1979) Leptospirosis in pigs: the effectiveness of streptomycin in stopping leptospiruria. NZ Vet J 27:124–126

Hyakutake S, Biasi PD, Belluomini HE, Santa Rosa CA (1980) Leptospiroses in Brazilian snakes. Int J Zoon 7:73–77

Ibanez-Contreras A, Hernandez-Godinez B, Torres-Barranca JI, Melendez-Velez P (2010) Antibodies findings against *Leptospira* spp., of the serovars Panama, Lai, Australis, Shermani, and Patoc, in a group of rhesus monkeys (*Macaca mulatto*) in conditions of captivity. Archivos De Medicina Veterinaria 42:101–104

Jaffe JE, Hartskeerl RA, Bolhuis HGH, Ahmed A, Houwers DJ (2007).Serological survey of leptospirosis in a Dutch primate colony and the local rodent population. In: Erkrankungen der Zootiere Verhandlungsbericht des 43 Internationalen Symposiums uber die Erkrankungen der Zoo- und Wildtiere, Edinburgh, 19–20 May 2007, pp 257–258

Jagun AT, Ajayi OL, Ilugbo MO, Olugasa BO (2011) Isolation and prevalence of pathogenic *Leptospira interrogans* in slaughtered cattle in two abattoirs in southwestern Nigeria. In: Animal hygiene and sustainable livestock production. In: Proceedings of the 15th international congress of the international society for animal hygiene, vol 1. Vienna, 3–7 July 2011, pp 235–237

Jamshidi S, Akhavizadegan MA, Bokaie S, Maazi N, Ali AG (2009) Serologic study of feline leptospirosis in Tehran, Iran. Iranian J Microbiol 1:32–36

Jiang L, Lu Q, Luo Y, Ye J, Zhang Z, Xu B, Jiang LP, Lu QY, Luo Y, Ye JL, Zhang Z, Xu BX (2011) Application of a *lipL32*-PCR method for detection of *Leptospira interrogans*. Chinese J Vector Biol Cont 22:388–392

Jimenez MA, Sanchez B, Pena L (2013) Itistopathological detection of subclinical leptospirosis in free-ranging Iberian Lynxes (Lynx pardinus). J Comp Pathol 148:55

Johnson RC, Seiter CW (1976) *Leptospira* and their cultivation. Monograph Reheis Chem Co. Phoenix, Arizona, pp :1–13

Kalsow CM, Dwyer AE (1998) Retinal immunopathology in horses with uveitis. Ocul Immunol Inflamm 6:239–251

Kemenes F, Suveges T (1976) Leptospira—induced repeated abortion in sows. Acta Vet Acad Sci Hung 26:395–403

Khalacheva M, Sherkov SH (1981) Outbreak of leptospirosis among buffaloes in Bulgaria. Veterinarna Sbirka 79:33–36

Khbou MK, Hammami S, Kodjo A (2010) Anti-leptospires antibodies seroprevalence in sheep from the Fahs region, Tunisia. Revue De Medecine Veterinaire 161:185–192

Kinde H, Hietala SK, Bolin CA, Dowe JT (1996) Leptospiral abortion in horses following a flooding incident. Equine Vet J 28:327–330

Kingscote B (1988) Leptospiral antibodies in cattle in Alberta and evidence of an emerging serovar. Can Vet J 29:647–653

Klaasen HLBM, van der Veen M, Molkenboer MJCH, Sutton D (2013) A novel tetravalent *Leptospira* bacterin protects against infection and shedding following challenge in dogs. Vet Rec 172:181

Koizumi N, Muto M, Yamamoto S, Baba Y, Kudo M, Tamae Y, Shimomura K, Takatori I, Iwakiri A, Ishikawa K, Soma H, Watanabe H (2008) Investigation of reservoir animals of *Leptospira* in the northern part of Miyazaki prefecture. Jap J Infect Dis 61:465–468

Koizumi N, Muto MM, Akachi S, Okano S, Yamamoto S, Horikawa K, Harada S, Funatsumaru S, Ohnishi M (2013) Molecular and serological investigation of *Leptospira* and leptospirosis in dogs in Japan. J Med Microbiol 62:630–636

Kohm A (1988) Death of a polar bear cub from *Leptospira autumnalis* infection. Erkrankungen der Zootiere Verhandlungsbericht des 30 Internationalen Symposiums uber die Erkrankungen der Zoo und Wildtiere, Sofia 1988 Berlin, German Democratic Republic; Akademie, pp 298–300

Kulbrock M, Mv B, Rohn K, Distl O, Ohnesorge B (2013) Occurrence and severity of equine recurrent uveitis in warmblood horses—a comparative study. Pferdeheilkunde 29:27–36

La-ard A, Amavisit P, Sukpuaram T, Wajjwalku W (2011) Evaluation of recombinant lig antigen-based ELISA for detection of leptospiral antibodies in canine sera. Southeast Asian J Trop Med Public Health 42:128–137

Larsson CE, Santa RCA, Larsson M, Birgel EH, Fernandes WR, Paim GV (1985) Laboratory and clinical features of experimental feline leptospirosis. Int J Zoonoses 12:111–119

Leon VL, Hermoso DMM, Garrido F (1987) Incidence of abortions caused by leptospirosis in sheep and goats in Spain. Comp Immunol Microbiol Infect Dis 10:149–153

Leonard F, Quinn PJ, Ellis WA (1992) Possible effect of ph on the survival of leptospires in cattle urine. Vet Rec 131:53–54

Levett PN (2001) Leptospirosis. Clin Microbiol Rev 14:296–328

Lilenbaum W, Morais ZM, Goncales AP, de Souza GO, Richtzenhain L, Vasconcellos SA (2007) First isolation of leptospires from dairy goats in Brazil. Brazil J Microbiol 38:507–510

Lilenbaum W, Varges R, Brandao FZ, Cortez A, de Souza SO, Brandao PE, Richtzenhain LJ, Vasconcellos SA (2008) Detection of *Leptospira* spp. in semen and vaginal fluids of goats and sheep by polymerase chain reaction. Theriogenol 69:837–842

Lilenbaum W, Varges R, Ristow P, Cortez A, Souza SO, Richtzenhain LJ, Vasconcellos SA (2009) Identification of *Leptospira* spp. carriers among seroreactive goats and sheep by polymerase chain reaction. Res Vet Sci 87:16–19

Lilenbaum W, Varges R, Moraes IA, Ferreira AM, Pissinatti A (2005) Leptospiral antibodies in captive Lion tamarins (*Leontopithecus* sp.) in Brazil. Vet J 169:462–464

Little TWA, Parker BNJ, Stevens AE, Hathaway SC, Markson LM (1981) Inapparent infection of sheep in Britain by leptospires of the Australis serogroup. Res Vet Sci 31:386–387

Llorente P, Leoni L, Vivot MM (2002) Leptospirosis in South-American Camelids: a study on the serological prevalence in different regions of Argentina. Archivos De Medicina Veterinaria 34:59–68

Mancia A, Ryan JC, Chapman RW, Wu QZ, Warr GW, Gulland FMD, Van Dolah FM (2012) Health status, infection and disease in California sea lions (*Zalophus californianus*) studied using a canine microarray platform and machine-learning approaches. Dev Comp Immunol 36:629–637

Marianelli C, Tarantino M, Astarita S, Martucciello A, Capuano F, Galiero G (2007) Molecular detection of *Leptospira* species in aborted fetuses of water Buffalo. Vet Rec 161:310–312

Marin RE, Brihuega B, Romero G (2008) Seroprevalence of infectious diseases in Llamas from Jujuy province, Argentina. Vet Argent 25:281–287

Martins G, Penna B, Hamond C, Leite RCK, Silva A, Ferreira A, Brandao F, Oliveira F, Lilenbaum W (2012) Leptospirosis as the most frequent infectious disease impairing productivity in small ruminants in Rio de Janeiro, Brazil. Trop Anim Health Prod 44:773–777

Masuzawa T, Hashiguchi NR, Suzuki R, Shimizu T, Iwamoto Y, Morita T, Yanagihara Y (1991) Experimental lethal infection of *Leptospira interrogans* in mice treated with cyclophosphamide. Can J Microbiol 37:312–315

Mathur KN, Khanna VK, Purohit AK (1984) Macroscopic plate agglutination results of serological examination of camels, cattle and goats for leptospirosis in Rajasthan. [Abstract]. Indian J Pub Hlth 28:61

Matthias MA, Diaz MM, Campos KJ, Calderon M, Willig MR, Pacheco V, Gotuzzo E, Gilman RH, Vinetz JM (2005) Diversity of Bat-associated *Leptospira* in the Peruvian Amazon inferred by Bayesian phylogenetic analysis of 16S ribosomal DNA sequences. Am J Trop Med Hyg 73:964–974

Matthews A (1999) Equine recurrent uveitis—an update. In Practice 21:370–376

Mayer-Scholl A, Luge E, Draeger A, Nockler K, Kohn B (2013) Distribution of *Leptospira* serogroups in dogs from Berlin, Germany. Vector Borne Zoon Dis 13:200–202

McKeown JD, Ellis WA (1986) *Leptospira* hardjo agalactia in sheep. Vet Rec 118:482

McTague T (1997) Outbreak of *Leptospira* hardjo abortion in a lowland flock. Irish Vet J 50:128

Michna SW (1970) Leptospirosis. Vet Rec 86:484–496

Michna SW, Campbell RSF (1969) The isolation of *Leptospira* sejroe from the kidney of aborting cattle. Vet Rec 84:83–86

Mitchell D, Robertson A, Corner AH, Boulanger P (1966) Some observations on the diagnosis and epidemiology of leptospirosis in swine. Can J Comp Med Vet Sci 30:211–217

Modric Z, Knezevic N (1997) Leptospirosis in domestic cats (*Felis domestica* Briss.) in the Sisak area. Veterinarska Stanica 28:261–265

Monahan AM, Callanan JJ, Nally JE (2008) Proteomic analysis of *Leptospira interrogans* shed in urine of chronically infected hosts. Infect Immun 76:4952–4958

Monteiro RV, Fedullo LPL, Albuquerque CE, Lilenbaum W (2003) Leptospirosis in a giant anteater (*Myrmecophaga tridactyla*, Linnaeus, 1758) in Rio de Janeiro Zoo, Brazil. Revista Brasileira de Ciencia Veterinaria 10:126–127

Moore GE, Guptill LF, Glickman NW, Caldanaro RJ, Aucoin D, Glickman LT (2006) Canine Leptospirosis, United States, 2002–2004. Emerg Infect Dis 12:501–503

Moreira EC (1994) Avaliação de métodos para erradicação de leptospirosis em bovinos leiteiros. Tese de Doutorado Escola de Veterinária, Universidade Federal de Minas Gerais, Belo Horizonte, p 93

Morse EV, Langham RF (1958) Experimental leptospirosis. III. Caprine *Leptospira pomona* infection. Am J Vet Res 19:139–144

Moshkelani S, Javaheri-Koupaei M, Rabiee S, Moazeni M (2011) Detection of *Brucella* spp. and *Leptospira* spp. by multiplex polymerase chain reaction (PCR) from aborted bovine, ovine and caprine fetuses in Iran. Afr J Microbiol Res 5:4627–4630

Muehldorfer K (2013) Bats and bacterial pathogens: a review. Zoonoses Public Health 60:93–103

Mylonakis ME, Bourtzi-Hatzopoulou E, Koutinas AF, Petridou E, Saridomichelakis MN, Leontides L, Siochu A (2005) Leptospiral seroepidemiology in a feline hospital population in Greece. Vet Rec 156:615–616

Nally JE, Monahan AM, Miller IS, Bonilla-Santiago R, Souda P, Whitelegge JP (2011) Comparative proteomic analysis of differentially expressed proteins in the urine of reservoir hosts of leptospirosis. PLoS ONE 6:26046

Natarajaseenivasan K, Ratnam S (1999) Isolation of *Leptospira* javanica from sheep. Indian J Anim Sci 69:759–761

Neiffer DL, Klein EC, Wallace-Switalski C (2001) Leptospira infection in two black Rhinoceroses (Diceros bicornis Michaeli). J Zoo Wildl Med 32:476–486

Nervig RM, Garrett LA (1979) Use of furosemide to obtain bovine urine samples for leptospiral isolation. Am J Vet Res 40:1197–1200

Oliveira SJD, Bortolanza F, Passos DT, Pires Neto JAS, Fallavena LCB, TdA W (2007) Molecular diagnosis of *Leptospira* spp. in culled sows. Brazil J Vet Res Anim Sci 44:18–23

Oliveira FCS, Azevedo SS, Pinheiro SR, Batista CSA, Moraes ZM, Souza GO, Goncales AP, Vasconcellos SA (2010) Risk factors associated with leptospirosis in cows in the state of Bahia, northeastern Brazil. Pesquisa Veterinaria Brasileira 30:398–402

Oliveira ST, Messick JB, Biondo AW, dos Santos AP, Stedile R, Dalmolin ML, de Sa Guimaraes AM, Mohamed AS, Riediger IN, Diaz Gonzalez FH (2012) Exposure to *Leptospira* spp. in sick dogs, shelter dogs and dogs from an endemic area: points to consider. Acta Scientiae Veterinariae 40:1056

Otaka DY, Martins G, Hamond C, Penna B, Medeiros MA, Lilenbaum W (2012) Serology and PCR for bovine leptospirosis: herd and individual approaches. Vet Rec 170:338

Pande PG, Sekariah PC, Ramachandra Iyer PK, Shukla RR (1961) Cerebrospinal leptospirosis in Buffalo Calves due to *Leptospira hebdomadis*. Curr Sci 30:147–148

Pekelder JJ, Westenbrink F, Vellema P, Peterse DJ, Bokhout BA, Franken P (1993) Serological study of the occurrence of *L. hardjo* in sheep in The Netherlands. Tijdschr Diergeneeskd 118:433–443

Perea A, Garcia R, Maldonado A, Tarradas MC, Luque I, Astorga R, Arenas A (1994) Prevalence of antibodies to different *Leptospira interrogans* serovars in pigs on large farms. J Vet Med Series-B 41:512–516

Pereira MM, Da Silva JJ, Pinto MA, Da Silva MF, Machado MP, Lenzi HL, Marchevsky RS (2005) Experimental leptospirosis in marmoset monkeys (*Callithrix jacchus*): a new model for studies of severe pulmonary leptospirosis. Am J Trop Med Hyg 72:13–20

Perez J, Goarant C (2010) Rapid *Leptospira* identification by direct sequencing of the diagnostic PCR products in New Caledonia. BMC Microbiol 10:325

Perolat P, Poingt JP, Vie JC, Jouaneau C, Baranton G, Gysin J (1992) Occurrence of severe leptospirosis in a breeding colony of Squirrel monkeys. Am J Trop Med Hyg 46:538–545

Picardeau M (2013) Diagnosis and epidemiology of leptospirosis. Medecine et Maladies Infectieuses 43:1–9

Pinna MH, Martins G, Pinheiro ACO, Almeida DS, Oria AP, Lilenbaum W (2012) Detection of anti-*Leptospira* antibodies in captive nonhuman primates from Salvador, Brazil. Am J Primatol 74:8–11

Pintore A, Palmas B, Noworol M, Canu M, Fiori E, Picardeau M, Tola A, Piredda I, Ponti MN (2012) First record of *Leptospira* isolation from wild boars of Sardinia. European Leptospirosis Conference, Dubrovnik

Poonacha KB, Donahue JM, Giles RC, Hong CB, Petritesmurphy MB, Smith BJ, Swerczek TW, Tramontin RR, Tuttle PA (1993) Leptospirosis in equine fetuses, stillborn foals, and placentas. Vet Pathol 30:362–369

Power SB (1991) Diagnosing *Leptospira* in pigs. Vet Rec 128:43

Pritchard GC (1999) Bulk milk antibody testing for *Leptospira* hardjo infection. cattle Practice 7:59–61

Pumarola A, Mora R, Pumarola T (1987). A serological survey on *Leptospira* infections of pigs and cattle in the province of Barcelona (Spain). Trop Geogr Med 39:S7; Proceedings of 5th Mtg Europ *Leptospira* Workers, Amsterdam

Rapley WA, Cranfield MR, Mehren KG, Vas SI, Barker IK, Lathe F (1981) A natural outbreak of leptospirosis in a captive black tailed deer (*Odocoileus heminonus* columbianus) herd and in Dall's sheep (*Ovis dalli*) at the Metropolitan Toronto zoo. In: American Association of Zoo Veterinarians Annual proceedings, Seattle, Washington, USA, pp 115–120

Reid AC, Herron AJ, Hines ME, Orchard EA, Altman NH (1993) Leptospirosis in a white lipped Tamarin (*Saguinus labiatus*). Lab Anim Sci 43:258–259

Reilly GAC, Bailie NC, Morrow WT, McDowell SWJ, Ellis WA (1994) Feline stillbirths associated with mixed Salmonella typhimurium and *Leptospira* infection. Vet Rec 135:608

Renaud C, Andrews S, Djelouadji Z, Lecheval S, Corrao-Revol N, Buff S, Demont P, Kodjo A (2013) Prevalence of the *Leptospira* serovars Bratislava, Grippotyphosa, Mozdok and Pomona in French dogs. Vet J 196:126–127

Ribotta M, Higgins R, Perron D (1999) Swine leptospirosis: low risk of exposure for humans. Can Vet J 40:809–810

Ridler A, Heuer C, West D, Dorjee S (2005). Leptospirosis in sheep in New Zealand. In: Proceedings of 6th international sheep veterinary congress, Crete, Greece, June 2005, pp 270–271

Rinehart CL, Zimmerman AD, Buterbaugh RE, Jolie RA, Chase CCL (2012a) Efficacy of vaccination of cattle with the *Leptospira interrogans* serovar hardjo type hardjoprajitno component of a pentavalent *Leptospira* bacterin against experimental challenge with *Leptospira borgpetersenii* serovar hardjo type hardjo-bovis. Am J Vet Res 73:735–740

Rinehart CL, Jolie RA, Zimmerman AD, Buterbaugh RE, Chase CCL (2012b) Concerns about *Leptospira* vaccine efficacy study. Response. Am J Vet Res 73:929

Rocha T (1990) Isolation of *Leptospira interrogans* serovar mozdok from aborted swine fetuses in Portugal. Vet Rec 126:602

Rodrigues ALB, Girio RJS, Esper CR, Rodrigues LH, Magajevski FS, Oliveira MA (2003) *Leptospira interrogans* serovar pomona bovine semen survive contaminated experimentally. Revista Brasileira de Reproducao Animal 27:636–643

Romberg J, Lang S, Balks E, Kamphuis E, Duchow K, Loos D, Rau H, Motitschke A, Jungbäck C (2012) Potency testing of veterinary vaccines: the way from in vivo to in vitro. Biologicals 40:100–106

Romero PM, Astudillo HM, Sanchez VJ, Gonzalez GL, Varela AN (2012) Antibody titers against *Leptospira* sp., in primates from Matecana zoo, Pereira, Colombia. Revista MVZ Cordoba 17:3224–3230

Rosadio AR, Veliz AA, Castillo DH, Yaya LK, Rodriguez HA, Rivera GH, Wheeler JC (2012) Seroprevalence to pathogenic *Leptospira* in alpacas and vicunas from Huancavelica and Ayacucho, Peru. Revista de Investigaciones Veterinarias del Peru 23:350–356

Ross L, Jakowski R, Bolin C, Kiupel M (2011) Retrospective immunohistochemical detection of *Leptospira* in dogs with renal pathology. Int J Appl Res Vet Med 9:324–331

Roth EE, Adams WV, Sanford GE, Newman K, Moore M, Greer B (1964) Isolation of *Leptospira pomona* from white tailed deer in Louisiana. Am J Vet Res 25:259–261

Ryan EG, Leonard N, O'Grady L, Doherty ML, More SJ (2012) Herd-level risk factors associated with *Leptospira* Hardjo seroprevalence in Beef/Suckler herds in the Republic of Ireland. Vet Ireland J 2:449–458

Sanhueza JM, Heuer C, West D (2013) Contribution of *Leptospira*, *Neospora caninum* and bovine viral diarrhea virus to fetal loss of beef cattle in New Zealand. Prev Vet Med 112:90–98

Scarcelli E, Piatti RM, Fedullo JDL, Simon F, Cardoso MV, Castro V, Miyashiro S, Genovez ME (2003) *Leptospira* spp. detection by polymerase chain reaction (pcr) in clinical samples of captive black-capped capuchin monkey (*Cebus apella*). Brazil J Microbiol 34:143–146

Schollum LM, Blackmore DK (1981) The serological and cultural prevalence of leptospirosis in a sample of feral goats. NZ Vet J 29:104–106

Schonberg A, Hahnhey B, Kampe U, Schmidt K, Ellis WA (1992) The isolation and identification of *Leptospira interrogans* serovar bratislava from a pig in Germany. J Vet Med Series B 39:362–368

Sebastian M, Giles R, Roberts J, Poonacha K, Harrison L, Donahue J, Benirschke K (2005) Funisitis associated with leptospiral abortion in an equine placenta. Vet Pathol 42:659–662

Shigidi MTA (1974) Animal leptospirosis in the Sudan. Brit Vet J 130:528–531

Shive RJ, Green SS, Evans LB, Garner FM (1969) Leptospirosis in barbary Apes (*Macaca sylvana*). J Am Vet Med Assoc 155:1176–1178

Silva EF, Brod CS, Cerqueira GM, Bourscheidt D, Seyffert N, Queiroz A, Santos CS, Ko AI, Dellagostin OA (2007) Isolation of *Leptospira noguchii* from sheep. Vet Microbiol 121:144–149

Smith CR, Corney BG, McGowan MR, McClintock CS, Ward W, Ketterer PJ (1997) Amoxycillin as an alternative to dihydrostreptomycin sulphate for treating cattle infected with *Leptospira borgpetersenii* serovar hardjo. Aust Vet J 75:818–821

Smyth JA, Fitzpatrick DA, Ellis WA (1999) Stillbirth/perinatal weak Calf syndrome: a study of Calves infected with *Leptospira*. Vet Rec 145:539–542

Spiess BM (2008) New findings on the treatment of periodic ophthalmia. Praktische Tierarzt 89:648–650

Stasilevich ZK, Dzhikidze EK, Anisimova TA, Krylova RI (2000) Serological investigations for leptospirosis in monkeys of the Adler monkey colony. Baltic J Lab Anim Sci 10:33–38

Stokes WS, Kulpa-Eddy J, Brown K, Srinivas G, McFarland R (2012) Recent progress and future directions for reduction, refinement, and replacement of animal use in veterinary vaccine potency and safety testing: a report from the 2010 NICEATM-ICCVAM International Vaccine Workshop. Dev Biol (Basel) 134:9–21

Subathra M, Senthilkumar TMA, Ramadass P (2013) Recombinant OmpL1 protein as a diagnostic antigen for the detection of canine leptospirosis. Appl Biochem Biotechnol 169:431–437

Subharat S, Wilson PR, Heuer C, Collins-Emerson JM (2010) Investigation of localisation of *Leptospira* spp. in uterine and fetal tissues of non-pregnant and pregnant farmed deer. NZ Vet J 58:281–285

Subharat S, Wilson PR, Heuer C, Collins-Emerson JM (2011) Vaccination for leptospirosis improved the weaning percentage of 2-year-old farmed red deer hinds in New Zealand. NZ Vet J 59:191–196

Subharat S, Wilson PR, Heuer C, Collins-Emerson JM (2012a) Growth response and shedding of *Leptospira* spp. in urine following vaccination for leptospirosis in young farmed deer. NZ Vet J 60:14–20

Subharat S, Wilson PR, Heuer C, Collins-Emerson JM (2012b) Longitudinal serological survey and herd-level risk factors for *Leptospira* spp. serovars Hardjo-bovis and Pomona on deer farms with sheep and/or beef cattle. NZ Vet J 60:215–222

Szonyi B, Agudelo-Flórez P, Ramírez M, Moreno N, Ko AI (2011) An outbreak of severe leptospirosis in capuchin (*Cebus*) monkeys. Vet J 188:237–239

Tangeman LE, Littman MP (2013) Clinicopathologic features and atypical presentations of naturally occurring canine leptospirosis: 51 cases (2000–2010). J Am Vet Med Assoc 243:1316–1322

Thaipadungpanit J, Chierakul W, Wuthiekanun V, Limmathurotsakul D, Amornchai P, Boonslip S, Smythe LD, Limpaiboon R, Hoffmaster AR, Day NPJ, Peacock SJ (2011) Diagnostic accuracy of real-time PCR assays targeting 16S *rRNA* and *lipL32* genes for human leptospirosis in Thailand: a case-control study. PLoS ONE 6:16236

Thiermann AB (1982) Experimental leptospiral infections in pregnant cattle with organisms of the hebdomadis serogroup. Am J Vet Res 43:780–784

Thorne T (1985) Experimental *Leptospira interrogans* serovar hardjo in pronghorn antelope. In: Proceedings of 88th annual meeting USAHA 1984 Fort Worth Texas 1984, p 634

Timoney JF, Kalimuthusamy N, Velineni S, Donahue JM, Artiushin SC, Fettinger M (2011) A unique genotype of *Leptospira interrogans* serovar Pomona type kennewicki is associated with equine abortion. Vet Microbiol 150:349–353

Tochetto C, Flores MM, Kommers GD, Barros CSL, Fighera RA (2012) Pathological aspects of leptospirosis in dogs: 53 cases (1965–2011). Pesquisa Vet Bras 32:430–443

Tomordy E, Hassig M, Spiess BM (2010) The outcome of pars plana vitrectomy in horses with equine recurrent uveitis with regard to the presence or absence of intravitreal antibodies against various serovars of *Leptospira interrogans*. Pferdeheilkunde 26:251–254

Torten, M (1979) Leptopsirosis. In: Stoenner H, Kaplan W, Torten M (eds) A.C.R.C. Handbook series in Zoonoses, vol 1. C.R.C. Press, Boca Rato

Trap D, Garin BB (1988) Leptospirosis in sheep. Bulletin Mensuel de la Societe Veterinaire Pratique de France 72(283–286):288–292

Tripathy DN, Hanson LE, Bedoya M, Mansfield ME (1985) Experimental infection of pregnant and lactating goats with *Leptospira interrogans* serovars hardjo and szwajizak. Am J Vet Res 46:2515–2518

Tucunduva de Faria M, Athanazio DA, Goncalves Ramos EA, Silva EF, Reis MG, Ko AI (2007) Morphological alterations in the kidney of Rats with natural and experimental *Leptospira* infection. J Comp Pathol 137:231–238

Tulsiani SM, Cobbold RN, Graham GC, Dohnt MF, Burns MA, Leung LKP, Field HE, Smythe LD, Craig SB (2011) The role of fruit Bats in the transmission of pathogenic leptospires in Australia. Ann Trop Med Parasitol 105:71–84

Twigg GI, Hughes DM, McDairmid A (1971) Occurrence of leptospirosis in thoroughbred horses. Equine Vet J 2:52–55

Upadhye AS, Rajasekhar M, Ahmed SN, Krishnappa G (1983) Isolation of *Leptospira* Andaman from an active clinical case of jaundice in a Buffalo. Indian Vet J 60:319–320

Van Schaik G, Schukken YH, Nielen M, Dijkhuizen AA, Barkema HW, Benedictus G (2002) Probability of and risk factors for introduction of infectious diseases into Dutch SPF dairy farms: a cohort study. Prev Vet Med 54:279–289

Verma A, Kumar P, Babb K, Timoney JF, Stevenson B (2010) Cross-reactivity of antibodies against leptospiral recurrent uveitis-associated proteins A and B (LruA and LruB) with eye proteins. PLoS Negl Trop Dis 4:778

Verma A, Stevenson B, Adler B (2013) Leptospirosis in horses. Vet Microbiol 167:61–66

Vermunt JJ, West DM, Cooke MM, Alley MR, Collins Emerson J (1994) Observations on three outbreaks of *Leptospira interrogans* serovar pomona infection in lambs. NZ Vet J 42:133–136

Vijayachari P, Sugunan AP, Sehgal SC (2001) Evaluation of microscopic agglutination test as a diagnostic tool during acute stage of leptospirosis in high and low endemic areas. Indian J Med Res 114:99–106

Vijayarani K, Reghana J, Sridhar R, Jayathangaraj MG, Thirumurugan R, Raj GD, Kumanan K (2010) A report on leptospirosis in a wild dog. Indian Vet J 87:497–498

Weber MFVJ, Verhoeff J (2001) Integrated disease control in dairy herds: a case study from the veterinarians' viewpoint. Tijdschr Diergeneeskd 126:340–345

Wernery U, Thomas R, Raghavan R, Syriac G, Joseph S, Georgy N (2008) Seroepidemiological studies for the detection of antibodies against 8 infectious diseases in dairy dromedaries of the United Arab Emirates using modern laboratory techniques—Part II. J Camel Pract Res 15:139–145

Wood JLN, Townsend HGG (1999) Leptospiral infections associated with disease and fertility in horses. J Anim Breed 3:39–45

Zieris H (1991) Epidemiology of *Leptospira interrogans* serovar mozdok in former GDR. Monatsh Veterinarmed 46:355–358

The Molecular Basis of Leptospiral Pathogenesis

Gerald L. Murray

Abstract The mechanisms of disease pathogenesis in leptospirosis are poorly defined. Recent developments in the application of genetic tools in the study of *Leptospira* have advanced our understanding by allowing the assessment of mutants in animal models. As a result, a small number of essential virulence factors have been identified, though most do not have a clearly defined function. Significant advances have also been made in the in vitro characterization of leptospiral interaction with host structures, including extracellular matrix proteins (such as laminin, elastin, fibronectin, collagens), proteins related to hemostasis (fibrinogen, plasmin), and soluble mediators of complement resistance (factor H, C4b-binding protein), although none of these in vitro findings has been translated to the host animal. Binding to host structures may permit colonization of the host, prevention of blood clotting may contribute to hemorrhage, while interaction with complement resistance mediators may contribute to survival in serum. While not a classical intracellular pathogen, the interaction of leptospires and phagocytic cells appears complex, with bacteria surviving uptake and promoting apoptosis; mutants relating to these processes (such as cell invasion and oxidative stress resistance) are attenuated in vivo. Another feature of leptospiral biology is the high degree of functional redundancy and the surprising lack of attenuation of mutants in what appear to be certain virulence factors, such as LipL32 and LigB. While many advances have been made, there remains a lack of understanding of how *Leptospira* causes tissue pathology. It is likely that leptospires have many novel pathogenesis mechanisms that are yet to be identified.

Contents

G.L. Murray (✉)
Department of Microbiology, Monash University, Melbourne, Australia
e-mail: gerald.murray@monash.edu

© Springer-Verlag Berlin Heidelberg 2015
B. Adler (ed.), *Leptospira and Leptospirosis*, Current Topics in Microbiology and Immunology 387, DOI 10.1007/978-3-662-45059-8_7

1 Introduction to the Pathogenesis of Leptospirosis

The molecular basis of leptospiral pathogenesis remains poorly understood. Leptospires lack classical virulence factors due to the large phylogenetic distance to well-studied, prototypic, bacterial pathogens. This indicates that *Leptospira* likely has novel virulence mechanisms, a notion supported by the over representation of "hypothetical" open reading frames in the group of genes specific to pathogenic *Leptospira interrogans*; 78 % of pathogen-specific genes have no defined function, compared to 40 % of the whole genome (Adler et al. 2011).

Recent advances in genetics, including the construction of the first defined mutants by transposon mutagenesis (Bourhy et al. 2005), and directed mutagenesis (Croda et al. 2008), combined with the increase in available genomic sequences (see the chapter by M. Picardeau, this volume) have led to progress in the identification and characterization of virulence factors. Virulence factors that are required for disease in animal models, identified through mutagenesis, are summarized in Tables 1 and 2. An overview of the stages of acute infection is illustrated in Fig. 1; the virulence factors essential for acute disease and their probable role in disease are indicated. Clearly, most disease processes occur by mechanisms that are yet to be fully defined.

This chapter covers recent research into known and predicted virulence factors, redundancy of virulence mechanisms, molecular mechanisms of damage to the

Table 1 *Leptospira interrogans* virulence factors with a confirmed role in acute disease[a]

Name[b]	Mutated gene[c]	Description/function	Possible role in virulence	Distribution[d]	Serovar	Animal model	Renal colonization of acute host[e]	References[f]
Loa22*	la0222	Outer membrane lipoprotein, OmpA domain	Unknown	P, I, S	Lai	Guinea pig, hamster	Yes	Ristow et al. (2007)
HemO	lb186	Heme oxygenase, degrades heme	Iron acquisition	P, I, S	Manilae	Hamster	Yes	Murray et al. (2009b)
FliY	la2613	Flagellar motor switch, motility	Dissemination	P, I, S	Lai	Guinea pig	NA	Liao et al. (2009)
LPS†	la1641	LPS synthesis	Unknown	P	Manilae	Hamster	No	Marcsisin et al. (2013), Murray et al. (2010)
LPS†	lman_1408 HQ127382	Potential methyltransferase, LPS synthesis	Unknown	P, I	Manilae	Hamster	No	Marcsisin et al. (2013), Murray et al. (2010)
ClpB*	la1879/ licl2017	Molecular chaperone	Resist heat and oxidative stress, nutrient restriction	P, I	Kito	Gerbil	NA	Lourdault et al. (2011)
FlaA2	la3380	Probable flagellar sheath protein, motility	Dissemination	P, I, S	Manilae	Hamster	No	Lambert et al. (2012a)
KatE†	la1859	Catalase, degrades hydrogen peroxide	Resist oxidative stress	P, I	Pomona, Manilae	Hamster	NA	Eshghi et al. (2012)
Mce**	la2055	Mce, cell adhesion and entry	Cell entry	P, I, S	Lai	Hamster	Yes	Zhang et al. (2012)

(continued)

Table 1 (continued)

Name[b]	Mutated gene[c]	Description/function	Possible role in virulence	Distribution[d]	Serovar	Animal model	Renal colonization of acute host[e]	References[f]
LruA	la3097	Lipoprotein, may be involved in leptospiral interaction with apolipoprotein A-I	Unknown	P, I, S	Manilae	Hamster	Yes	Zhang et al. (2013)
HtpG**	lb058	Probable chaperone, function not defined	Unknown	P, I, S	Manilae	Hamster	Yes	King et al. (2013), Marcsisin et al. (2013)
ColA**	la0872	Collagenase	Dissemination, tissue damage	P	Lai	Hamster	Yes	Kassegne et al. (2014)
LB139	lb139	Sensor protein	Motility, protein expression	P	Manilae	Hamster	No	Eshghi et al. (2014)

[a] Based on animal survival. Tissue pathology such as lung hemorrhage and kidney colonization by *Leptospira* generally still observed. LPS mutants were attenuated by both intraperitoneal injection and conjunctival infection. All other mutants were tested by intraperitoneal infection route only
[b] Partial (*) or full (**) restoration of virulence after complementation, attenuation found in independent mutants of the same gene or pathway (†)
[c] Locus tag from Lai and/or Copenhageni indicated where available. GenBank accession number indicated in parentheses, if appropriate
[d] Distribution of genes across species determined by BLASTp search (NCBI) and/or analysis of gene synteny. P, found in pathogenic strains (*L. kirschneri, L. noguchii, L. interrogans, L. borgpetersenii, L. weilii, L. santarosai, L. alexanderi, L. kmetyi, L. alstonii*); I, found in intermediate pathogenicity species (*L. broomii, L. licerasiae, L. inadai, L. fainei, L. wolffii*); S, found in saprophytic species (*L. biflexa, L. meyeri, L. vanthielii, L. terpstrae*)
[e] NA Not assessed
[f] Further references relating to these factors may be found in the text

Table 2 *Leptospira interrogans* virulence factors with a confirmed role in carrier host colonization

Name[a]	Mutated gene[b]	Description/function	Possible role in virulence	Distribution[c]	Serovar	Renal colonization of mouse	Attenuated in acute model[d]	References[e]
LPS†	la1641	LPS synthesis	Unknown	P	Manilae	No	Yes	Marcsisin et al. (2013), Murray et al. (2010)
LPS†	lman_1408 HQ127382	Potential methyltransferase, LPS synthesis	Unknown	P, I	Manilae	No	Yes	Marcsisin et al. (2013), Murray et al. (2010)
HbpA	lb191	TonB-dependent receptor, binds hemin	Iron acquisition	P, I, S	Manilae	No	No	Marcsisin et al. (2013)
LruA	la3097	Lipoprotein, may be involved in leptospiral interaction with apolipoprotein A-I	Unknown	P, I, S	Manilae	No	Yes	Zhang et al. (2013)
HtpG	lb058	Probable chaperone, function not defined	Unknown	P, I, S	Manilae	No	Yes	King et al. (2013), Marcsisin et al. (2013)
LB194	lb194	Hypothetical protein, iron utilization locus	Unknown	P, I, S	Manilae	No	No	Marcsisin et al. (2013)

(continued)

Table 2 (continued)

Name[a]	Mutated gene[b]	Description/function	Possible role in virulence	Distribution[c]	Serovar	Renal colonization of mouse	Attenuated in acute model[d]	References[e]
LA2786	la2786	Hypothetical	Unknown	P	Manilae	No	No	Marcsisin et al. (2013)
LA0589	la0589	Hypothetical, family of paralogous proteins	Unknown	P	Manilae	No	No	Marcsisin et al. (2013)

[a] Attenuation found in independent mutants of the same gene or pathway (†)

[b] Locus tag from Lai and/or Copenhageni indicated where available. GenBank accession number indicated in parentheses, if appropriate

[c] Distribution of genes across species determined by BLASTp search (NCBI) and/or analysis of gene synteny. P, found in pathogenic strains (*L. kirschneri, L. noguchii, L. interrogans, L. borgpetersenii, L. weilii, L. santarosai, L. alexanderi, L. kmetyi, L. alstonii*); I, found in intermediate pathogenicity species (*L. broomii, L. licerasiae, L. inadai, L. fainei, L. wolffii*); S, found in saprophytic species (*L. biflexa, L. meyeri, L. vanthielii, L. terpstrae*)

[d] Based on animal survival. Tissue pathology such as lung hemorrhage and kidney colonization by *Leptospira* generally still observed. LPS mutants were attenuated by both intraperitoneal injection and conjunctival infection. All other mutants were tested by intraperitoneal infection route only

[e] Further references relating to these factors may be found in the text

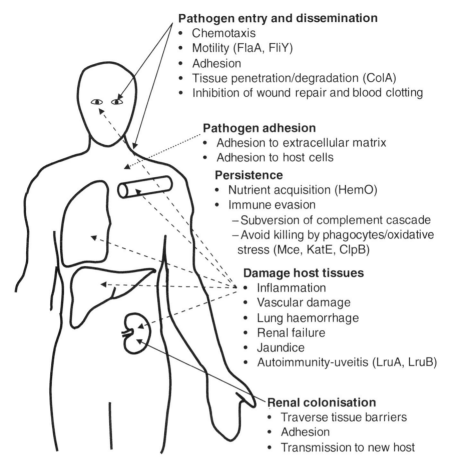

Pathogen entry and dissemination
- Chemotaxis
- Motility (FlaA, FliY)
- Adhesion
- Tissue penetration/degradation (ColA)
- Inhibition of wound repair and blood clotting

Pathogen adhesion
- Adhesion to extracellular matrix
- Adhesion to host cells

Persistence
- Nutrient acquisition (HemO)
- Immune evasion
  - Subversion of complement cascade
  - Avoid killing by phagocytes/oxidative stress (Mce, KatE, ClpB)

Damage host tissues
- Inflammation
- Vascular damage
- Lung haemorrhage
- Renal failure
- Jaundice
- Autoimmunity-uveitis (LruA, LruB)

Renal colonisation
- Traverse tissue barriers
- Adhesion
- Transmission to new host

Fig. 1 Stages of the leptospirosis infection process. Probable virulence mechanisms are indicated along with associated virulence factors experimentally confirmed to be required for disease (see text for references). The pronounced lack of confirmed virulence factors for various aspects of infection highlights our limited understanding of the pathogenesis of leptospirosis. Additional virulence factors, without defined function, include Loa22, LPS, LB139, and the heat shock protein HtpG. LruA is also essential for virulence (unrelated to the role in *Leptospira*-induced uveitis)

host, and the molecular basis of host specificity. The term virulence factor is used to describe proteins, structures (e.g., LPS), or phenotypes (e.g., motility) that are required to cause disease, or have been demonstrated to interact with host proteins in a way that may potentiate disease.

1.1 Methods for the Identification and Characterization of Virulence Factors

Virulence factors can be predicted bioinformatically or identified experimentally. Bioinformatics approaches include identification of sequences similar to known virulence factors in other species, and genomic comparisons, especially between pathogenic and saprophytic species (Adler et al. 2011). Few confirmed leptospiral virulence factors have been identified by bioinformatics, with the exception of catalase, collagenase, heme oxygenase, and Mce (Table 1). Genomes of pathogenic leptospires also encode sphingomyelinases and phospholipase, other proteases and TlyABC-like hemolysins, though a definitive role in virulence for these has not been established (Nascimento et al. 2004). Pathogenic leptospiral genomes also encode an unusually large number of leucine-rich repeat proteins, containing a motif often associated with pathogen–host interaction. Notably, leptospires lack recognized systems for translocation of effectors into host cells such as non-flagellar type III, and types IV and VI secretion systems (Nascimento et al. 2004). In vitro experimental approaches for identification of virulence factors include prospecting for interactions between a substrate and leptospiral proteins by ligand blots (Hoke et al. 2008; Verma et al. 2006), "pull down" or column extraction experiments (Asuthkar et al. 2007), analysis of leptospiral cells that have interacted with host proteins (Zhang et al. 2013), protein arrays (Pinne et al. 2012), and phage display (Ching et al. 2012). Potential virulence factors have also been inferred through comparison of the genomic and transcriptional changes between a virulent strain of *L. interrogans* and a culture-attenuated derivative (Zhong et al. 2011; Lehmann et al. 2013; Toma et al. 2014).

Characterization of putative virulence factors can be conducted in vitro or in vivo. In vitro demonstration of interaction between recombinant leptospiral protein and host proteins is commonly used, though this does not prove a role in vivo and is subject to artifacts that may be introduced in vitro, such as protein misfolding and possible lack of appropriate post-translational modifications. Whole, live cells can also be used in in vitro assays such as binding experiments; interactions can be blocked with specific antibodies or by competitive inhibition with the protein of interest (Choy et al. 2007), but it may be difficult to isolate the role of a particular factor due to functional redundancy (Murray et al. 2009c). "Gain of function" studies involve transfer of genes from pathogens to saprophytes and measurement of virulence characteristics such as adhesion (Figueira et al. 2011). In these experiments, a protein is more likely to be expressed with "normal" conformation, post-translational modifications and context, such as lipidation or membrane insertion, and also have the advantage of excluding functionally analogous proteins of pathogens that may confound results.

The only definitive method to determine that a factor is required for virulence is by mutagenesis followed by testing in vivo; factors essential for virulence identified by this methodology are detailed in Tables 1 and 2. It is important to stress that the majority of putative virulence factors have not been shown to have a role in the host. Notably, mutagenesis and in vivo testing may not identify virulence factors with redundant function. The readout for these experiments is usually animal survival, though as a crude measure of virulence this may not identify subtle attenuation (Adler et al. 2011). Other useful readouts include tissue pathology (e.g., frequency and severity of macroscopic lung hemorrhage, histopathology of various tissues), renal colonization, and bacterial burden in tissues (measured by quantitative PCR) (King et al. 2014; Lambert et al. 2012a). Recently, a high throughput method for screening mutants for attenuation was described (Marcsisin et al. 2013). Tables 1 and 2 should be viewed with the following caveats. Only mutants in *L. interrogans* have been tested, mainly in serovars Manilae and Lai. This may not be representative of pathogenic strains generally, and what is true for one strain may not necessarily be extrapolated to other strains [e.g., the *clpB* mutant is avirulent in serovar Kito but retains virulence in serovar Manilae (Lourdault et al. 2011)]. The intraperitoneal challenge route does not test aspects of disease such as host entry, meaning that factors with a key role in these aspects of disease may not be identified. For some of the attenuated mutants, the challenge strain retained sufficient virulence to cause pathology and kidney colonization, and with sufficient dose, host death. Finally, the majority of mutants have been tested in the acute models of gerbils, hamsters, and guinea pigs, neglecting carrier hosts which are the reservoir from which humans are infected.

Complementation is a cornerstone of microbiological studies that rely on mutagenesis to prove phenotype (Falkow 1988); however, due to the lack of replicating plasmids for pathogenic leptospires this is difficult and few mutants have been successfully complemented (Table 1). This has been achieved by transforming bacteria a second time with the *himar*1 transposon with an alternative selective marker and intact gene with promoter (King et al. 2014; Lourdault et al. 2011; Ristow et al. 2007), or through integrating an intact copy of the gene onto the chromosome by homologous recombination (Zhang et al. 2012; Kassegne et al. 2014). In the absence of complementation use of a second, independent mutant in the gene or pathway of interest (Eshghi et al. 2012; Murray et al. 2010; Lambert et al. 2012a) or whole genome sequencing (Zhang et al. 2013) can be used to rule out other attenuating mutations.

It should be noted that many "virulence factors" are also found in the saprophytes. In some cases, a role in virulence overlaps with normal cell metabolism; for example, heme oxygenase is presumably useful for the degradation of heme from endogenous or exogenous sources in both saprophyte and pathogen (Guégan et al. 2003). Other "virulence factors" in saprophytes may have roles in environmental survival; for example, saprophytes and pathogens can degrade the lipids in cell membranes (Kasărov 1970) which could be used to obtain lipids from environmental organisms as well as animal hosts.

1.2 Redundancy of Leptospiral Virulence Mechanisms

Pathogenic leptospires possess extensive genetic and functional redundancy. This may be a result of a process of genomic expansion through gene duplication (Bulach et al. 2006, Chap. 4). Groups of functionally similar, paralogous genes such as the *lig* and *len* families abound; LigA and LigB both bind collagen, laminin, fibrinogen, fibronectin, and numerous soluble regulators of the complement system (Choy et al. 2007), while LenABCDEF all bind laminin and fibronectin (Barbosa et al. 2006; Stevenson et al. 2007). There is also considerable functional overlap between proteins without sequence similarity, particularly adhesins and proteins that bind complement regulatory proteins. For example, LipL32, LigA, LenABC-DEF, TlyC are among more than 25 proteins reported to bind to laminin (Carvalho et al. 2009; Hoke et al. 2008; Stevenson et al. 2007, Table 3).

The maintenance of redundant factors in the leptospiral genome is difficult to explain. Functionally redundant proteins may operate at different stages of disease, in different tissues, or work synergistically. Multiple leptospiral receptors targeting a particular host substrate may also permit leptospires to infect a diverse repertoire of mammalian hosts where the target molecule may vary in structure. It is plausible that the numerous receptors for soluble proteins such as fibronectin and plasminogen (Tables 3 and 4) may coat the surface of leptospires with host proteins in a form of immune evasion, masking the underlying antigens.

The flipside of functional redundancy is the surprising lack of attenuation for specific mutants. There are several proteins, such as LipL32, LipL41, and LigB that appear to be obvious virulence factors by way of in vitro functional characterization, conservation, and expression profiles. However, mutants in genes encoding these proteins retain full virulence (Croda et al. 2008; King et al. 2013; Murray et al. 2009c). Notably, LipL32 and LigB mutants retained virulence in both acute disease and animal colonization models. Other notable mutants that retained virulence include *L. interrogans* serovar Manilae mutants in *ligC*, *lenB*, and *lenE* (Murray et al. 2009a). Presumably the loss of these putative virulence factors is covered by other functionally related proteins (Adler et al. 2011).

2 Pathogen Entry

Human infection with *Leptospira* occurs upon contact with contaminated environmental reservoirs (water, soil) or animal sources (urine, animal tissues). Bacteria breach mucosal membranes or enter transdermally through wet or abraded skin (Adler and de la Peña Moctezuma 2010). The molecular mechanisms by which entry occurs are currently unknown.

Table 3 Leptospiral proteins that interact with extracellular matrix proteins

Name(s)	Locus tag	Description	Collagen I	Collagen III	Collagen IV	Collagen V	Elastin	Tropoelastin	Heparan sulfate	Laminin	Fibronectin[a]	Location[b]	Function verified[c]	References
EF-Tu	LIC12875, LA0737	Elongation factor (protein synthesis)	Y		Y		Y			Y	Y	OM		Wolff et al. (2013)
LenA/ Lsa24/ LfhA	LIC12906, LA0695	Endostatin-like protein								Y	Y	OM	Y	Barbosa et al. (2006), Stevenson et al. (2007), Verma et al. (2006, 2010a)
LenB	LIC10997, LA3103	Endostatin-like protein								Y	Y	NA		Stevenson et al. (2007)
LenC	LIC13006, LA0563	Endostatin-like protein								Y	Y	NA		Stevenson et al. (2007)
LenD	LIC12315, LA1433	Endostatin-like protein								Y	Y	OM		Stevenson et al. (2007)
LenE	LIC13467, LA4324	Endostatin-like protein								Y	Y	NA		Stevenson et al. (2007)
LenF	LIC13248, LA4073	Endostatin-like protein								Y	Y	NA		Stevenson et al. (2007)
LIC12976	LIC12976, LA0602	NAD/FAD-binding protein								Y		NA		Lima et al. (2013)
LigA	LIC10465	Bacterial immunoglobulin-like repeat protein	Y		Y					Y	Y	OM	Y	Choy et al. (2007), Figueira et al. (2011)
LigB	LIC10464, LA3778	Bacterial immunoglobulin-like repeat protein	Y	Y	Y		Y	Y	Y	Y	Y	OM	Y	Ching et al. (2012), Choy et al. (2007, 2011), Figueira et al. (2011), Lin et al. (2009), Toma et al. (2014)

(continued)

Table 3 (continued)

Name(s)	Locus tag	Description	Collagen I	Collagen III	Collagen IV	Collagen V	Elastin	Tropelastin	Heparan sulfate	Laminin	Fibronectin[a]	Location[b]	Function verified[c]	References
LipL32	LIC11352, LA2637	Major outer membrane protein	Y		Y	Y				Y	Y	OM	Y	Hauk et al. (2008), Hoke et al. (2008), Vieira et al. (2010a)
LipL53	LIC12099, LA1691	Hypothetical protein			Y					Y	Y	I		Oliveira et al. (2010)
LMB216	LB216, LIC20172										Y	OM		Toma et al. (2014)
Lp30	LIC12880, LA0730	Hypothetical protein										I		Oliveira et al. (2011)
Lp95	LIC12690, LA0962	Hypothetical protein								Y	Y	NA		Atzingen et al. (2009)
Lsa20	LIC11469, LA2496	Hypothetical protein								Y		OM	Y	Mendes et al. (2011)
Lsa21	LIC10368, LA0419	Hypothetical protein			Y					Y	Y	OM		Atzingen et al. (2008)
Lsa25	LIC12253, LA1508	Hypothetical protein								Y		OM	Y	Domingos et al. (2012)
Lsa27	LIC12895, LA0710	Hypothetical protein								Y		I		Longhi et al. (2009)
Lsa30	LIC11087, LA2975									Y	Y	OM		Souza et al. (2012)
Lsa33	LIC11834, LA2083	LipL45-related protein, FecR domain								Y		I	Y	Domingos et al. (2012)

(continued)

Table 3 (continued)

Name(s)	Locus tag	Description	Collagen I	Collagen III	Collagen IV	Collagen V	Elastin	Tropoelastin	Heparan sulfate	Laminin	Fibronectin[a]	Location[b]	Function verified[c]	References
Lsa63	LIC10314, LA0365	Hypothetical protein			Y					Y		OM	Y	Vieira et al. (2010b)
Lsa66, MFn8	LIC10258, LA0301	OmpA-related protein								Y	Y	I	Y	Oliveira et al. (2011), Pinne et al. (2012)
MFn1	LIC11612, LA2330	Hypothetical protein									Y	OM	Y	Pinne et al. (2012)
MFn10	LIC11755, LA2167	Hypothetical protein									Y	NA		Pinne et al. (2012)
MFn11	LIC11028, LA3067	Tol transport system component									Y	NA		Pinne et al. (2012)
MFn12	LIC12952, LA0635	Hypothetical protein									Y	NA		Pinne et al. (2012)
MFn13	LIC11893, LA2014	CreD-like protein									Y	NA		Pinne et al. (2012)
MFn14, LruB	LIC10713, LA3469	Lipoprotein LruB									Y	NA		Pinne et al. (2012)
MFn15	LIC13066, LA3834	Hypothetical protein, beta propeller domains									Y	NA		Pinne et al. (2012)
MFn2	LIC10714, LA3468	TonB-dependent receptor									Y	NA		Pinne et al. (2012)
MFn3, Sph3	LIC13198, LA4004	Sphingomyelinase 3									Y	NA		Pinne et al. (2012)
MFn4, Sph2	LIC12631, LA1029	Sphingomyelinase 2									Y	NA	Y	Pinne et al. (2012)

(continued)

152   G.L. Murray

Table 3 (continued)

Name(s)	Locus tag	Description	Collagen I	Collagen III	Collagen IV	Collagen V	Elastin	Tropoelastin	Heparan sulfate	Laminin	Fibronectin[a]	Location[b]	Function verified[c]	References
MFn5	LIC13135, LA3927	TolC family protein									Y	NA		Pinne et al. (2012)
MFn6	LIC11051, LA3028	Leucine-rich repeat protein									Y	NA		Pinne et al. (2012)
MFn7	LIC11436, LA2537	LipL45-related protein									Y	OM	Y	Pinne et al. (2012)
MFn9	LIC10537, LA3685	OmpA family protein									Y	OM		Pinne et al. (2012)
OmpL1	LIC10973, LA3138	Transmembrane protein								Y	Y	OM	Y	Fernandes et al. (2012)
OmpL37	LIC12263, LA1495	Transmembrane protein					Y			Y	Y	OM		Pinne et al. (2010)
OmpL47	LIC13050, LA0505	Transmembrane protein		Y			Y			Y	Y	OM		Pinne et al. (2010)
TlyC	LIC13143, LA3937	Hemolysin-like protein			Y					Y	Y	OM	Y	Carvalho et al. (2009)

[a] Indicates binding to cellular fibronectin, plasma fibronectin, or both
[b] Location confirmed experimentally. *OM* Located in outer membrane and/or surface exposed; *I* Inconclusive evidence of surface exposure; *NA* Data not available
[c] Function(s) verified by one or more of the following: independent study, inhibition of binding by antibodies or purified protein, gain of function after expression in *L. biflexa*. See text for further details

Table 4 Leptospiral proteins that interact with plasma proteins and soluble mediators of complement resistance

Name	Locus tag	Fibrinogen	Plasminogen	Factor H	Factor H-related protein 1	Factor H-like protein 1	C4b-binding protein	Location[a]	References
Enolase	LIC11954, LA1951		Y					OM	Nogueira et al. (2013)
EF-Tu	LIC12875, LA0737	Y	Y	Y				OM	Wolff et al. (2013)
LcpA	LIC11947, LA1957						Y	OM	Barbosa et al. (2010)
LenA/ Lsa24/ LfhA	LIC12906, LA0695		Y	Y	Y			OM	Stevenson et al. (2007), Verma et al. (2006, 2010a)
LenB	LIC10997, LA3103			Y				NA	Stevenson et al. (2007)
LIC10494	LA3735		Y					I	Vieira et al. (2010a)
LIC11360	LA2626	Y						NA	Oliveira et al. (2013)
LIC11975	LA1931	Y						NA	Oliveira et al. (2013)
LIC12238	LA1523	Y	Y					I	Oliveira et al. (2013), Vieira et al. (2010a)
LIC12730	LA0913		Y					I	Vieira et al. (2010a)
LigA	LIC10465	Y		Y	Y	Y	Y	OM	Castiblanco-Valencia et al. (2012), Choy et al. (2007)
LigB	LIC10464, LA3778	Y		Y	Y	Y	Y	OM	Castiblanco-Valencia et al. (2012), Choy et al. (2007)
LipL32	LIC11352, LA2637		Y					OM	Vieira et al. (2010a)

(continued)

Table 4 (continued)

Name	Locus tag	Fibrinogen	Plasminogen	Factor H	Factor H-related protein 1	Factor H-like protein 1	C4b-binding protein	Location[a]	References
LipL40	LIC10091, LA0103		Y					I	Vieira et al. (2010a)
Lp29	LIC12892		Y					OM	Vieira et al. (2010a)
Lp30	LIC12880, LA070		Y					I	Oliveira et al. (2011)
Lp49	LIC10793, LA3370		Y					I	Vieira et al. (2010a)
Lsa20	LIC11469, LA2496		Y					OM	Mendes et al. (2011)
Lsa25	LIC12253, LA1508	Y					Y	I	Domingos et al. (2012), Oliveira et al. (2013)
Lsa30	LIC11087, LA2975	Y	Y				Y	OM	Oliveira et al. (2013), Souza et al. (2012)
Lsa33	LIC11834, LA2083	Y	Y				Y	I	Domingos et al. (2012); Oliveira et al. (2013)
Lsa66	LIC10258, LA0301		Y					I	Oliveira et al. (2011)
MPL36	LIC10054, LA0061		Y					I	Vieira et al. (2010a)
OmpL1	LIC10973, LA3138	Y	Y					OM	Fernandes et al. (2012), Oliveira et al. (2013)
OmpL37	LIC12263, LA1495	Y						OM	Pinne et al. (2010)
OmpL47	LIC13050, LA0505	Y						OM	Pinne et al. (2010)

[a] Location confirmed experimentally. *OM*, Located in outer membrane and/or surface exposed; *I* Inconclusive evidence of surface exposure; *NA* Data not available

2.1 Motility

Leptospires are highly motile as a result of two periplasmic flagella that are inserted subterminally and wrap around the protoplasmic cylinder (see the chapter by C.E. Cameron, this volume); loss of flagella results in loss of motility (Picardeau et al. 2001). Flagella are thought to comprise a core containing FlaB (encoded by four *flaB* genes), a sheath composed of FlaA (encoded by two *flaA* genes), and possibly other proteins yet to be identified (Lambert et al. 2012a). Leptospiral motility is more effective in viscous substrates (Berg and Turner 1979; Kaiser and Doetsch 1975), which may allow penetration of substrates such as collagen and hyaluronic acid found in tissues that would stall externally flagellated bacteria (reviewed in Charon and Goldstein 2002).

In the initial stages of leptospirosis, motility is most likely necessary to breach the mucosal membranes or enter the tissues through damaged skin, though this has not been directly demonstrated. An undefined motility mutant of *L. interrogans* (with defective translational motility, loss of hooked ends) was attenuated in hamsters (Faine and van der Hoeden 1964). Similar motility mutants had reduced adhesion to primary murine renal epithelial cells and a murine fibroblast cell line (Ballard et al. 1986; Vinh et al. 1984). More recently two defined mutants, in *fliY* and *flaA2*, that lack motility were attenuated in acute models of infection. Together these studies indicate that once inside the host motility is essential for disease.

A *fliY* (flagella motor switch) mutant exhibited reduced motility, although polar effects on the expression of multiple downstream flagellar genes were noted (Liao et al. 2009). The *fliY* mutant was attenuated in guinea pigs and showed reduced adhesion to macrophages and reduced induction of macrophage apoptosis (Table 1). The authors speculate that this may result from reduced export of adhesins and toxins through the flagella apparatus (Liao et al. 2009). As an alternative explanation, lack of motility may reduce encounters between leptospires and macrophages, giving the appearance of a less adhesive strain and reduced apoptosis; attenuation in vivo maybe a consequence of reduced dissemination in the host.

A *flaA2* transposon mutant has been described which did not express FlaA1 nor FlaA2 (Lambert et al. 2012a). This mutant had altered flagella structure (loss of helical shape), altered cell morphology (loss of hooked/helical cell ends), and lacked translational motility, similar to motility mutants described earlier (Faine and van der Hoeden 1964). The *flaA2* mutant was highly attenuated in hamsters, which survived $>10^5$ LD$_{50}$ with no detectable kidney colonization 25 days after infection (Table 1). Interestingly, the *flaA2* mutant was present in far lower numbers or undetectable in liver and kidney 5 days post infection compared to very high numbers of WT bacteria (Lambert et al. 2012a), suggesting that motility is necessary for the ubiquitous tissue distribution of leptospires found in acute hosts (Faine 1957).

A mutant in a gene encoding a putative sensor protein, *lb139*, showed down regulation of 115 genes; of these, genes encoding regulatory proteins, putative secreted proteins, and motility and chemotaxis proteins were over represented (Eshghi et al. 2014). The mutant was highly attenuated in the hamster model of infection by both conjunctival and intraperitoneal routes. While the down regulated secreted proteins may have a direct role in virulence, reduced motility (observed in plate and video microscope assays) may also explain the attenuation of this strain.

2.2 Chemotaxis

Leptospires possess the majority of the key chemotaxis genes found in other bacteria, with approximately 12 methyl-accepting chemotaxis proteins (MCPs) encoded in the genomes of pathogens (Nascimento et al. 2004; Ren et al. 2003). This indicates that leptospires respond to a wide range of chemical stimuli, though the ligand for each receptor is unknown. One suggested chemical attractant is hemoglobin (Yuri et al. 1993), although hemoglobin is too large to cross the outer membrane and be detected in the periplasm by an MCP (Lambert et al. 2012b); perhaps in these experiments bacteria were attracted to a smaller, readily diffusible breakdown product. Nevertheless, this result indicates chemotaxis toward blood, suggesting that leptospires are attracted to the host at the site of injury where tissue barriers have already been degraded.

Other leptospiral chemoattractants include glucose, sucrose, pyruvate, and Tween 80 (a source of oleic acid) (Lambert et al. 2012b). As a synthetic compound, Tween 80 would have no role in leptospirosis per se, although chemotaxis toward Tween 80 may indicate a tendency to move toward nutritional sources of fatty acids, even though the level of lipids such as triglycerides in blood is low (approximately 1 mM). Likewise, the significance of chemotaxis toward glucose is unknown as leptospires do not utilize this sugar as an energy source, and the concentration of glucose in blood is around 5 mM, lower than the tested concentration (100 mM).

The importance of chemotaxis in leptospiral infection has not been thoroughly investigated. Mutants in putative chemotaxis genes *cheB* and *cheX* were not attenuated in hamsters when infected intraperitoneally (Murray et al. 2009a), although a role for these proteins in leptospiral chemotaxis is yet to be established and there are multiple *cheB* genes encoded in leptospiral genome (Dong et al. 2010). Additionally, it is possible that chemotaxis is not required once the host has been invaded; therefore mutants should also be tested via "natural" routes of infection (conjunctiva, dermal abrasion). It is tempting to speculate that chemotaxis is important for tissue tropisms, but apparent tissue tropisms such as localization in the renal tubules may alternatively be the result of immune clearance of leptospires from some sites but not others.

2.3 Crossing Host Tissue Barriers

In order to disseminate throughout the host, leptospires must cross many barriers including extracellular matrix, basement membranes, and cell layers. The mechanisms by which leptospires cross tissue layers occurs remain unknown, but motility is likely to play a key role (Lambert et al. 2012a).

Treponema pallidum is thought to cross cell layers through cell junctions (Thomas et al. 1988), while *Borrelia burgdorferi* had been reported to cross cell layers by invading the cell cytoplasm (Comstock and Thomas 1989) or at cell junctions (Moriarty et al. 2008; Szczepanski et al. 1990). In a mouse infection model, leptospires were observed to cross into the kidney lumen between cells (Marshall 1976). In contrast, two studies examining transcytosis of leptospires across the polarized Madin-Darby canine kidney (MDCK) cell line found evidence of transit through cells (Barocchi et al. 2002; Thomas and Higbie 1990); leptospires crossed layers rapidly without major disruption of tight junctions and were observed intracellularly, presumably in transit across the cell layer. Intracellular bacteria were sometimes surrounded by a host cell membrane, but were also free in the cytoplasm. Many pathogens such as *Salmonella* spp. and *Yersinia* spp. enter host cells through specific interactions that cause perturbations in cellular architecture. By contrast, during leptospiral "invasion" of the monolayer, cells remained intact and there was no evidence of cytoskeletal rearrangements. The results suggest a novel mechanism of cell invasion as a means of crossing tissue barriers. Interestingly, *Leptospira biflexa* was also observed to cross layers (though less efficiently than pathogenic leptospires) (Barocchi et al. 2002); perhaps transcytosis is a result of the thin, helical morphology and vigorous motility shared between pathogen and saprophyte rather than a specific molecular mechanism. Experiments could be repeated with motility mutants to test this theory.

Proteases may also contribute to the crossing of cell layers. Transcytosis across human umbilical vein endothelial cell (HUVEC) monolayers was enhanced when leptospires were coated with plasminogen or plasmin, suggesting a proteolytic mechanism (Vieira et al. 2013). A collagenase mutant also had reduced ability to cross HUVEC and human renal tubular epithelial cell line (HEK293) cell layers, and in vivo the same mutant had reduced distribution in tissues in hamsters, indicating that collagenase may assist with bacterial dissemination (Kassegne et al. 2014).

3 Pathogen Adhesion and Dissemination

3.1 Adhesion to Host Cells

Adhesion to host surfaces is an important step in bacterial pathogenesis (Kline et al. 2009). In animals, close association of leptospires with microvilli of proximal renal tubules has been observed in hamsters and sheep, but generally without obvious cytopathology (Faine et al. 1999; Marshall 1974). In vitro, adhesion to various host cells has been observed, including MDCK and primary dog kidney cell lines (Thomas and Higbie 1990; Tsuchimoto et al. 1984), mouse fibroblast cells (Vinh et al. 1984), mouse renal tubular epithelial cells (Ballard et al. 1998), human umbilical vein endothelial cells, and porcine kidney epithelial cells (Thomas and Higbie 1990). Adhesion levels correlated with strain virulence (Tsuchimoto et al. 1984). Leptospiral adherence to cells is diminished after pretreatment of monoloayers with proteases, indicating probable protein receptors (Breiner et al. 2009; Thomas and Higbie 1990). Cellular fibronectin and glycosaminoglycans are potential host receptors participating in this binding.

3.2 Glycosaminoglycans

Glycosaminoglycans (GAGs) are unbranched, long polymers of disaccharides that may be sulfated. GAGs form part of the extracellular matrix, and when bound to proteins, they constitute proteoglycans and are located on the surface of cells. *Leptospira* binds to GAGs, chondroitin sulfate B and C, though specific unknown receptors (Breiner et al. 2009); in the absence of GAGs significant binding to host cells occurred, implying that additional adhesin targets exist. The authors speculated that GAGs present on cells at mucosal surfaces may be involved in initial host colonization, while GAGs expressed in the renal tubule and released in the urine may facilitate renal colonization and shedding (Breiner et al. 2009). In a phage display experiment, LigB was found to bind to the heparin sulfate, which could mediate binding to host cells (Ching et al. 2012), although a *ligB* mutant bound to MDCK cells at the same rate as WT leptospires (Croda et al. 2008).

During the hematogenous spread, pathogenic leptospires most likely adhere to the endothelium of the blood vessel under fluid shear forces and then penetrate the cell layer to enter tissues. The mechanism by which this occurs is unknown, but studies in *B. burgdorferi* may provide clues. *B. burgdorferi* exits from post-capillary venules through a sequence of interactions with the vessel endothelium: transient interactions, dragging interactions, adhesion, then transmigration into surrounding tissues, mainly through cell junctions (Moriarty et al. 2008). The *B. burgdorferi* protein BBK32 is thought to play a role in this process by mediating direct and indirect interaction via fibronectin with GAGs of endothelial cells (Moriarty et al. 2012). A similar process of escape from the microvasculature may occur in leptospirosis, facilitated by direct interaction with GAGs or indirect interaction via numerous fibronectin receptors with different affinity for fibronectin.

3.3 Adhesion to Extracellular Matrix

The extracellular matrix (ECM) is a complex mixture of fibrous proteins and other components such as GAGs that supports the architecture of tissues, as well as contributing to cell viability, development, differentiation, and motility. Components include 28 types of collagen (with I, III, IV, and VI being most prominent), laminin, fibronectin, and proteoglycans (Batzios et al. 2013). Early studies identified that pathogenic leptospires can bind to ECM components, including fibronectin, collagen, laminin, and hyaluronic acid (Ito and Yanagawa 1987). Adhesion to ECM molecules is enhanced after incubation at physiological osmolarity, simulating the transition from environment to host (Matsunaga et al. 2007).

Proteins that bind to host structures are often termed Microbial Surface Components Recognizing Adhesive Matrix Molecules (MSCRAMMs). The first indication of a specific leptospiral protein that binds ECM components was the finding that a 36-kDa outer membrane protein binds fibronectin, though the identity of this protein is unknown (Merien et al. 2000). Subsequently, a very large number of leptospiral proteins have been reported to bind to components of the ECM (Table 3). Despite the identification of many potential adhesins, none has been shown to be essential for virulence, a possible consequence of functional redundancy.

The majority of studies characterizing the interaction of leptospiral proteins with ECM components have used recombinant protein in in vitro assays. It is therefore difficult to translate the meaning of these findings to natural infection. This difficulty is compounded when the exposure of the protein of interest on the leptospiral cell is either not investigated (Lima et al. 2013), is inconclusive, or cannot be verified (Oliveira et al. 2011; Pinne et al. 2012, Table 3). The use of recombinant protein also presents a number of problems. Some leptospiral proteins undergo post-translational modification, such as lipidation, sialylation, glycosylation, phosphorylation, methylation, and proteolysis (Cao et al. 2010; Cullen et al. 2002; Ricaldi et al. 2012). Recombinant proteins produced in *Escherichia coli* are unlikely to have appropriate modifications. Furthermore, the majority of putative leptospiral membrane proteins are insoluble when expressed in *E. coli* in high quantities (Murray et al. 2013). Refolding of proteins is difficult and may result in formation of soluble multimers of protein which may not produce obvious solution turbidity but participate in non-specific ionic interactions (Burgess 2009). It is unlikely that leptospires require more than 25 laminin-binding proteins and more than 30 fibronectin-binding proteins, leading to the conclusion that some findings may be in vitro artifacts.

In some studies, protein function has been verified through alternative assays (Table 3), adding confidence to the results of the study. For example, the binding of leptospiral cells to host protein substrates was competitively inhibited by the addition of recombinant leptospiral proteins including LigA and LigB (inhibited leptospiral binding to fibronectin) (Choy et al. 2007), TlyC (ECM) (Carvalho et al. 2009), enolase (plasminogen) (Nogueira et al. 2013), Lsa20, Lsa25, and Lsa33 (laminin and plasminogen) (Domingos et al. 2012; Mendes et al. 2011), Lsa66 (ECM and plasminogen) (Oliveira et al. 2011), Lsa63 (collagen IV and laminin) (Vieira et al. 2010b), and OmpL1 (laminin, plasminogen, fibronectin) (Fernandes et al. 2012). In a similar confirmatory process, leptospiral attachment to laminin was blocked by antibody to Lsa24/lenA/LfhA (Barbosa et al. 2006), and binding to plasminogen was reduced by antibodies to enolase (Nogueira et al. 2013). In each of these studies, *Leptospira*–substrate interaction was only partially inhibited by antibody or recombinant protein, supporting the notion of multiple, redundant adhesins sharing the same substrate specificity. In some studies, the use of specific antibodies or excess recombinant protein resulted in no inhibition. For example, leptospiral binding to ECM was not inhibited by specific antibody to LipL32 (Hoke et al. 2008). In the case of OmpL37, cell adhesion to elastin was not inhibited by excess recombinant protein and, surprisingly, was enhanced in the presence of specific antiserum (Pinne et al. 2010). In another approach to confirmation of protein function, the ability of LigA and LigB to bind to fibronectin and laminin and the properties of fibronectin-binding proteins Mfn1, Mfn4, and Mfn7 were confirmed through gain of function studies using the saprophyte *L. biflexa* (Figueira et al. 2011; Pinne et al. 2012; Toma et al. 2014). In contrast, the mutants in *lipL32* and *ligB* displayed normal binding to ECM and MDCK cells, respectively (Croda et al. 2008; Murray et al. 2009c).

3.3.1 Fibronectin-Binding Proteins

Fibronectin exists both as a major component of the extracellular matrix and in soluble form in plasma. A large number of leptospiral proteins have fibronectin-binding properties in in vitro binding experiments (Table 3). Binding interactions with different affinities play a part in the slowing and exit of *B. burdorferi* from blood vessels (Moriarty et al. 2012); hence multiple proteins with different affinities may potentially be involved in the attachment, dragging, and arrest of leptospires in the blood vessel endothelium. Leptospiral fibronectin binding may also mediate binding to host cells via the I domain of the CR3 complement receptor (found on polymorphonuclear leucocytes, mononuclear phagocytes, and natural killer cells), potentially increasing phagocytosis in the absence of specific opsonins (Cinco et al. 2002).

The identification of fibronectin-binding proteins highlights how different methods of analysis do not always correlate. Merien et al. (2000) found one fibronectin-binding protein by ligand blot, yet subsequent studies have found more than 30 such proteins in *Leptospira* (Table 3). When a protein array comprising 401 predicted leptospiral outer membrane proteins was used to screen for fibronectin-binding proteins (Pinne et al. 2012), of the top 15 fibronectin-binding proteins only one had previously been identified (Lsa66). Notable fibronectin-binding proteins LigB (repeat domains 8–12) had 34th highest affinity for fibronectin, while LipL32 was 169th on the list. Regardless of this, fibronectin binding was validated by ligand blot for six of the top 15 proteins, and expression of three proteins in

L. biflexa conferred the ability to bind soluble fibronectin (Pinne et al. 2012). While different experimental approaches may have contributed to the different outcomes from these and other studies, the lack of correlation is surprising and suggests that some binding affinities identified in vitro are artifacts.

3.3.2 Laminin-Binding Proteins

Laminin is an important component of basement membranes of epithelial and endothelial surfaces. Ability to bind to laminin may enhance the ability of lepto-spires to invade and cross tissue layers. A remarkably large number of leptospiral proteins have been found to bind laminin in in vitro assays. One group of proteins is the Len protein paralogs; all of the Len proteins bind to laminin with varying degrees of affinity (Stevenson et al. 2007).

3.3.3 Elastin-Binding Proteins

Elastin fibers composed of the soluble protein tropoelastin confer elasticity to tis-sues, and are found in ECM of numerous tissues including the lung, skin, arteries, uterus, and placenta. Leptospirosis has an impact on many of these tissues; hence elastin-binding properties of LigB and OmpL37 and OmpL47 (Lin et al. 2009; Pinne et al. 2010) may assist with the initial stages of colonization in the skin, or facilitate pathogen adherence and damage to the lungs and blood vessel endothe-lium resulting in lung hemorrhage and vessel damage, or contribute to abortion. Interestingly, all three of these proteins bind specifically to numerous other host ligands (Table 3). LigB was observed to bind to elastin, and binding was localized to certain LigB domains (Lin et al. 2009). LigB also bound tropoelastin, potentially inhibiting tissue repair by preventing formation of elastin fibers (Lin et al. 2009). OmpL37 had high affinity for skin elastin. Rather than inhibit adhesion, antibodies to OmpL37 enhanced OmpL37 binding to elastin but not to other ECM proteins, suggesting that the host immune response to this protein may specifically promote adhesion to elastin (Pinne et al. 2010).

3.4 Disruption of Hemostasis and Wound Repair

3.4.1 Leptospiral Binding of Fibrinogen

Leptospirosis is characterized by thrombocytopenia, hemorrhage, and vascular injury. Some of these pathologies may be explained by the ability of leptospires to bind fibrinogen (Choy et al. 2007) with subsequent inhibition of fibrin formation (Oliveira et al. 2013). This may assist bacterial dissemination and contribute directly to hemorrhage. Numerous fibrinogen-binding proteins have been identified

(Table 4). Of these, LigB, Lsa33, LIC12238, LIC11975, and OmpL1 inhibited thrombin-catalyzed fibrin formation in vitro (Choy et al. 2011; Lin et al. 2011; Oliveira et al. 2013). LigB binding to the C-terminal αC domain of fibrinogen also inhibited platelet adhesion and aggregation in vitro (Lin et al. 2011). Some of the leptospiral proteins caused a slight decrease in the binding of leptospiral cells to fibrinogen in a competitive binding assay (Oliveira et al. 2013). However, none of these proteins has a confirmed role in disease, and as stated above, a *ligB* mutant retains normal virulence (Croda et al. 2008).

Notably, while other fibrinogen-binding proteins such as *Streptococcus epidermidis* SdrG completely inhibit fibrin formation (Davis et al. 2001), inhibition by leptospiral proteins was incomplete. This may indicate that leptospiral proteins are more important as adhesins, or work in concert for an additive effect. LigA also binds fibrinogen and is released from the leptospiral cell; this may inhibit blood coagulation beyond the immediate proximity of the leptospiral cell, though this has not been demonstrated (Choy et al. 2007). In addition to a role in prevention of hemostasis, LigB binds to collagen type III, fibroblast fibronectin and tropoelastin, which are all involved in tissue repair (Choy et al. 2011; Lin et al. 2009). This may allow leptospires to attach to a fresh wound for initial colonization, and may potentiate the formation of lesions and hemorrhage during systemic disease.

It should be noted that in one study, *L. biflexa* serovar Patoc also bound fibrinogen to about 75 % of the level seen in a virulent *L. interrogans* strain; *L. biflexa*-bound fibrinogen was able to inhibit thrombin-dependent fibrin formation to the same degree as *L. interrogans* strains (Oliveira et al. 2013). This finding questions the relevance of in vitro fibrinogen binding to pathogenesis.

3.4.2 Leptospiral Binding of Plasminogen

Plasminogen is a proenzyme found in extracellular fluid and plasma that can be converted to the enzyme plasmin by proteases such as urokinase plasminogen activator (uPA). Active plasmin may degrade numerous substrates, including fibrin clots, ECM proteins such as fibronectin and laminin, and immunoglobulins. Many pathogens bind to plasminogen, which is activated by endogenous or host proteases to produce the active protease plasmin. Surface-bound plasmin is involved in pathogenesis through degradation of ECM, complement components and antibodies, and the activation of matrix metalloproteases (Lähteenmäki et al. 2001) and plays an important role in the pathogenesis of bacteria such as streptococci (Li et al. 1999; Sanderson-Smith et al. 2008; Svensson et al. 2002).

Leptospires bind plasminogen in vitro, and bound plasminogen can be converted to plasmin in the presence of uPA (Verma et al. 2010a; Vieira et al. 2009). In vitro, *Leptospira*-bound plasmin degrades ECM components such as fibronectin (Vieira et al. 2009) and human fibrinogen (Oliveira et al. 2013), and may activate host matrix metalloproteases which in turn could contribute to tissue degradation. Plasmin-coated leptospires also crossed human umbilical vein epithelial cell monolayers more efficiently than normal leptospires, although the precise mechanism was not investigated (Vieira et al. 2013). Taken together these data suggest that surface-bound plasmin may facilitate crossing of ECM and tissue barriers and degradation of fibrin clots by leptospires, resulting in dissemination throughout the host. As found in other pathogens (Lähteenmäki et al. 2001), leptospires may up regulate activators of plasminogen in host cells (Vieira et al. 2013). However, one study reported that saprophytic *L. biflexa* acquired more plasmin activity in vitro than some pathogenic strains, tempering these observations and complicating extrapolation to a host infection scenario (Vieira et al. 2009).

In vitro, leptospiral surface-bound plasmin also interferes with the deposition of C3b and immunoglobulin on the cell surface (Vieira et al. 2011). The elongation factor Tu (EF-Tu), involved in protein synthesis but also found to moonlight as a surface protein, binds plasminogen which may be activated to cleave C3b (Wolff et al. 2013). Reduced binding to C3b may diminish opsonization for phagocytosis and decrease the activation of the complement cascade at the cell surface by both the classical and alternative pathways. Plasmin-coated *L. interrogans* serovar Pomona displayed enhanced serum survival (Vieira et al. 2011).

Numerous leptospiral receptors for plasminogen have been identified. LenA binds plasminogen and it can be converted to plasmin to degrade fibronectin (Verma et al. 2010a). Enolase, a recognized plasminogen-binding protein of other bacterial pathogens, also binds plasminogen in *Leptospira* (Nogueira et al. 2013). Interestingly, leptospiral enolase is secreted and then associates with the leptospiral surface. More than a dozen additional receptors, including LipL32, have been reported to bind plasminogen and allow conversion to active plasmin in the presence of uPA, although evidence of surface localization for many of these proteins was inconclusive (Table 4). The significance of plasmin binding in vivo by these receptors is yet to be demonstrated.

3.5 Notable Proteins with Multiple Binding Affinities

Some leptospiral proteins bind to a remarkable number of diverse host proteins, potentially playing a role in varied aspects of pathogenesis. There are precedents for such proteins in the spirochetes; for example, the *Treponema denticola* protein OppA binds to plasminogen and fibronectin (Fenno et al. 2000), while Msp binds to fibronectin, keratin, laminin, collagen type I, fibrinogen, hyaluronic acid, and heparin (Edwards et al. 2005). Outside the spirochetes examples include Emp of *Staphylococcus aureus*, which interacts with fibronectin, fibrinogen, collagen, and vitronectin (Hussain et al. 2001).

3.5.1 Lig Proteins

The leptospiral Lig proteins are a group of three proteins (LigABC) that belong to a family of bacterial immunoglobulin-like proteins (Bigs) containing 12–13 immunoglobulin-like repeats (Matsunaga et al. 2003; Palaniappan et al. 2002). Bigs such as *E. coli* intimin and *Yersinia pseudotuberculosis* invasin mediate adhesion and invasion of host cells (Hamburger et al. 1999; Luo et al. 2000). The *ligA* gene is found in *L. interrogans*, *L. kirschneri*, and *L. santarosai*, although it is not yet clear whether it is universally present in all serovars and strains. LigA is one of the few promising vaccine candidate molecules for which statistically significant protection against acute leptospirosis has been demonstrated (see the chapter by B. Adler). *ligA* appears to have evolved from a partial gene duplication of *ligB* (McBride et al. 2009), and LigA is released from cells for an unknown purpose (Matsunaga et al. 2005). LigB is widely distributed in pathogenic leptospires. Many strains only have *ligB*, suggesting that it may be sufficient for pathogenesis. LigC has a wider distribution than LigA but is a pseudogene in multiple strains that retain virulence, indicating that it is unnecessary in these strains for disease pathogenesis (Cerqueira et al. 2009; McBride et al. 2009). LigC has not been functionally characterized.

Many factors indicate that Lig proteins are virulence factors. Lig proteins are significantly induced under conditions of increased osmolarity, emulating the transition from an environmental source to the host (Choy et al. 2007). Prolonged in vitro culture of leptospires leads to loss of Lig expression, correlating with a loss of virulence (Matsunaga et al. 2003). LigA and LigB bind to numerous host proteins and may play a role in disease by binding host ECM molecules at different stages (Choy et al. 2007, Table 3). Lig proteins also bind complement regulatory proteins (Table 4) and may play a role in potentiating tissue damage through binding fibrinogen and matrix components associated with wound healing (Choy et al. 2011). When *ligA* or *ligB* were expressed from a plasmid in the saprophyte strain *L. biflexa*, the resulting strain exhibited enhanced binding to some ECM components (fibronectin and laminin), but not others (Figueira et al. 2011). Lig proteins contribute to binding to host cells (Figueira et al. 2011; Lin et al. 2010; Toma et al. 2014). Lig proteins bind to complement regulatory proteins factor H and C4-binding protein (Castiblanco-Valencia et al. 2012), and LigB appears to contribute to serum resistance by inhibiting the alternative pathway of complement activation (Choy 2012).

However, evidence of an essential role in disease, or otherwise, for Lig proteins is inconclusive as a strain lacking all three Lig proteins has not been assessed in vivo. *L. interrogans* serovar Lai lacks *ligA* but retains *ligB* and *ligC* and is virulent (Ristow et al. 2007). A *ligB* mutant in *L. interrogans* serovar Copenhageni also retained virulence, but this strain still possessed *ligA* (*ligC* is a pseudogene in this strain) (Croda et al. 2008). Likewise, an *L. interrogans* serovar Manilae *ligC* mutant caused disease, but this strain retains *ligA* and *ligB* (Murray et al. 2009a). Given the extensive number of host substrates with which Lig proteins interact, in pathways including host matrix adhesion, complement resistance, and blood coagulation pathways, it seems likely that at least one Lig protein is required to cause disease.

3.5.2 The Len Proteins

This group of six proteins with similarity to human endostatins is found in pathogenic leptospires. It may have arisen through a process of gene duplication and recombination events, resulting in some overlap and some unique functions in the group (Stevenson et al. 2007). All of the Len proteins bind fibronectin and laminin. LenA (also known as LfhA/Lsa24) also binds plasminogen, factor H, and factor H-related protein, while LenB binds factor H (Verma et al. 2006, 2010a). Mutants in *lenB* and *lenE* retained virulence, but this is understandable given the functional redundancy of these proteins (Murray et al. 2009a).

3.5.3 LipL32

LipL32, also known as Hap1, is a dominant lipoprotein of the leptospiral outer membrane (Haake et al. 2000). It is the most abundant protein in *Leptospira* with an estimated 38,000 copies per cell (Malmstrom et al. 2009). The prominence of LipL32 combined with a high degree of conservation in pathogens and leptospires of intermediate pathogenicity, absence in saprophytic leptospires, and demonstrated expression in vivo make this protein a likely virulence factor (Murray 2013). An earlier indication that LipL32 may be associated with hemolysis has not been confirmed (Lee et al. 2000). Studies using recombinant LipL32 have identified binding substrates, including laminin, collagen I and V (Hoke et al. 2008), collagen IV and plasma fibronectin (Hauk et al. 2008). Notably, these studies had conflicting findings regarding laminin and collagen I binding by LipL32. Although reported binding strengths were moderate, the sheer number of LipL32 molecules on the surface may markedly increase the avidity of interaction (Vivian et al. 2009). LipL32 has also been reported to bind to plasminogen (Vieira et al. 2010a).

Despite all the indications of a role in virulence, a *lipl32* mutant remained virulent in both the hamster acute and rat colonization models of infection (Murray et al. 2009c). Notably, hamsters were challenged by both intraperitoneal and mucosal infection routes. The lack of attenuation of the *lipL32* mutant may be a result of functional redundancy, as many proteins share substrate specificity with LipL32 (Tables 3 and 4). Interestingly, while LipL32 is found in leptospires that are pathogenic or of intermediate pathogenicity, there are LipL32 orthologs in environmental organisms outside *Leptospira* (Murray 2013) including the marine organism *Pseudoalteromonas tunicata* (Hoke et al. 2008); perhaps this indicates a role for this LipL32 in transmission and environmental survival, two factors not assessed in current animal models. Furthermore, recent evidence using immunofluorescence and surface proteolysis suggests that LipL32 may not in fact be exposed on the surface of the cell (Pinne and Haake 2013). This may explain the general lack of protection conferred by immunization with LipL32 and naturally acquired immunity to LipL32 (Murray 2013, Chap. 10). As a result of this finding, it is advisable not to use LipL32 as a surface marker control when performing immunofluorescence and surface proteolysis experiments (see the chapter by D.A. Haake and W.R. Zückert, this volume).

4 Persistence

4.1 Evasion of Host Immunity

Phagocytes help to control the early stages of leptospiral infection, while protective acquired immunity is humoral in the vast majority of animal species and can be transferred passively by serum (Jost et al. 1986; Masuzawa et al. 1990; Schoone et al. 1989). Protective immunity is usually directed against lipopolysaccharides, and so is restricted to related serovars (Adler and de la Peña Moctezuma 2010) (see the chapter by R.L. Zuerner, this volume). Numerous interesting interactions have been characterized between leptospires and the immune system, which may increase the disease-causing potential of *Leptospira*.

4.1.1 Interaction with the Complement Cascade

During the initial stages of leptospirosis, bacteria are found in the blood for up to 2 weeks (Faine et al. 1999), necessitating a high degree of resistance to serum complement. Complement resistance distinguishes pathogenic leptospires from the highly susceptible saprophytes (Cinco and Banfi 1983). The difference between pathogen and saprophytes appears to be at the level of C3 deposition and this correlates with pathogen binding of host complement regulatory proteins factor H (Meri et al. 2005) and C4-binding protein (C4BP) (Barbosa et al. 2009). The consequence of inhibition of the complement cascade is not only reduced bacterial cell lysis, but also potentially diminished recruitment and activation of phagocytes (through reduced release of anaphylotoxins C3a and C5a) and reduced opsono-phagocytosis (via phagocyte C3b receptors) (Blom et al. 2009).

Numerous proteins bind to the soluble host regulators of serum resistance factor H (and related proteins) and C4BP (Table 4). As most findings have only identified binding affinities using recombinant proteins, further work is required to elucidate the role of these proteins in serum resistance; for example, can binding to respective regulatory proteins be inhibited (by antibodies or ligand peptides), thereby enhancing complement sensitivity, or do mutants in these factors have enhanced serum sensitivity? Only *ligB* has been demonstrated to partially contribute to serum resistance when expressed in *L. biflexa* (Choy 2012). As is the case for ECM-binding proteins, a definitive in vivo role for complement pathway-interacting proteins in Table 4 is yet to be established. Mutants in genes encoding LenB (binds to factor H) and LigB (binds to factor H and C4BP) retained virulence, indicating that these proteins are not essential for disease (Croda et al. 2008; Murray et al. 2009a).

In alternative strategies for serum resistance, leptospires may inactivate bound complement proteins by proteases; plasmin-mediated reduction in C3b deposition and enhanced serum survival has been reported (Vieira et al. 2011), while secreted leptospiral proteases appear to degrade complement components (Fraga et al. 2014).

There is also evidence that leptospires can synthesize sialic acid and related non-ulosonic acids that may be added to surface proteins to promote serum resistance (Ricaldi et al. 2012), though further investigation is necessary.

4.1.2 Interaction with Phagocytic Immune Cells

Leptospires are not classical intracellular pathogens. However, recent discoveries suggest that intracellular phases may play a role in pathogenesis. In vitro studies have found leptospires maybe transiently intracellular when passing through cell layers (Barocchi et al. 2002; Thomas and Higbie 1990), and appear to persist in macrophages (Li et al. 2010; Toma et al. 2011).

In the murine macrophage/monocyte-like cell line J774A.1, internalization of leptospires occurred by receptor-mediated endocytosis rather than phagocytosis (Merien et al. 1997), suggesting entry into phagocytic cells by a non-phagocytic mechanism is beneficial to leptospires. A possible mechanism for this is via a mammalian cell entry (Mce) protein. Mce proteins are a group of proteins identified in *Mycobacterium tuberculosis* that mediate attachment and entry into host cells (Arruda et al. 1993). Pathogenic leptospires have an *mce*-like gene; when disrupted leptospiral adhesion and entry into macrophage-like cells was significantly reduced, and these capacities were restored upon complementation (Zhang et al. 2012). Adhesin and cell entry properties were conferred to *L. biflexa* upon complementation with the Mce protein and to Mce-coated latex beads. RGD protein motifs bind to integrins (Ruoslahti 1996) and this may be exploited by bacterial pathogens for cell adhesion and entry (Hauck et al. 2006). Binding of Mce to integrins $\alpha5\beta1$ and $\alpha_V\beta3$ was demonstrated, and when the RGD motif of Mce was modified, binding of *L. biflexa* to host cells was lost (Zhang et al. 2012). The *mce* mutant had a modest attenuation upon infection of hamsters compared to the parent strain and complemented mutant (50-fold increase in LD_{50}) (Table 1) (Zhang et al. 2012), suggesting this entry mechanism is somewhat important for virulence. Leptospiral proteins LMB216 and LigB also contribute to the uptake of leptospires by phagocytic cells, as shown through analysis of *L. interrogans* mutants and by heterologous protein expression in *L. biflexa* (Toma et al. 2014).

Phagocytosis is an important immune control mechanism during leptospirosis (Faine 1957, 1964), therefore subversion of phagocytic outcomes may be an important mechanism of immune evasion. The production of reactive oxygen species is an important microbicidal mechanism for phagocytes. Catalase (KatE) found in pathogenic leptospires is required for resistance to hydrogen peroxide (Eshghi et al. 2012). While the role of KatE in survival in macrophages has not been directly tested, hamsters infected with *katE* mutants of *L. interrogans* serovars Pomona or Manilae survived challenge without signs of disease, indicating that oxidative stress resistance is essential for virulence (Table 1). Another mediator of resistance to oxidative stress is the molecular chaperone ClpB; this protein is also required for growth under nutrient restriction and heat stress (Lourdault et al. 2011). A *clpB* mutant was also highly attenuated; gerbils receiving a very high dose survived infection with no clinical signs of leptospirosis and no macroscopic lesions normally associated with disease (Table 1). Restoration of growth under oxidative, heat, and nutrient stress conditions was achieved by complementation with an intact copy of *clpB*, along with partial restoration of virulence (Lourdault et al. 2011). The precise cause of attenuation of the *clpB* mutant is unknown, but may be due to altered expression of virulence factors, in vivo growth deficiency, or increased susceptibility to stress conditions including oxidative stress (Lourdault et al. 2011). Interestingly, a second chaperone, HtpG, has been shown to be required for virulence, but the mechanism of attenuation is yet to be determined (Tables 1 and 2).

Apoptosis is another potential mechanism for pathogens to escape killing in phagocytes, but paradoxically may also be a host mechanism to contain infection. Numerous potential mechanisms have been suggested for apoptosis observed in vitro (Jin et al. 2009; Hu et al. 2013), including the involvement of sphingomyelinase 2 in a human liver cell line (Zhang et al. 2008) and by calcium ion flux initiated by leptospiral phospholipase C (LB361) in human and murine macrophage cell lines (Zhao et al. 2013). However, it remains unclear what role macrophage apoptosis plays in leptospirosis as other studies have reported no evidence of apoptosis in vitro (Toma et al. 2011). Additionally, evidence of apoptosis in animal infection is limited, being reported in hepatocytes of laboratory infected guinea pigs (Merien et al. 1998).

4.2 Nutrient Acquisition

The nutritional requirements of *Leptospira* are relatively simple, comprising a source of B vitamins, iron, ammonium, and long chain fatty acids as an energy source for β-oxidation (see the chapter by C.E. Cameron, this volume). Leptospires have approximately 12 predicted TonB-dependent receptors that may be responsible for active nutrient import (Nascimento et al. 2004; Ren et al. 2003). However, little is known about the substrates for these receptors.

Fatty acids for β-oxidation may be obtained through degradation of host cells membranes by phospholipases or sphingomyelinases (Kasărov 1970; Narayanavari et al. 2012). Sphingomyelinases catalyze the hydrolysis of sphingomyelin into ceramide and phosphorylcholine and may be responsible for hemolysis and damage to host tissues. *L. interrogans* has five predicted sphingomyelinases (Sph1, Sph2, Sph3, Sph4, SphH) while *L. borgpetersenii* has three (SphA, SphB, Sph4), although only Sph2 and SphA are predicted to have complete catalytic sites (Narayanavari et al. 2012). The sphingomyelinase activities of SphA and Sph2 have been demonstrated (del Real et al. 1989; Segers et al. 1992), and Sph2 has cytotoxic effects on cultured cells (Artiushin et al. 2004), while the activities of the remaining enzymes are not fully resolved (Narayanavari et al. 2012). As noted in Table 3, Sph2 may be an adhesin binding to fibronectin (Pinne et al. 2012) and may initiate signaling that leads to cellular apoptosis (Zhang et al. 2008). It is hypothesized that the sphingomyelinases lacking key amino acid residues in catalytic sites may still bind to sphingomyelin of the host cell followed by another effector function (Narayanavari et al. 2012). Sphingomyelinases may contribute directly to endothelial damage leading to hemorrhage, but this remains speculative. Sublytic properties of sphingomyelinases may also be important in disease; the generation of excess ceramide in the host cell membrane may lead to perturbations in cell biology in different tissues leading to different pathologies (Narayanavari et al. 2012).

Leptospires require iron for growth (Faine 1959). In vivo, free iron is scarce due to the rapid formation of oxidized forms under physiological conditions, and due to host sequestration of iron by iron-binding proteins, especially as a defense against pathogens during infection (Wooldridge and Williams 1993). The majority of iron in the mammalian host (74 %) is in the form of heme in the protein hemoglobin (Wooldridge and Williams 1993). Heme and hemoglobin are sufficient to support leptospiral growth as sole iron sources (Guégan et al. 2003). In vivo, hemoglobin may be obtained by lysis of erythrocytes by sphingomyelinases. There are orthologs of the *tlyABC* hemolysins of *Brachyspira hyodysenteriae* encoded on the leptospiral genome, but TlyB and TlyC do not appear to have hemolytic activity (Carvalho et al. 2009). Efficient use of hemoglobin requires heme oxygenase to liberate ferrous iron from the tetrapyrrole ring for use by the leptospires (Murray et al. 2008). A heme oxygenase mutant was moderately attenuated for virulence in the acute model of disease, confirming that heme is an important iron source in vivo (Murray et al. 2009b, Table 1).

Leptospira interrogans has one characterized heme import mechanism. HbpA is a TonB-dependent receptor that binds heme (Asuthkar et al. 2007). A mutant in *hbpA* was unable to colonize mice but was still virulent in the hamster model of infection (Marcsisin et al. 2013). LipL41 was also reported to bind to heme but there are conflicting findings regarding this potential function (Asuthkar et al. 2007; King et al. 2013; Lin et al. 2013).

5 Mechanisms of Damage to Host Tissues

Leptospirosis is characterized by various symptoms, including vasculitis, acute renal failure, jaundice, thrombocytopenia, pulmonary hemorrhage, myocarditis, conjunctival suffusion, and uveitis (Levett 2001, Chap. 5). The mechanisms by which damage occurs are not conclusively known. Injury to the endothelium of small blood vessels may contribute to ischemia and dysfunction of multiple organs, while circulating toxic cellular components or undefined toxins may contribute to tissue damage (Adler and de la Peña Moctezuma 2010). Disruption of tissue integrity may occur by activity of leptospiral sphingomyelinases and phospholipase D. Leptospires also encode multiple proteases that may damage host tissues (collagenase, metalloproteases, and multiple thermolysins) (Nascimento et al. 2004). While the virulence properties of most of these remain to be fully characterized, a collagenase mutant was recently reported to have modestly reduced virulence in the hamster model of infection (25-fold increase in LD_{50}), though it should be noted that the challenge strain had an extremely high LD_{50} of around 10^6 leptospires (Table 1) (Kassegne et al. 2014). Decreased tissue distribution and reduced tissue pathology were also reported in animals infected with the mutant (Kassegne et al. 2014), though it is unclear if the reduced pathology was a direct result of the loss of collagenase activity. Activation of host proteases such as plasminogen and matrix metalloproteases may also contribute to host tissue destruction and bacterial dissemination. Hemorrhage may be a result from a combination of tissue damage, disruption of hemostatic mechanisms, and interference of wound repair.

Fever is a key feature of leptospirosis, and many pathologies associated with leptospirosis may result from inflammation. Inflammation may be a consequence of tissue damage rather than be directly mediated by bacterial factors (Faine et al. 1999), as leptospiral LPS has remarkably low pyrogenicity compared to the LPS of other bacteria; LPS extracts injected into rabbits were non-pyrogenic in doses up to 5 μg/kg, had reduced activity in *Limulus* lysate assay (Vinh et al. 1986), and 500-fold less acute lethality in mice and 20-fold less mitogenicity when compared to *Salmonella typhimurium* LPS (Shimizu et al. 1987). In contrast to LPS, glycolipoprotein extracts (containing polysaccharides, lipids and proteins) had cytotoxic activity (Vinh et al. 1986). Low LPS toxicity may contribute to the ability of leptospires to achieve high numbers in vivo, and may be a consequence of an unusual lipid A structure (Que-Gewirth et al. 2004). It should be noted that biological properties of leptospiral LPS have been elucidated from in vitro-grown bacteria and it is possible that LPS is modified in vivo (Nally et al. 2005), conferring different pyrogenic properties. Leptospiral LPS also signals via TLR2 (rather than the normal TLR4) in human macrophages, while signaling via TLR2 and TLR4 in murine cells (Nahori et al. 2005), which may also contribute to different outcomes in disease depending on host species.

Renal pathology during leptospirosis is associated with interstitial nephritis and cellular infiltrates containing neutrophils and monocytes, suggesting an inflammatory mechanism. Leptospiral membrane protein extracts induced inflammatory response in cultured murine proximal tubule cells (Yang et al. 2002) signaling through TLR2 (Yang et al. 2006); this activity may play a role in interstitial nephritis. It was found that LipL32 plays a role in this stimulation via TLR2 (Hsu et al. 2010; Yang et al. 2006). However, these experiments were performed using extracted proteins with cell lines in vitro; an in vivo role for LipL32 signaling via TLR2 is less clear as LipL32 in intact organisms may not be surface-exposed (Pinne and Haake 2013), and hamsters infected with a LipL32 mutant had the same renal pathology as hamsters infected with wild-type bacteria, indicating a role for other processes in renal pathology (Murray et al. 2009c). The leptospiral outer membrane protein Loa22 has also been implicated in causing necrosis of a rat proximal tubule cell line and inducing an inflammatory response (Zhang et al. 2010). An alternative inflammatory mechanism has recently been described, by down regulation of the Na/K-ATPase pump by leptospiral glycolipoprotein, thereby activating the NLRP3 inflammasome (Lacroix-Lamande et al. 2012). Inhibition of the Na/K-ATPase pump may also contribute to loss of lung integrity and kidney dysfunction, leading to hypokalemia (Goncalves-de-Albuquerque et al. 2012).

Uveitis is another complication of leptospirosis that may occur weeks to years after initial infection. The condition may result from a breakdown in the immune privilege status of the eye with a combination of inflammation and autoimmunity (Verma and Stevenson 2012). Self-reactive antibodies have been found in uveitic eyes, including antibodies to leptospiral proteins LruA that cross-react with lens proteins α-crystallin B and vimentin, and antibodies to LruB that cross-react to retinal protein β-crystallin B2 (Verma et al. 2010b).

6 Virulence-Associated Factors Without a Defined Function

The role in pathogenesis has not been determined for a significant number of virulence factors identified by mutagenesis and in vivo screening.

6.1 Loa22

Loa22 is a probable lipoprotein with an OmpA domain and peptidoglycan-binding domain, indicating that it could be both surface exposed and interact with the peptidoglycan layer. Loa22 was the first virulence factor identified by mutagenesis and testing in vivo (Ristow et al. 2007). A *loa22* mutant was attenuated in guinea pigs and hamsters; virulence was partially restored upon complementation. Guinea pigs infected with the *loa22* mutant showed little or no tissue pathology, but bacteremia was detected on day 3 and renal colonization was detected upon termination of the experiment at day 21. The level of attenuation for the *loa22* mutant was moderate given that at doses of approximately 10^8 leptospires not all animals in the control group died, while some animals challenged with the *loa22* mutant died; this may be due to the use of strain *L. interrogans* serovar Lai strain Lai 56601 which has reduced virulence.

The function of Loa22 remains unknown. Given that Loa22 is the second most abundant protein of the cell envelope of *L. interrogans* after LipL32 (Malmstrom et al. 2009), it may play an essential structural or other role in the cell not directly related to virulence (reviewed in Confer and Ayalew 2013). Surface exposure raises the possibility that it may interact directly with host proteins/structures (Ristow et al. 2007); in many bacterial species, OmpA proteins have been identified as adhesins for host cells and extracellular proteins (Confer and Ayalew 2013) and moderate binding to collagen type I, collagen type IV, and plasma fibronectin has been reported for Loa22 (Barbosa et al. 2006). OmpA domains are a pathogen-associated molecular pattern, thereby recognized by pattern recognition molecules such as TLR2, and OmpA proteins activate dendritic cells (Torres et al. 2006). Recombinant Loa22 was cytotoxic to a rat proximal tubule cell line and induced an inflammatory response via TLR2 (Zhang et al. 2010), even in the absence of protein lipidation. OmpA family proteins have a diverse array of other virulence properties, including promoting invasion, intracellular survival, and evasion of host immune defenses such as complement (by binding fluid phase complement regulatory proteins) and antimicrobial peptides (Confer and Ayalew 2013).

6.2 LruA

LruA is a lipoprotein that is conserved across the different classes of leptospires and contains a LysM domain, suggesting that it binds to peptidoglycan. While LruA is at least partly surface exposed (Zhang et al. 2013) the majority remains cell-associated after TritonX 114 extraction (Verma et al. 2005), suggesting that the protein either has an unusual membrane topology or multiple subcellular locations; although unusual, lipoproteins with multiple subcellular locations have been described (Michel et al. 2013). LruA is a probable inducer of autoimmunity that causes reactive uveitis; antibodies to this protein cross-react with α-crystallin B and vimentin of the ocular lens (Verma et al. 2010b). Independent of this property, a recent study also identified this protein as essential for virulence (Zhang et al. 2013). Mutation of *lruA* led to a moderate attenuation; infection with a dose 100 times the estimated LD_{50} for serovar Manilae led to the death of 10 % of hamsters across two experiments. Interestingly, a second mutant with a minor truncation of LruA (Δ525-556) retained virulence, suggesting that the functional domains are not present at the carboxy terminus of the protein.

The mechanism of attenuation of the *lruA* mutant is unknown, but may be related to the interaction with host serum protein apolipoprotein A-I (Apo A-I). Apo A-I is involved in lipid transport, but can also play a role in LPS detoxification and inflammation during sepsis (Guo et al. 2013) and has been implicated in the killing of *Yersinia enterocolitica* by serum complement (Biedzka-Sarek et al. 2011). The LruA mutant bound considerably more Apo A-I than WT bacteria, but the significance of this is yet to be determined, and it did not increase susceptibility to killing by serum complement (Zhang et al. 2013). Given that LruA is a lipoprotein and therefore membrane bound, and binds to peptidoglycan, it may have a structural role not directly related to virulence.

6.3 Lipopolysaccharide (LPS)

Leptospires have unusually large LPS synthesis loci of approximately 100 genes, all encoded on the same DNA strand (Bulach et al. 2006; Nascimento et al. 2004; Ren et al. 2003). The structure of LPS is unknown, as are the roles of individual proteins in LPS synthesis. During a mutagenesis study of *L. interrogans*, relatively few mutants disrupted in the LPS locus were identified, implying an essential role in the biology of *Leptospira* (Murray et al. 2009a).

In many pathogenic bacteria, LPS is essential for virulence. Two leptospiral mutants with modified LPS were highly attenuated in the acute model of infection even at very high dose (10^7 leptospires, more than 10^6 times estimated LD_{50}). No disease pathology and no symptoms of infection or tissue pathology were observed (Murray et al. 2010; Srikram et al. 2011). The first LPS mutant (M895) had a mutation in a gene of unknown function resulting in truncated LPS. The second mutant had no obvious change in molecular mass but different reaction with antibodies to LPS; subsequent bioinformatics analysis suggests that this gene may encode a methyltransferase of the LIC12133 family (NCBI Conserved Domain Database), which may explain the lack of a detectable mass difference by SDS PAGE. Both of these strains with modified LPS also failed to colonize the mouse maintenance host model (Marcsisin et al. 2013). The precise mechanism of attenuation is unknown, but was not due to increased susceptibility to complement-killing (Murray et al. 2010). It is predicted that the LPS locus contains long transcripts, raising the possibility that the mutations may affect the transcription of downstream LPS synthesis genes.

6.4 Bacterial Chaperone HtpG

Bacterial chaperone HtpG is a homolog of the eukaryotic Hsp90. It has been attributed variable roles in different bacteria, including resistance to heat and oxidative stress and survival in macrophages (Dang et al. 2011; Weiss et al. 2007). Attenuated *htpG* mutants have been described for *Edwardsiella tarda* (Dang et al. 2011) and *Francisella tularensis* (Weiss et al. 2007). A leptospiral *htpG* (*lb058/ lic20044*) mutant was highly attenuated in hamsters, with animals surviving a dose of >10^6 times LD_{50} and lower bacterial burdens detected in tissues (King et al. 2014), although the *htpG* mutant colonized hamster kidneys. Additionally, microscopic and macroscopic pathology was observed in hamsters infected with the mutant. Virulence of the *htpG* mutant was fully restored upon complementation.

The mechanism of attenuation of the leptospiral *htpG* mutant is unknown, as bacteria displayed no increase in susceptibility to physical and chemical stresses (heat, osmolarity, and oxidative) and exhibited essential virulence phenotypes (LPS expression, motility, expression of Loa22, survival in macrophages) (King et al. 2014). The ClpB chaperone contributes to resistance to oxidative and heat stress (Lourdault et al. 2011) and there is a second *htpG* paralog (LA1231/LIC12469) encoded in the leptospiral genome that may also account for some of these properties, although a mutant in this gene retained virulence (King et al. 2014). It is difficult to predict what role HtpG plays in virulence as the substrates of this bacterial chaperone are poorly defined (Buchner 2010). Disruption of *htpG* may result in modulation of the expression of virulence factors and further characterization of this mutant may identify novel virulence processes.

6.5 Other Attenuated Mutants

Mutants in genes encoding *lb194*, *la2786*, and *la0589* (all of unknown function) were colonization-deficient in the mouse colonization model (Marcsisin et al. 2013). LB194 may be involved in iron utilization; it is up regulated under low iron conditions and is located in a preserved locus with HbpA (hemin-binding TonB-dependent receptor) in both pathogenic and saprophytic species of *Leptospira*. LA2786 is also marginally up regulated under low iron conditions (Lo et al. 2010).

LA0589 is one of around 12 highly similar paralogous proteins encoded in the *L. interrogans* genome. Of note, these genes are highly up regulated in vivo and point mutations in paralogs *la3490 la3388* were identified in a culture-attenuated leptospiral strain (Lehmann et al. 2013), further suggesting a role in virulence for this gene family. Interestingly, there are similar sets of paralogous proteins in *Bartonella* spp. Further work is required to elucidate the role of these proteins in host colonization.

7 The Renal Carrier State

Depending on the host and infecting serovar, leptospiral infection may cause a spectrum of syndromes from an asymptomatic carriage to a fulminant, acute disease. A carrier host, also termed maintenance, reservoir or chronically infected host, may be defined as a host in which infection is endemic, disease is mild or asymptomatic, and transmission occurs back to the same host species (Blackmore and Hathaway 1979). Carrier hosts are often rodents. Hosts that suffer acute disease such as humans are incidental hosts that are unlikely to serve as a source of transmission, constituting a dead end infection.

Upon infection, bacteria disseminate throughout the carrier host and are most likely cleared by the immune system from all tissues except the kidney. In the renal tubules, bacteria continue to multiply and are excreted in the urine at concentrations of as high as 10^7 leptospires/ml (Faine 1962; Monahan et al. 2008). While carrier hosts may become lifetime shedders of *Leptospira*, acute hosts become temporary urinary shedders, in the case of humans for 2 weeks to 1 month (Faine et al. 1999). The carrier host has a long-term evolutionary association with leptospires where equilibrium has been reached between virulence and host response, making the organism almost commensal. The contrast with an acute host can be remarkable; *L. interrogans* serovar Manilae has an LD_{50} of <10 bacteria in hamsters but a dose of 10^8 does not cause any overt signs of disease in rats apart from renal colonization (Murray et al. 2009c). Experimentally infected rats also display no tissue pathology apart from possible interstitial nephritis (Monahan et al. 2008; Tucunduva de Faria et al. 2007). It is feasible that incidental hosts become maintenance hosts over time, concomitant with a reduction in leptospiral virulence for the particular host. For example, in an area of high transmission rates in the Peruvian Amazon, around 5 %

of people may become long-term renal shedders of *Leptospira* suggesting host adaptation, although direct human to human transmission is yet to be demonstrated (Ganoza et al. 2010).

While the carrier state is required for leptospiral transmission cycle, and carrier animals are the exclusive reservoir for human infection, very little is known about the molecular basis for development of the carrier state. Specific mechanism may be required to cross into the lumen of proximal renal tubules, adhere to renal epithelial cells, evade antibodies in the filtrate, and to acquire nutrients. Some studies have analyzed antigenic properties relating to the carrier state. When compared to bacteria from an acute guinea pig model, leptospires derived from rat urine had comparatively more LPS present, although the significance of this is unknown (Nally et al. 2005). Furthermore, urine-derived bacteria exhibit reduced reactivity to host-derived antibodies (Faine 1962). This may avoid the activity of antibodies that leak into the tubule as a result of renal injury during infection (Lane and Faine 1963), possibly in part due to down regulation of proteins to which the host has mounted an immune response (Monahan et al. 2008).

Analysis of defined mutants may give insights into the molecular basis for the carrier state. Only a handful of mutants has been studied in carrier models of disease. LipL32 and LigB were found to be unnecessary for renal colonization of rats (Croda et al. 2008; Murray et al. 2009c). A third study analyzed 28 mutants for virulence in a mouse carrier host (Marcsisin et al. 2013). Two virulence factors required to cause disease in the acute model, LPS and HtpG, were also required to colonize mouse kidneys. An additional five mutants were unable to colonize the carrier host but still caused disease in the acute host (Marcsisin et al. 2013). These colonization-deficient leptospires had mutations in genes encoding several proteins of unknown function and with two proteins with potential roles in iron transport (Table 2), thus identifying the first colonization-specific virulence factors.

While bacterial factors may contribute to the outcome of infection, there are likely to be host factors that are also important, such as immune recognition of leptospires. Leptospiral LPS signals via TLR2 in human macrophages (rather than the more usual LPS receptor, TLR4), while signaling via TLR2 and TLR4 in murine cells (Nahori et al. 2005). Recognition of leptospires through TLR4 is important for the resistance of mice to acute leptospirosis, as mice defective in TLR4 are susceptible to acute leptospirosis (Chassin et al. 2009; Viriyakosol et al. 2006, Chap. 9). This point of difference between human and murine recognition of *Leptospira* may contribute to the contrasting disease outcomes (Werts 2010).

8 Future Directions

In the past decade, significant advances have been made in the understanding of the pathogenesis of leptospirosis. However, the molecular basis of disease remains poorly elucidated. For example, the molecular basis for the pathology of leptospirosis is largely unknown. Additionally, the functions of numerous essential virulence factors (Tables 1 and 2) are either uncharacterized or poorly defined. The secretome also remains to be fully explored. It is likely that many more virulence factors remain to be discovered and considering the overrepresentation of hypothetical genes in those genes exclusively found in pathogenic leptospires, it is likely that these will be novel. Hence, unbiased screening experiments for attenuated mutants will be very useful (Marcsisin et al. 2013). Exclusively in vitro findings also require consolidation with the understanding in animal models; the plethora of leptospiral proteins with an in vitro-characterized function needs to be translated into the host, and any in vitro artefactual findings need to be identified and discarded. Finally, the elucidation of colonization mechanisms in the carrier host will be important in understanding human disease and may lead to methods of disease prevention.

References

Adler B, de la Peña Moctezuma A (2010) *Leptospira* and leptospirosis. Vet Microbiol 140:287–296

Adler B, Lo M, Seemann T, Murray GL (2011) Pathogenesis of leptospirosis: the influence of genomics. Vet Microbiol 153:73–81

Arruda S, Bomfim G, Knights R, Huima-Byron T, Riley LW (1993) Cloning of an *Mycobacterium tuberculosis* DNA fragment associated with entry and survival inside cells. Science 261:1454–1457

Artiushin S, Timoney JF, Nally J, Verma A (2004) Host-inducible immunogenic sphingomye-linase-like protein, Lk73.5, of *Leptospira interrogans*. Infect Immun 72:742–749

Asuthkar S, Velineni S, Stadlmann J, Altmann F, Sritharan M (2007) Expression and characterization of an iron-regulated hemin-binding protein, HbpA, from *Leptospira interrogans* serovar Lai. Infect Immun 75:4582–4591

Atzingen MV, Barbosa AS, De Brito T, Vasconcellos SA, de Morais ZM, Lima DM, Abreu PA, Nascimento AL (2008) Lsa21, a novel leptospiral protein binding adhesive matrix molecules and present during human infection. BMC Microbiol 8:70

Atzingen MV, Gomez RM, Schattner M, Pretre G, Goncales AP, de Morais ZM, Vasconcellos SA, Nascimento AL (2009) Lp95, a novel leptospiral protein that binds extracellular matrix components and activates e-selectin on endothelial cells. J Infect 59:264–276

Ballard SA, Williamson M, Adler B, Vinh T, Faine S (1986) Interactions of virulent and avirulent leptospires with primary cultures of renal epithelial cells. J Med Microbiol 21:59–67

Ballard SA, Go M, Segers RP, Adler B (1998) Molecular analysis of the dnaK locus of *Leptospira interrogans* serovar Copenhageni. Gene 216:21–29

Barbosa AS, Abreu PA, Neves FO, Atzingen MV, Watanabe MM, Vieira ML, Morais ZM, Vasconcellos SA, Nascimento AL (2006) A newly identified leptospiral adhesin mediates attachment to laminin. Infect Immun 74:6356–6364

Barbosa AS, Abreu PA, Vasconcellos SA, Morais ZM, Goncales AP, Silva AS, Daha MR, Isaac L (2009) Immune evasion of *Leptospira* species by acquisition of human complement regulator C4BP. Infect Immun 77:1137–1143

Barbosa AS, Monaris D, Silva LB, Morais ZM, Vasconcellos SA, Cianciarullo AM, Isaac L, Abreu PA (2010) Functional characterization of LcpA, a surface-exposed protein of *Leptospira* spp. that binds the human complement regulator C4BP. Infect Immun 78:3207–3216

Barocchi MA, Ko AI, Reis MG, McDonald KL, Riley LW (2002) Rapid translocation of polarized MDCK cell monolayers by *Leptospira interrogans*, an invasive but nonintracellular pathogen. Infect Immun 70:6926–6932

Batzios SP, Zafeiriou DI, Papakonstantinou E (2013) Extracellular matrix components: an intricate network of possible biomarkers for lysosomal storage disorders? FEBS Lett 587:1258–1267

Berg HC, Turner L (1979) Movement of microorganisms in viscous environments. Nature 278:349–351

Biedzka-Sarek M, Metso J, Kateifides A, Meri T, Jokiranta TS, Muszynski A, Radziejewska-Lebrecht J, Zannis V, Skurnik M, Jauhiainen M (2011) Apolipoprotein A-I exerts bactericidal activity against *Yersinia enterocolitica* serotype O:3. J Biol Chem 286:38211–38219

Blackmore DK, Hathaway SC (1979) The nidality of zoonoses. In: Proceedings of the 2nd international symposium on veterinary epidemiology and economics, pp 207–213

Blom AM, Hallström T, Riesbeck K (2009) Complement evasion strategies of pathogens-acquisition of inhibitors and beyond. Mol Immunol 46:2808–2817

Bourhy P, Louvel H, Saint Girons I, Picardeau M (2005) Random insertional mutagenesis of *Leptospira interrogans*, the agent of leptospirosis, using a mariner transposon. J Bacteriol 187:3255–3258

Breiner DD, Fahey M, Salvador R, Novakova J, Coburn J (2009) *Leptospira interrogans* binds to human cell surface receptors including proteoglycans. Infect Immun 77:5528–5536

Buchner J (2010) Bacterial Hsp90–desperately seeking clients. Mol Microbiol 76:540–544

Bulach DM, Zuerner RL, Wilson P, Seemann T, McGrath A, Cullen PA, Davis J, Johnson M, Kuczek E, Alt DP, Peterson-Burch B, Coppel RL, Rood JI, Davies JK, Adler B (2006) Genome reduction in *Leptospira borgpetersenii* reflects limited transmission potential. Proc Natl Acad Sci USA 103:14560–14565

Burgess RR (2009) Refolding solubilized inclusion body proteins. Methods Enzymol 463:259–282

Cao XJ, Dai J, Xu H, Nie S, Chang X, Hu BY, Sheng QH, Wang LS, Ning ZB, Li YX, Guo XK, Zhao GP, Zeng R (2010) High-coverage proteome analysis reveals the first insight of protein modification systems in the pathogenic spirochete *Leptospira interrogans*. Cell Res 20:197–210

Carvalho E, Barbosa AS, Gomez RM, Cianciarullo AM, Hauk P, Abreu PA, Fiorini LC, Oliveira ML, Romero EC, Goncales AP, Morais ZM, Vasconcellos SA, Ho PL (2009) Leptospiral TlyC is an extracellular matrix-binding protein and does not present hemolysin activity. FEBS Lett 583:1381–1385

Castiblanco-Valencia MM, Fraga TR, Silva LB, Monaris D, Abreu PA, Strobel S, Jozsi M, Isaac L, Barbosa AS (2012) Leptospiral immunoglobulin-like proteins interact with human complement regulators factor H, FHL-1, FHR-1, and C4BP. J Infect Dis 205:995–1004

Cerqueira GM, McBride AJ, Picardeau M, Ribeiro SG, Moreira AN, Morel V, Reis MG, Ko AI, Dellagostin OA (2009) Distribution of the leptospiral immunoglobulin-like (lig) genes in pathogenic *Leptospira* species and application of *ligB* to typing leptospiral isolates. J Med Microbiol 58:1173–1181

Charon NW, Goldstein SF (2002) Genetics of motility and chemotaxis of a fascinating group of bacteria: the spirochetes. Ann Rev Genet 36:47–73

Chassin C, Picardeau M, Goujon JM, Bourhy P, Quellard N, Darche S, Badell E, d'Andon MF, Winter N, Lacroix-Lamande S, Buzoni-Gatel D, Vandewalle A, Werts C (2009) TLR4- and TLR2-mediated B cell responses control the clearance of the bacterial pathogen, *Leptospira interrogans*. J Immunol 183:2669–2677

Ching AT, Favaro RD, Lima SS, Chaves Ade A, de Lima MA, Nader HB, Abreu PA, Ho PL (2012) *Leptospira interrogans* shotgun phage display identified LigB as a heparin-binding protein. Biochem Biophys Res Comm 427:774–779

Choy HA, Kelley MM, Chen TL, Moller AK, Matsunaga J, Haake DA (2007) Physiological osmotic induction of *Leptospira interrogans* adhesion: LigA and LigB bind extracellular matrix proteins and fibrinogen. Infect Immun 75:2441–2450

Choy HA, Kelley MM, Croda J, Matsunaga J, Babbitt JT, Ko AI, Picardeau M, Haake DA (2011) The multifunctional LigB adhesin binds homeostatic proteins with potential roles in cutaneous infection by pathogenic *Leptospira interrogans*. PLoS ONE 6:e16879

Choy HA (2012) Multiple activities of LigB potentiate virulence of *Leptospira interrogans*: inhibition of alternative and classical pathways of complement. PLoS ONE 7:e41566

Cinco M, Banfi E (1983) Activation of complement by leptospires and its bactericidal activity. Zentralbl Bakteriol Mikrobiol Hyg A 254:261–265

Cinco M, Cini B, Perticarari S, Presani G (2002) *Leptospira interrogans* binds to the CR3 receptor on mammalian cells. Microb Pathog 33:299–305

Comstock LE, Thomas DD (1989) Penetration of endothelial cell monolayers by *Borrelia burgdorferi*. Infect Immun 57:1626–1628

Confer AW, Ayalew S (2013) The OmpA family of proteins: roles in bacterial pathogenesis and immunity. Vet Microbiol 163:207–222

Croda J, Figueira CP, Wunder EA Jr, Santos CS, Reis MG, Ko AI, Picardeau M (2008) Targeted mutagenesis in pathogenic *Leptospira* species: disruption of the LigB gene does not affect virulence in animal models of leptospirosis. Infect Immun 76:5826–5833

Cullen PA, Cordwell SJ, Bulach DM, Haake DA, Adler B (2002) Global analysis of outer membrane proteins from *Leptospira interrogans* serovar Lai. Infect Immun 70:2311–2318

Dang W, Hu YH, Sun L (2011) HtpG is involved in the pathogenesis of *Edwardsiella tarda*. Vet Microbiol 152:394–400

Davis SL, Gurusiddappa S, McCrea KW, Perkins S, Hook M (2001) SdrG, a fibrinogen-binding bacterial adhesin of the microbial surface components recognizing adhesive matrix molecules subfamily from *Staphylococcus epidermidis*, targets the thrombin cleavage site in the Bβ chain. J Biol Chem 276:27799–27805

del Real G, Segers RP, van der Zeijst BA, Gaastra W (1989) Cloning of a hemolysin gene from *Leptospira interrogans* serovar Hardjo. Infect Immun 57:2588–2590

Domingos RF, Vieira ML, Romero EC, Goncales AP, de Morais ZM, Vasconcellos SA, Nascimento AL (2012) Features of two proteins of *Leptospira interrogans* with potential role in host-pathogen interactions. BMC Microbiol 12:50

Dong K, Li Q, Liu C, Zhang Y, Zhao G, Guo X (2010) Cloning and characterization of three *cheB* genes in *Leptospira interrogans*. Acta Biochim Biophys Sinica 42:216–223

Edwards AM, Jenkinson HF, Woodward MJ, Dymock D (2005) Binding properties and adhesion-mediating regions of the major sheath protein of *Treponema denticola* ATCC 35405. Infect Immun 73:2891–2898

Eslghi A, Becam J, Lambert A, Sismeiro O, Dillies MA, Jagla B, Wunder EA Jr, Ko AI, Coppee JY, Goarant C, Picardeau M (2014) A putative regulatory genetic locus modulates virulence in the pathogen *Leptospira interrogans*. Infect Immun 82:2542–2552

Eshghi A, Lourdault K, Murray GL, Bartpho T, Sermswan RW, Picardeau M, Adler B, Snarr B, Zuerner RL, Cameron CE (2012) *Leptospira interrogans* catalase is required for resistance to H₂O₂ and for virulence. Infect Immun 80:3892–3899

Faine S (1957) Virulence in *Leptospira*. I. Reactions of guinea-pigs to experimental infection with *Leptospira icterohaemorrhagiae*. Br J Exp Pathol 38:1–7

Faine S (1959) Iron as a growth requirement for pathogenic *Leptospira*. J Gen Microbiol 20:246–251

Faine S (1962) The growth of *Leptospira australis* B in the kidneys of mice in the incipient experimental carrier state. J Hyg (Lond) 60:435–442

Faine S (1964) Reticuloendothelial phagocytosis of virulent leptospires. Am J Vet Res 25:830–835

Faine S, van der Hoeden J (1964) Virulence-linked colonial and morphological variation in *Leptospira*. J Bacteriol 88:1493–1496

Faine S, Adler B, Bolin C, Perolat P (1999) *Leptospira* and leptospirosis. MediSci, Melbourne

Falkow S (1988) Molecular Koch's postulates applied to microbial pathogenicity. Rev Infect Dis 10(Suppl 2):S274–S276

Fenno JC, Tamura M, Hannam PM, Wong GW, Chan RA, McBride BC (2000) Identification of a *Treponema denticola* OppA homologue that binds host proteins present in the subgingival environment. Infect Immun 68:1884–1892

Fernandes LG, Vieira ML, Kirchgatter K, Alves IJ, de Morais ZM, Vasconcellos SA, Romero EC, Nascimento AL (2012) OmpL1 is an extracellular matrix- and plasminogen-interacting protein of *Leptospira* spp. Infect Immun 80:3679–3692

Figueira CP, Croda J, Choy HA, Haake DA, Reis MG, Ko AI, Picardeau M (2011) Heterologous expression of pathogen-specific genes *ligA* and *ligB* in the saprophyte *Leptospira biflexa* confers enhanced adhesion to cultured cells and fibronectin. BMC Microbiol 11:129

Fraga TR, Courrol DD, Castiblanco-Valencia MM, Hirata IY, Vasconcellos SA, Juliano L, Barbosa AS, Isaac L (2014) Immune evasion by pathogenic *Leptospira* strains: the secretion of proteases that directly cleave complement proteins. J Infect Dis 209:876–886

Ganoza CA, Matthias MA, Saito M, Cespedes M, Gotuzzo E, Vinetz JM (2010) Asymptomatic renal colonization of humans in the peruvian Amazon by *Leptospira*. PLoS Negl Trop Dis 4:e612

Goncalves-de-Albuquerque CF, Burth P, Silva AR, Younes-Ibrahim M, Castro-Faria-Neto HC, Castro-Faria MV (2012) *Leptospira* and inflammation. Mediators Inflamm 2012:317950

Guégan R, Camadro JM, Saint Girons I, Picardeau M (2003) *Leptospira* spp. possess a complete haem biosynthetic pathway and are able to use exogenous haem sources. Mol Microbiol 49:745–754

Guo L, Ai J, Zheng Z, Howatt DA, Daugherty A, Huang B, Li XA (2013) High density lipoprotein protects against polymicrobe-induced sepsis in mice. J Biol Chem 288:17947–17953

Haake DA, Chao G, Zuerner RL, Barnett JK, Barnett D, Mazel M, Matsunaga J, Levett PN, Bolin CA (2000) The leptospiral major outer membrane protein LipL32 is a lipoprotein expressed during mammalian infection. Infect Immun 68:2276–2285

Hamburger ZA, Brown MS, Isberg RR, Bjorkman PJ (1999) Crystal structure of invasin: a bacterial integrin-binding protein. Science 286:291–295

Hauck CR, Agerer F, Muenzner P, Schmitter T (2006) Cellular adhesion molecules as targets for bacterial infection. Eur J Cell Biol 85:235–242

Hauk P, Macedo F, Romero EC, Vasconcellos SA, de Morais ZM, Barbosa AS, Ho PL (2008) LipL32, the major leptospiral lipoprotein: the C-terminus is the primary immunogenic domain and mediates interaction with collagen IV and plasma fibronectin. Infect Immun 76:2642–2650

Hoke DE, Egan S, Cullen PA, Adler B (2008) LipL32 is an extracellular matrix-interacting protein of *Leptospira* spp. and *Pseudoalteromonas tunicata*. Infect Immun 76:2063–2069

Hsu SH, Lo YY, Tung JY, Ko YC, Sun YJ, Hung CC, Yang CW, Tseng FG, Fu CC, Pan RL (2010) Leptospiral outer membrane lipoprotein LipL32 binding on toll-like receptor 2 of renal cells as determined with an atomic force microscope. Biochemistry 49:5408–5417

Hu W, Ge Y, Ojcius DM, Sun D, Dong H, Yang XF, Yan J (2013) p53 signalling controls cell cycle arrest and caspase-independent apoptosis in macrophages infected with pathogenic *Leptospira* species. Cell Microbiol 15:1624–1659

Hussain M, Becker K, von Eiff C, Schrenzel J, Peters G, Herrmann M (2001) Identification and characterization of a novel 38.5-kilodalton cell surface protein of *Staphylococcus aureus* with extended-spectrum binding activity for extracellular matrix and plasma proteins. J Bacteriol 183:6778–6786

Ito T, Yanagawa R (1987) Leptospiral attachment to four structural components of extracellular matrix. Nihon Juigaku Zasshi 49:875–882

Jin D, Ojcius DM, Sun D, Dong H, Luo Y, Mao Y, Yan J (2009) *Leptospira interrogans* induces apoptosis in macrophages via caspase-8- and caspase-3-dependent pathways. Infect Immun 77:799–809

Jost BH, Adler B, Vinh T, Faine S (1986) A monoclonal antibody reacting with a determinant on leptospiral lipopolysaccharide protects guinea pigs against leptospirosis. J Med Microbiol 22:269–275

Kaiser GE, Doetsch RN (1975) Enhanced translational motion of *Leptospira* in viscous environments. Nature 255:656–657

Kasǎrov LB (1970) Degradiation of the erythrocyte phospholipids and haemolysis of the erythrocytes of different animal species by leptospirae. J Med Microbiol 3:29–37

Kassegne K, Hu W, Ojcius DM, Sun D, Ge Y, Zhao J, Yang XF, Li L, Yan J (2014) Identification of collagenase as a critical virulence factor for invasiveness and transmission of pathogenic *Leptospira* species. J Infect Dis 209:1105–1115

King AM, Bartpho T, Sermswan RW, Bulach DM, Eshghi A, Picardeau M, Adler B, Murray GL
(2013) Leptospiral outer membrane protein LipL41 is not essential for acute leptospirosis, but
requires a small chaperone, Lep, for stable expression. Infect Immun 8:2768–2776
King AM, Pretre G, Bartpho T, Sermswan RW, Toma C, Suzuki T, Eshghi A, Picardeau M, Adler
B, Murray GL (2014) High temperature protein G (HtpG) is an essential virulence factor of
Leptospira interrogans. Infect Immun 82:1123–1131
Kline KA, Falker S, Dahlberg S, Normark S, Henriques-Normark B (2009) Bacterial adhesins in
host-microbe interactions. Cell Host Microbe 5:580–592
Lacroix-Lamande S, d'Andon MF, Michel E, Ratet G, Philpott DJ, Girardin SE, Boneca IG,
Vandewalle A, Werts C (2012) Downregulation of the Na/K-ATPase pump by leptospiral
glycolipoprotein activates the NLRP3 inflammasome. J Immunol 188:2805–2814
Lähteenmäki K, Kuusela P, Korhonen TK (2001) Bacterial plasminogen activators and receptors.
FEMS Microbiol Rev 25:531–552
Lambert A, Picardeau M, Haake DA, Sermswan RW, Srikram A, Adler B, Murray GL (2012a)
FlaA proteins in *Leptospira interrogans* are essential for motility and virulence but are not
required for formation of the flagellum sheath. Infect Immun 80:2019–2025
Lambert A, Takahashi N, Charon NW, Picardeau M (2012b) Chemotactic behavior of pathogenic
and nonpathogenic *Leptospira* species. Appl Environ Microbiol 78:8467–8469
Lane GK, Faine S (1963) Urinary antibody during renal damage due to leptospiral infection in
mice. J Infect Dis 113:110–112
Lee SH, Kim KA, Park YG, Seong IW, Kim MJ, Lee YJ (2000) Identification and partial
characterization of a novel hemolysin from *Leptospira interrogans* serovar lai. Gene 254:19–28
Lehmann JS, Fouts DE, Haft DH, Cannella AP, Ricaldi JN, Brinkac L, Harkins D, Durkin S,
Sanka R, Sutton G, Moreno A, Vinetz JM, Matthias MA (2013) Pathogenomic inference of
virulence-associated genes in *Leptospira interrogans*. PLoS Negl Trop Dis 7:e2468
Levett PN (2001) Leptospirosis. Clin Microbiol Rev 14:296–326
Li S, Ojcius DM, Liao S, Li L, Xue F, Dong H, Yan J (2010) Replication or death: distinct fates of
pathogenic *Leptospira* strain Lai within macrophages of human or mouse origin. Innate Immun
16:80–92
Li Z, Ploplis VA, French EL, Boyle MD (1999) Interaction between group A streptococci and the
plasmin(ogen) system promotes virulence in a mouse skin infection model. J Infect Dis
179:907–914
Liao S, Sun A, Ojcius DM, Wu S, Zhao J, Yan J (2009) Inactivation of the *fliY* gene encoding a
flagellar motor switch protein attenuates mobility and virulence of *Leptospira interrogans*
strain Lai. BMC Microbiol 9:253
Lima SS, Ching AT, Favaro RD, Da Silva JB, Oliveira ML, Carvalho E, Abreu PA, Vasconcellos
SA, Ho PL (2013) Adhesin activity of *Leptospira interrogans* lipoprotein identified by in vivo
and in vitro shotgun phage display. Biochem Biophys Res Comm 431:342–347
Lin MH, Chang YC, Hsiao CD, Huang SH, Wang MS, Ko YC, Yang CW, Sun YJ (2013) LipL41,
a hemin binding protein from *Leptospira santarosai* serovar Shermani. PLoS ONE 8:e83246
Lin YP, Lee DW, McDonough SP, Nicholson LK, Sharma Y, Chang YF (2009) Repeated
domains of *Leptospira* immunoglobulin-like proteins interact with elastin and tropoelastin.
J Biol Chem 284:19380–19391
Lin YP, McDonough SP, Sharma Y, Chang YF (2010) The terminal immunoglobulin-like repeats
of LigA and LigB of *Leptospira* enhance their binding to gelatin binding domain of fibronectin
and host cells. PLoS ONE 5:e11301
Lin YP, McDonough SP, Sharma Y, Chang YF (2011) *Leptospira* immunoglobulin-like protein B
(LigB) binding to the C-terminal fibrinogen alphaC domain inhibits fibrin clot formation,
platelet adhesion and aggregation. Mol Microbiol 79:1063–1076
Lo M, Murray GL, Khoo CA, Haake DA, Zuerner RL, Adler B (2010) Transcriptional response of
Leptospira interrogans to iron limitation and characterization of a PerR homolog. Infect
Immun 78:4850–4859

Longhi MT, Oliveira TR, Romero EC, Goncales AP, de Morais ZM, Vasconcellos SA, Nascimento AL (2009) A newly identified protein of *Leptospira interrogans* mediates binding to laminin. J Med Microbiol 58:1275–1282

Lourdault K, Cerqueira GM, Wunder EA Jr, Picardeau M (2011) Inactivation of *clpB* in the pathogen *Leptospira interrogans* reduces virulence and resistance to stress conditions. Infect Immun 79:3711–3717

Luo Y, Frey EA, Pfuetzner RA, Creagh AL, Knoechel DG, Haynes CA, Finlay BB, Strynadka NC (2000) Crystal structure of enteropathogenic *Escherichia coli* intimin-receptor complex. Nature 405:1073–1077

Malmstrom J, Beck M, Schmidt A, Lange V, Deutsch EW, Aebersold R (2009) Proteome-wide cellular protein concentrations of the human pathogen *Leptospira interrogans*. Nature 460:762–765

Marcsisin RA, Bartpho T, Bulach DM, Srikram A, Sermswan RW, Adler B, Murray GL (2013) Use of a high-throughput screen to identify *Leptospira* mutants unable to colonise the carrier host or cause disease in the acute model of infection. J Med Microbiol 62:1601–1608

Marshall RB (1974) Ultrastructural changes in renal tubules of sheep following experimental infection with *Leptospira interrogans* serotype Pomona. J Med Microbiol 7:505–508

Marshall RB (1976) The route of entry of leptospires into the kidney tubule. J Med Microbiol 9:149–152

Masuzawa T, Nakamura R, Hashiguchi Y, Shimizu T, Iwamoto Y, Morita T, Yanagihara Y (1990) Immunological reactivity and passive protective activity of monoclonal antibodies against protective antigen (PAg) of *Leptospira interrogans* serovar lai. Zentralbl Bakteriol 272:328–336

Matsunaga J, Barocchi MA, Croda J, Young TA, Sanchez Y, Siqueira I, Bolin CA, Reis MG, Riley LW, Haake DA, Ko AI (2003) Pathogenic *Leptospira* species express surface-exposed proteins belonging to the bacterial immunoglobulin superfamily. Mol Microbiol 49:929–945

Matsunaga J, Sanchez Y, Xu X, Haake DA (2005) Osmolarity, a key environmental signal controlling expression of leptospiral proteins LigA and LigB and the extracellular release of LigA. Infect Immun 73:70–78

Matsunaga J, Lo M, Bulach DM, Zuerner RL, Adler B, Haake DA (2007) Response of *Leptospira interrogans* to physiologic osmolarity: relevance in signaling the environment-to-host transition. Infect Immun 75:2864–2874

McBride AJ, Cerqueira GM, Suchard MA, Moreira AN, Zuerner RL, Reis MG, Haake DA, Ko AI, Dellagostin OA (2009) Genetic diversity of the leptospiral immunoglobulin-like (Lig) genes in pathogenic *Leptospira* spp. Infect Genet Evol 9:196–205

Mendes RS, Von Atzingen M, de Morais ZM, Goncales AP, Serrano SM, Asega AF, Romero EC, Vasconcellos SA, Nascimento AL (2011) The novel leptospiral surface adhesin Lsa20 binds laminin and human plasminogen and is probably expressed during infection. Infect Immun 79:4657–4667

Meri T, Murgia R, Stefanel P, Meri S, Cinco M (2005) Regulation of complement activation at the C3-level by serum resistant leptospires. Microb Pathog 39:139–147

Merien F, Baranton G, Perolat P (1997) Invasion of Vero cells and induction of apoptosis in macrophages by pathogenic *Leptospira interrogans* are correlated with virulence. Infect Immun 65:729–738

Merien F, Truccolo J, Rougier Y, Baranton G, Perolat P (1998) In vivo apoptosis of hepatocytes in guinea pigs infected with *Leptospira interrogans* serovar icterohaemorrhagiae. FEMS Microbiol Lett 169:95–102

Merien F, Truccolo J, Baranton G, Perolat P (2000) Identification of a 36-kDa fibronectin-binding protein expressed by a virulent variant of *Leptospira interrogans* serovar icterohaemorrhagiae. FEMS Microbiol Lett 185:17–22

Michel LV, Snyder J, Schmidt R, Milillo J, Grimaldi K, Kalmeta B, Khan MN, Sharma S, Wright LK, Pichichero ME (2013) Dual orientation of the outer membrane lipoprotein P6 of nontypeable *Haemophilus influenzae*. J Bacteriol 195:3252–3259

Monahan AM, Callanan JJ, Nally JE (2008) Proteomic analysis of *Leptospira interrogans* shed in urine of chronically infected hosts. Infect Immun 76:4952–4958

Moriarty TJ, Norman MU, Colarusso P, Bankhead T, Kubes P, Chaconas G (2008) Real-time high resolution 3D imaging of the lyme disease spirochete adhering to and escaping from the vasculature of a living host. PLoS Pathog 4:e1000090

Moriarty TJ, Shi M, Lin YP, Ebady R, Zhou H, Odisho T, Hardy PO, Salman-Dilgimen A, Wu J, Weening EH, Skare JT, Kubes P, Leong J, Chaconas G (2012) Vascular binding of a pathogen under shear force through mechanistically distinct sequential interactions with host macromolecules. Mol Microbiol 86:1116–1131

Murray GL, Ellis KM, Lo M, Adler B (2008) *Leptospira interrogans* requires a functional heme oxygenase to scavenge iron from hemoglobin. Microbes Infect 10:791–797

Murray GL, Morel V, Cerqueira GM, Croda J, Srikram A, Henry R, Ko AI, Dellagostin OA, Bulach DM, Sermswan RW, Adler B, Picardeau M (2009a) Genome-wide transposon mutagenesis in pathogenic *Leptospira* species. Infect Immun 77:810–816

Murray GL, Srikram A, Henry R, Puapairoj A, Sermswan RW, Adler B (2009b) *Leptospira interrogans* requires heme oxygenase for disease pathogenesis. Microbes Infect 11:311–314

Murray GL, Srikram A, Hoke DE, Wunder EA Jr, Henry R, Lo M, Zhang K, Sermswan RW, Ko AI, Adler B (2009c) Major surface protein LipL32 is not required for either acute or chronic infection with *Leptospira interrogans*. Infect Immun 77:952–958

Murray GL, Srikram A, Henry R, Hartskeerl RA, Sermswan RW, Adler B (2010) Mutations affecting *Leptospira interrogans* lipopolysaccharide attenuate virulence. Mol Microbiol 78:701–709

Murray GL (2013) The lipoprotein LipL32, an enigma of leptospiral biology. Vet Microbiol 162:305–314

Murray GL, Lo M, Bulach DM, Srikram A, Seemann T, Quinsey NS, Sermswan RW, Allen A, Adler B (2013) Evaluation of 238 antigens of *Leptospira borgpetersenii* serovar Hardjo for protection against kidney colonisation. Vaccine 31:495–499

Nahori MA, Fournie-Amazouz E, Que-Gewirth NS, Balloy V, Chignard M, Raetz CR, Saint Girons I, Werts C (2005) Differential TLR recognition of leptospiral lipid A and lipopolysaccharide in murine and human cells. J Immunol 175:6022–6031

Nally JE, Chow E, Fishbein MC, Blanco DR, Lovett MA (2005) Changes in lipopolysaccharide O antigen distinguish acute versus chronic *Leptospira interrogans* infections. Infect Immun 73:3251–3260

Narayanavari SA, Sritharan M, Haake DA, Matsunaga J (2012) Multiple leptospiral sphingomyelinases (or are there?). Microbiol 158:1137–1146

Nascimento AL, Ko AI, Martins EA, Monteiro-Vitorello CB, Ho PL, Haake DA, Verjovski-Almeida S, Hartskeerl RA, Marques MV, Oliveira MC, Menck CF, Leite LC, Carrer H, Coutinho LL, Degrave WM, Dellagostin OA, El-Dorry H, Ferro ES, Ferro MI, Furlan LR, Gamberini M, Giglioti EA, Goes-Neto A, Goldman GH, Goldman MH, Harakava R, Jeronimo SM, Junqueira-de-Azevedo IL, Kimura ET, Kuramae EE, Lemos EG, Lemos MV, Marino CL, Nunes LR, de Oliveira RC, Pereira GG, Reis MS, Schriefer A, Siqueira WJ, Sommer P, Tsai SM, Simpson AJ, Ferro JA, Camargo LE, Kitajima JP, Setubal JC, Van Sluys MA (2004) Comparative genomics of two *Leptospira interrogans* serovars reveals novel insights into physiology and pathogenesis. J Bacteriol 186:2164–2172

Nogueira SV, Backstedt BT, Smith AA, Qin JH, Wunder EA Jr, Ko A, Pal U (2013) *Leptospira interrogans* enolase is secreted extracellularly and interacts with plasminogen. PLoS ONE 8: e78150

Oliveira R, de Morais ZM, Goncales AP, Romero EC, Vasconcellos SA, Nascimento AL (2011) Characterization of novel OmpA-like protein of *Leptospira interrogans* that binds extracellular matrix molecules and plasminogen. PLoS ONE 6:e21962

Oliveira R, Domingos RF, Siqueira GH, Fernandes LG, Souza NM, Vieira ML, de Morais ZM, Vasconcellos SA, Nascimento AL (2013) Adhesins of *Leptospira interrogans* mediate the interaction to fibrinogen and inhibit fibrin clot formation *in vitro*. PLoS Negl Trop Dis 7:e2396

Oliveira TR, Longhi MT, Goncales AP, de Morais ZM, Vasconcellos SA, Nascimento AL (2010) LipL53, a temperature regulated protein from *Leptospira interrogans* that binds to extracellular matrix molecules. Microbes Infect 12:207–217

Palaniappan RU, Chang YF, Jusuf SS, Artiushin S, Timoney JF, McDonough SP, Barr SC, Divers TJ, Simpson KW, McDonough PL, Mohammed HO (2002) Cloning and molecular characterization of an immunogenic LigA protein of *Leptospira interrogans*. Infect Immun 70:5924–5930

Picardeau M, Brenot A, Saint Girons I (2001) First evidence for gene replacement in *Leptospira spp*. Inactivation of *L. biflexa flaB* results in non-motile mutants deficient in endoflagella. Mol Microbiol 40:189–199

Pinne M, Choy HA, Haake DA (2010) The OmpL37 surface-exposed protein is expressed by pathogenic *Leptospira* during infection and binds skin and vascular elastin. PLoS Negl Trop Dis 4:e815

Pinne M, Matsunaga J, Haake DA (2012) A novel approach to identification of host ligand-binding proteins: leptospiral outer-membrane protein microarray. J Bacteriol 194:6074–6087

Pinne M, Haake DA (2013) LipL32 is a subsurface lipoprotein of *Leptospira interrogans*: presentation of new data and reevaluation of previous studies. PLoS ONE 8:e51025

Que-Gewirth NL, Ribeiro AA, Kalb SR, Cotter RJ, Bulach DM, Adler B, Girons IS, Werts C, Raetz CR (2004) A methylated phosphate group and four amide-linked acyl chains in *Leptospira interrogans* lipid A. The membrane anchor of an unusual lipopolysaccharide that activates TLR2. J Biol Chem 279:25420–25429

Ren SX, Fu G, Jiang XG, Zeng R, Miao YG, Xu H, Zhang YX, Xiong H, Lu G, Lu LF, Jiang HQ, Jia J, Tu YF, Jiang JX, Gu WY, Zhang YQ, Cai Z, Sheng HH, Yin HF, Zhang Y, Zhu GF, Wan M, Huang HL, Qian Z, Wang SY, Ma W, Yao ZJ, Shen Y, Qiang BQ, Xia QC, Guo XK, Danchin A, Saint Girons I, Somerville RL, Wen YM, Shi MH, Chen Z, Xu JG, Zhao GP (2003) Unique physiological and pathogenic features of *Leptospira interrogans* revealed by whole-genome sequencing. Nature 422:888–893

Ricaldi JN, Matthias MA, Vinetz JM, Lewis AL (2012) Expression of sialic acids and other nonulosonic acids in *Leptospira*. BMC Microbiol 12:161

Ristow P, Bourhy P, da Cruz McBride FW, Figueira CP, Huerre M, Ave P, Girons IS, Ko AI, Picardeau M (2007) The OmpA-like protein Loa22 is essential for leptospiral virulence. PLoS Pathog 3:e97

Ruoslahti E (1996) RGD and other recognition sequences for integrins. Ann Rev Cell Dev Biol 12:697–715

Sanderson-Smith ML, Dinkla K, Cole JN, Cork AJ, Maamary PG, McArthur JD, Chhatwal GS, Walker MJ (2008) M protein-mediated plasminogen binding is essential for the virulence of an invasive *Streptococcus pyogenes* isolate. FASEB J 22:2715–2722

Schoone GJ, Everard CO, Korver H, Carrington DG, Inniss VA, Baulu J, Terpstra WJ (1989) An immunoprotective monoclonal antibody directed against *Leptospira interrogans* serovar Copenhageni. J Gen Microbiol 135:73–78

Segers RP, van Gestel JA, van Eys GJ, van der Zeijst BA, Gaastra W (1992) Presence of putative sphingomyelinase genes among members of the family Leptospiraceae. Infect Immun 60:1707–1710

Shimizu T, Matsusaka E, Takayanagi K, Masuzawa T, Iwamoto Y, Morita T, Mifuchi I, Yanagihara Y (1987) Biological activities of lipopolysaccharide-like substance (LLS) extracted from *Leptospira interrogans* serovar canicola strain moulton. Microbiol Immunol 31:727–735

Souza NM, Vieira ML, Alves IJ, de Morais ZM, Vasconcellos SA, Nascimento AL (2012) Lsa30, a novel adhesin of *Leptospira interrogans* binds human plasminogen and the complement regulator C4bp. Microb Pathog 53:125–134

Srikram A, Zhang K, Bartpho T, Lo M, Hoke DE, Sermswan RW, Adler B, Murray GL (2011) Cross-protective immunity against leptospirosis elicited by a live, attenuated lipopolysaccharide mutant. J Infect Dis 203:870–879

Stevenson B, Choy HA, Pinne M, Rotondi ML, Miller MC, Demoll E, Kraiczy P, Cooley AE, Creamer TP, Suchard MA, Brissette CA, Verma A, Haake DA (2007) *Leptospira interrogans* endostatin-like outer membrane proteins bind host fibronectin, laminin and regulators of complement. PLoS ONE 2:e1188

Svensson MD, Sjobring U, Luo F, Bessen DE (2002) Roles of the plasminogen activator streptokinase and the plasminogen-associated M protein in an experimental model for streptococcal impetigo. Microbiol 148:3933–3945

Szczepanski A, Furie MB, Benach JL, Lane BP, Fleit HB (1990) Interaction between *Borrelia burgdorferi* and endothelium in vitro. J Clin Invest 85:1637–1647

Thomas DD, Navab M, Haake DA, Fogelman AM, Miller JN, Lovett MA (1988) *Treponema pallidum* invades intercellular junctions of endothelial cell monolayers. Proc Natl Acad Sci USA 85:3608–3612

Thomas DD, Higbie LM (1990) In vitro association of leptospires with host cells. Infect Immun 58:581–585

Toma C, Okura N, Takayama C, Suzuki T (2011) Characteristic features of intracellular pathogenic *Leptospira* in infected murine macrophages. Cell Microbiol 13:1783–1792

Toma C, Murray GL, Nohara T, Mizuyama M, Koizumi N, Adler B, Suzuki T (2014) Leptospiral outer membrane protein LMB216 is involved in enhancement of phagocytic uptake by macrophages. Cell Microbiol 16:1366–1377

Torres AG, Li Y, Tutt CB, Xin L, Eaves-Pyles T, Soong L (2006) Outer membrane protein A of *Escherichia coli* O157:H7 stimulates dendritic cell activation. Infect Immun 74:2676–2685

Tsuchimoto M, Niikura M, Ono E, Kida H, Yanagawa R (1984) Leptospiral attachment to cultured cells. Zentralbl Bakteriol Mikrobiol Hyg A 258:268–274

Tucunduva de Faria M, Athanazio DA, Goncalves Ramos EA, Silva EF, Reis MG, Ko AI (2007) Morphological alterations in the kidney of rats with natural and experimental *Leptospira* infection. J Comp Pathol 137:231–238

Verma A, Artiushin S, Matsunaga J, Haake DA, Timoney JF (2005) LruA and LruB, novel lipoproteins of pathogenic *Leptospira interrogans* associated with equine recurrent uveitis. Infect Immun 73:7259–7266

Verma A, Hellwage J, Artiushin S, Zipfel PF, Kraiczy P, Timoney JF, Stevenson B (2006) LfhA, a novel factor H-binding protein of *Leptospira interrogans*. Infect Immun 74:2659–2666

Verma A, Brissette CA, Bowman AA, Shah ST, Zipfel PF, Stevenson B (2010a) Leptospiral endostatin-like protein A is a bacterial cell surface receptor for human plasminogen. Infect Immun 78:2053–2059

Verma A, Kumar P, Babb K, Timoney JF, Stevenson B (2010b) Cross-reactivity of antibodies against leptospiral recurrent uveitis-associated proteins A and B (LruA and LruB) with eye proteins. PLoS Negl Trop Dis 4:e778

Verma A, Stevenson B (2012) Leptospiral uveitis—there is more to it than meets the eye! Zoonoses Public Health 59(Suppl 2):132–141

Vieira ML, Vasconcellos SA, Goncales AP, de Morais ZM, Nascimento AL (2009) Plasminogen acquisition and activation at the surface of *Leptospira* species lead to fibronectin degradation. Infect Immun 77:4092–4101

Vieira ML, Atzingen MV, Oliveira TR, Oliveira R, Andrade DM, Vasconcellos SA, Nascimento AL (2010a) In vitro identification of novel plasminogen-binding receptors of the pathogen *Leptospira interrogans*. PLoS ONE 5:e11259

Vieira ML, de Morais ZM, Goncales AP, Romero EC, Vasconcellos SA, Nascimento AL (2010b) Lsa63, a newly identified surface protein of *Leptospira interrogans* binds laminin and collagen IV. J Infect 60:52–64

Vieira ML, de Morais ZM, Vasconcellos SA, Romero EC, Nascimento AL (2011) In vitro evidence for immune evasion activity by human plasmin associated to pathogenic *Leptospira interrogans*. Microb Pathog 51:360–365

Vieira ML, Alvarez-Flores MP, Kirchgatter K, Romero EC, Alves IJ, de Morais ZM, Vasconcellos SA, Chudzinski-Tavassi AM, Nascimento AL (2013) Interaction of *Leptospira interrogans* with human proteolytic systems enhances dissemination through endothelial cells and protease levels. Infect Immun 81:1764–1774

Vinh T, Faine S, Adler B (1984) Adhesion of leptospires to mouse fibroblasts (L929) and its enhancement by specific antibody. J Med Microbiol 18:73–85

Vinh T, Adler B, Faine S (1986) Glycolipoprotein cytotoxin from *Leptospira interrogans* serovar Copenhageni. J Gen Microbiol 132:111–123

Viriyakosol S, Matthias MA, Swancutt MA, Kirkland TN, Vinetz JM (2006) Toll-like receptor 4 protects against lethal *Leptospira interrogans* serovar icterohaemorrhagiae infection and contributes to *in vivo* control of leptospiral burden. Infect Immun 74:887–895

Vivian JP, Beddoe T, McAlister AD, Wilce MC, Zaker-Tabrizi L, Troy S, Byres E, Hoke DE, Cullen PA, Lo M, Murray GL, Adler B, Rossjohn J (2009) Crystal structure of LipL32, the most abundant surface protein of pathogenic *Leptospira* spp. J Mol Biol 387:1229–1238

Weiss DS, Brotcke A, Henry T, Margolis JJ, Chan K, Monack DM (2007) In vivo negative selection screen identifies genes required for *Francisella* virulence. Proc Natl Acad Sci USA 104:6037–6042

Werts C (2010) Leptospirosis: a toll road from B lymphocytes. Chang Gung Med J 33:591–601

Wolff DG, Castiblanco-Valencia MM, Abe CM, Monaris D, Morais ZM, Souza GO, Vasconcellos SA, Isaac L, Abreu PA, Barbosa AS (2013) Interaction of leptospira elongation factor Tu with plasminogen and complement Factor H: a metabolic leptospiral protein with moonlighting activities. PLoS ONE 8:e81818

Wooldridge KG, Williams PH (1993) Iron uptake mechanisms of pathogenic bacteria. FEMS Microbiol Rev 12:325–348

Yang CW, Wu MS, Pan MJ, Hsieh WJ, Vandewalle A, Huang CC (2002) The *Leptospira* outer membrane protein LipL32 induces tubulointerstitial nephritis-mediated gene expression in mouse proximal tubule cells. J Am Soc Nephrol 13:2037–2045

Yang CW, Hung CC, Wu MS, Tian YC, Chang CT, Pan MJ, Vandewalle A (2006) Toll-like receptor 2 mediates early inflammation by leptospiral outer membrane proteins in proximal tubule cells. Kidney Int 69:815–822

Yuri K, Takamoto Y, Okada M, Hiramune T, Kikuchi N, Yanagawa R (1993) Chemotaxis of leptospires to hemoglobin in relation to virulence. Infect Immun 61:2270–2272

Zhang K, Murray GL, Seemann T, Srikram A, Bartpho T, Sermswan RW, Adler B, Hoke DE (2013) Leptospiral LruA is required for virulence and modulates an interaction with mammalian Apolipoprotein A-I. Infect Immun 81:3872–3879

Zhang L, Zhang C, Ojcius DM, Sun D, Zhao J, Lin X, Li L, Yan J (2012) The mammalian cell entry (Mce) protein of pathogenic *Leptospira* species is responsible for RGD motif-dependent infection of cells and animals. Mol Microbiol 83:1006–1023

Zhang Y, Bao L, Zhu H, Huang B, Zhang H (2010) OmpA-like protein Loa22 from *Leptospira interrogans* serovar Lai is cytotoxic to cultured rat renal cells and promotes inflammatory responses. Acta Biochim Biophys Sin (Shanghai) 42:70–79

Zhang YX, Geng Y, Yang JW, Guo XK, Zhao GP (2008) Cytotoxic activity and probable apoptotic effect of Sph2, a sphigomyelinase hemolysin from *Leptospira interrogans* strain Lai. BMB Rep 41:119–125

Zhao JF, Chen HH, Ojcius DM, Zhao X, Sun D, Ge YM, Zheng LL, Lin X, Li LJ, Yan J (2013) Identification of *Leptospira interrogans* phospholipase C as a novel virulence factor responsible for intracellular free calcium ion elevation during macrophage death. PLoS ONE 8:e75652

Zhong Y, Chang X, Cao XJ, Zhang Y, Zheng H, Zhu Y, Cai C, Cui Z, Zhang Y, Li YY, Jiang XG, Zhao GP, Wang S, Li Y, Zeng R, Li X, Guo XK (2011) Comparative proteogenomic analysis of the *Leptospira interrogans* virulence-attenuated strain IPAV against the pathogenic strain 56601. Cell Res 21:1210–1229

The Leptospiral Outer Membrane

David A. Haake and Wolfram R. Zückert

Abstract The outer membrane (OM) is the front line of leptospiral interactions with their environment and the mammalian host. Unlike most invasive spirochetes, pathogenic leptospires must be able to survive in both free-living and host-adapted states. As organisms move from one set of environmental conditions to another, the OM must cope with a series of conflicting challenges. For example, the OM must be porous enough to allow nutrient uptake, yet robust enough to defend the cell against noxious substances. In the host, the OM presents a surface decorated with adhesins and receptors for attaching to, and acquiring, desirable host molecules such as the complement regulator, Factor H. On the other hand, the OM must enable leptospires to evade detection by the host's immune system on their way from sites of invasion through the bloodstream to the protected niche of the proximal tubule. The picture that is emerging of the leptospiral OM is that, while it shares many of the characteristics of the OMs of spirochetes and Gram-negative bacteria, it is also unique and different in ways that make it of general interest to microbiologists. For example, unlike most other pathogenic spirochetes, the leptospiral OM is rich in lipopolysaccharide (LPS). Leptospiral LPS is similar to that of Gram-negative bacteria but has a number of unique structural features that may explain why it is not recognized by the LPS-specific Toll-like receptor 4 of humans. As in other spirochetes, lipoproteins are major components of the leptospiral OM,

D.A. Haake (✉)
Division of Infectious Diseases, VA Greater Los Angeles Healthcare System,
Los Angeles, CA 90073, USA
e-mail: dhaake@ucla.edu

D.A. Haake
Departments of Medicine, Urology, and Microbiology, Immunology, and Molecular
Genetics, The David Geffen School of Medicine at UCLA, Los Angeles, CA 90095, USA

W.R. Zückert
Department of Microbiology, Molecular Genetics and Immunology, University of Kansas
School of Medicine, Kansas City, KS 66160, USA
e-mail: wzueckert@kumc.edu

© Springer-Verlag Berlin Heidelberg 2015
B. Adler (ed.), *Leptospira and Leptospirosis*, Current Topics in Microbiology
and Immunology 387, DOI 10.1007/978-3-662-45059-8_8

though their roles are poorly understood. The functions of transmembrane outer membrane proteins (OMPs) in many cases are better understood, thanks to homologies with their Gram-negative counterparts and the emergence of improved genetic techniques. This chapter will review recent discoveries involving the leptospiral OM and its role in leptospiral physiology and pathogenesis.

Contents

1 Lipopolysaccharide (LPS)

LPS is a major component of the leptospiral OM and its polysaccharides dominate the leptospiral surface. The degree to which LPS is exposed on the leptospiral surface is reflected in the abundance of electron-dense particles on the surface of *L. interrogans* after incubation with a gold-labeled anti-LPS monoclonal antibody (Fig. 1). Agglutination occurs within minutes in the presence of small concentrations of LPS-specific antibodies. Monoclonal antibodies to LPS mediate macrophage opsonization (Farrelly et al. 1987) and protect animals against challenge with pathogenic leptospires (Jost et al. 1989). LPS-specific immune responses are the basis for the sterilizing immunity elicited by whole cell vaccines (Midwinter et al. 1994). Given the sensitivity of leptospires to LPS-specific antibodies, it is not surprising that there is tremendous selective pressure to undergo genetic changes

Fig. 1 *Leptospira interrogans* coated with gold-labeled anti-LPS monoclonal antibodies. The number of electron-dense particles reflects the level of LPS exposure on the leptospiral surface

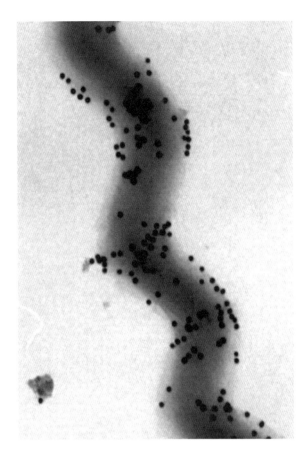

leading to O-antigen variation. Hundreds of leptospiral serovars have been defined, based on differential reactivity with antibodies or antisera in the microscopic agglutination test (MAT). The simple addition of LPS-antiserum to a leptospiral culture can result in the growth of escape mutants with altered LPS.

Despite its accessibility, LPS is by no means a liability for these organisms. Expression of intact LPS appears to be essential for leptospiral survival both inside and outside the mammalian host. This conclusion is based in part on the finding that the *rfb* locus encoding the enzymes responsible for LPS biosynthesis was relatively spared of insertions in a study of random transposon mutagenesis (Murray et al. 2009a), suggesting that most LPS mutants are nonviable for growth in culture. The rare mutants that did survive transposon insertion into the LPS locus were attenuated for virulence and were rapidly cleared after challenge (Murray et al. 2010). Interestingly, the LPS expressed by one of these LPS mutants, M1352, had little or no change in its molecular mass, suggesting that even subtle changes in LPS can result in a loss of virulence. Mutant M1352 was effective as a live attenuated vaccine, stimulating both homologous and heterologous immunity in the hamster model of leptospirosis (Srikram et al. 2011). Differential detection of organisms in the liver and kidney using serovar-specific monoclonal antibodies suggests that the O-antigen side chains of leptospiral LPS are not static and may undergo antigenic changes during infection (Nally et al. 2005a).

1.1 LPS Structure and Biosynthesis

As in Gram-negative bacteria, leptospiral LPS consists of three components: lipid A, the core, and polysaccharide. The *L. interrogans* genome contains homologs of all the genes required for lipid A biosynthesis (Ren et al. 2003). The structure of leptospiral lipid A has now been fully elucidated and found to contain both similarities with, and striking differences from, typical forms of lipid A (Que-Gewirth et al. 2004). The first key difference is that *L. interrogans* converts the usual GlcNAc (N-acetylglucosamine) disaccharide backbone of lipid A to GlcNAc3 N, so that each of the two sugars has two amino groups instead of one. Consequently, there are four amide-linked fatty acids in the *L. interrogans* lipid A instead of two. This is unusual, but has been observed in some environmental bacteria. In addition, the leptospiral fatty acids in leptospiral lipid A differ in length from those typically found in Gram-negative lipid A and some are unsaturated. An even more unusual aspect of *L. interrogans* lipid A involves the phosphate residue. *E. coli* lipid A has two phosphates, one on each end of the disaccharide, whereas leptospiral lipid A has a single phosphate, and that single phosphate is methylated. Methylated phosphates are extremely unusual in biology and have not been previously observed in lipid A.

1.2 Innate Immunity: TLR4 and TLR2

The structural differences between LPS of *E. coli* and *Leptospira* are of great interest because of their differential recognition by TLR4, the Toll-like receptor involved in the innate immune response to LPS. While human TLR 4 reacts with *E. coli* LPS at extremely low concentrations, it is unable to interact with leptospiral LPS (Werts et al. 2001). Failure of human TLR4 to recognize leptospiral LPS may be one reason why humans are accidental hosts in whom leptospirosis occasionally causes overwhelming, lethal infections. In contrast, murine TLR4 is able to recognize leptospiral LPS (Nahori et al. 2005) and mice are natural, reservoir hosts for pathogenic leptospires. This idea is consistent with the observation that while mice with intact Toll-like receptors are resistant to leptospiral infection, young (but not adult) C3H/ HeJ mice lacking TLR4 are susceptible to lethal infection with *L. interrogans* (Viriyakosol et al. 2006). Surprisingly, leptospiral LPS is recognized by both human and murine TLR2, the Toll-like receptor primarily involved in lipoprotein recognition. The importance of both TLR2 and TLR4 receptors in mice was highlighted by the finding that only when both of these receptors were knocked out did adult

C57BL/6 J mice develop lethal infections after leptospiral challenge (Nahori et al. 2005). Murine TLR4 and TLR2 appear to recognize different leptospiral LPS components: TLR4 recognizes leptospiral lipid A while TLR2 recognizes the polysaccharide or 2-keto-3-deoxyoctonoic acid (KDO) portion of leptospiral LPS (Nahori et al. 2005; Werts 2010).

1.3 LPS Assembly and Transport

Many of the genes involved in LPS export to the OM are present in leptospiral genomes, suggesting that the processes are similar to those in typical Gram-negative bacteria. A number of excellent reviews on the subject of LPS assembly and transport have recently been published (Ruiz et al. 2009; Sperandeo et al. 2009). The lipid A and core components of LPS are assembled on the cytoplasmic surface of the inner membrane. These rough LPS molecules (lacking the O-antigen) are transported to the periplasmic leaflet of the inner membrane by the ABC transporter, MsbA. It has not yet been determined which of the many *L. interrogans* ABC transporters is MsbA. O-antigen is assembled via the Wzy-dependent pathway in which polysaccharides are synthesized on the cytoplasmic surface of the inner membrane, followed by transport across the inner membrane by the Wzx flippase (LIC12135), where they are ligated to rough LPS by Wzy O-antigen ligase (LIC11753). After polysaccharide has been added to the LPS core, full-length (smooth) LPS is transported across the periplasm by LptA to the LPS assembly site on the OM formed by LptD (aka OstA, LIC11458) and LptE (11007). LptD is a porin-like molecule and appears to be involved in translocating LPS to the OM surface. Cryo-electron tomography has shown that the thickness of the *L. interrogans* LPS layer, and presumably the length of its polysaccharide, is 50 % greater than that of *L. biflexa* (Fig. 2), which again illustrates the importance of LPS for virulence (Raddi et al. 2012).

2 Outer Membrane Proteins (OMPs)

2.1 General Considerations

In recent years, much has been learned about the identity, expression, and functions of OMPs. The picture of the OM that has emerged (Fig. 3) is the result of improved methods for determining whether proteins are located in the OM and on its surface. A number of cell fractionation methods have been developed, including Triton X-114 fractionation (Haake et al. 1991; Zuerner et al. 1991), isolation of OM vesicles by sucrose density gradient fractionation (Haake and Matsunaga 2002; Nally et al. 2005b), and membrane fractionation (Matsunaga et al. 2002). Of particular

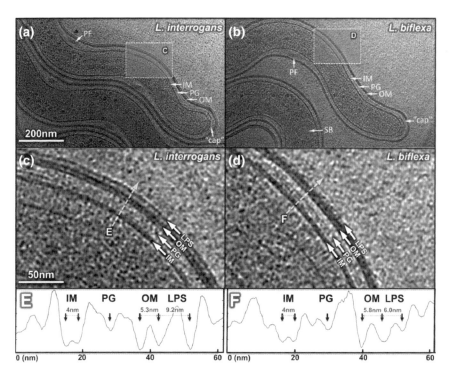

Fig. 2 Cryo-electron tomography of *L. interrogans* versus *L. biflexa*. The thickness of the LPS layer of *L. interrogans* is 9.2 nm versus 6.0 nm for *L. biflexa*. The increased thickness of the *L. interrogans* LPS layer is probably important for virulence. Reproduced from Raddi et al. (2012)

importance are methods to identify surface-exposed OMPs. Multiple assays should be applied, including surface and subsurface controls, before concluding whether a particular protein is surface exposed. The most accurate methods include surface immunoprecipitation (Haake et al. 1991), surface biotinylation (Cullen et al. 2003), surface proteolysis (Pinne and Haake 2009), and surface immunofluorescence (Pinne and Haake 2011).

Particularly useful has been the application of matrix-assisted laser desorption/ ionization time of flight (MALDI-TOF) to identification of surface-exposed (Cullen et al. 2005) and OM-associated proteins (Cullen et al. 2002; Nally et al. 2005b). More is now known about the absolute level of expression of leptospiral proteins than in almost any other bacterial species, thanks to the proteome-wide application of MALDI-TOF to identify and quantify leptospiral proteins (Malmström et al. 2009). Absolute quantification was achieved by inclusion of isotope-labeled reference peptides in leptospiral samples. DNA microarrays have been used to examine the response of leptospiral transcript levels to environmental signals including temperature upshift (Lo et al. 2006), osmolarity (Matsunaga et al. 2007a), iron levels (Lo et al. 2010), serum (Patarakul et al. 2010), and macrophage-derived

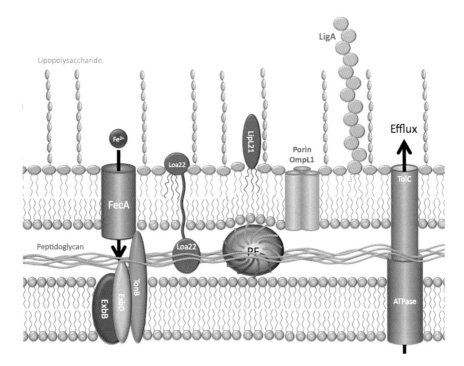

Fig. 3 Membrane architecture of *L. interrogans*. The outer membrane contains LPS, lipoproteins such as LipL21, Loa22, and LigA, and transmembrane proteins such as FecA, OmpL1, TolC, and possibly Loa22. Peptidoglycan and the periplasmic flagella *PF* are located in the periplasm

cells (Xue et al. 2010). Proteomic methods have also been used to examine thermoregulation (Lo et al. 2009) and posttranslational modification of OMPs (Cao et al. 2010; Eshghi et al. 2012). Proteome arrays have been used to identify fibronectin-binding OMPs (Pinne et al. 2012) and seroreactive OMPs (Lessa-Aquino et al. 2013).

2.2 *Lipoprotein OMPs*

Bacterial lipoproteins are proteins that have been posttranslationally modified by fatty acids (i.e., lipids) at a cysteine residue. This cysteine becomes the amino-terminal residue after the signal peptide has been removed by lipoprotein signal peptidase. Because the fatty acids of lipoproteins are extremely hydrophobic, they become embedded into membrane lipid bilayers and provide an anchor for lipoproteins to be tightly associated with the membrane. Treatments such as salt and urea that remove peripheral membrane proteins from membranes will not remove lipoproteins. This demonstrates that even though lipoproteins are generally not transmembrane proteins (Loa22 appears to be an exception), lipoproteins remain tightly associated with membranes, even after treatment with reagents that remove peripheral membrane proteins (Matsunaga et al. 2002). In contrast to the hydrophobicity of fatty acids, the protein components of most lipoproteins are typically hydrophilic and relatively soluble in aqueous buffers when expressed as recombinant proteins without their signal peptide. As such, the protein components of lipoproteins project out from membranes and decorate their surfaces. The first bacterial lipoprotein to be described was the Murein (or Braun's) lipoprotein, which is integrated into the inner leaflet of the *E. coli* OM by lipids at its amino terminus and covalently attached to peptidoglycan (PG) at its carboxy-terminal lysine. Murein lipoprotein is a major OM protein of *E. coli* and serves as an important structural role in maintaining cellular integrity by providing a link between the OM and the PG cell wall. The OM-PG linkage is so important that *E. coli* has a number of other proteins that play similar roles, including OmpA and Pal (peptidoglycan-associated lipoprotein). Leptospires also have a number of OmpA-related proteins, such as Loa22, that are presumed to play similar OM-anchoring roles.

2.3 Lipoprotein Lipidation and Export

The steps involved in lipoprotein lipidation and export are shown in Fig. 3. Proteins with amino-terminal signal peptides, including lipoproteins, are exported across the inner membrane by the Sec translocase complex. Orthologs of all essential components of the Sec translocase complex are present in *Leptospira*. Upon reaching the periplasm, lipoproteins of Gram-negative bacteria are processed by a series of three enzymes that remove the signal peptide and modify the new N-terminal cysteine with fatty acids. Each of these three lipoprotein processing enzymes is also present in *Leptospira* (Haake 2000; Nascimento et al. 2004). The first of these enzymes is lipoprotein diacylglyceryl transferase (Lgt), which attaches a diacyl group containing two fatty acids to the sulfhydryl residue of cysteine via a thioester linkage. Because Lgt is the first enzyme in the series, its active site is presumably responsible for identifying the "lipobox," which distinguishes the signal peptides of lipoproteins from those of other exported proteins. Lipoprotein signal peptidase (Lsp) is the second enzyme in the series, and is responsible for removing the signal peptide, so that cysteine becomes the N-terminal amino acid of the mature lipoprotein. The third enzyme in the series is lipoprotein N-acyl transferase (Lnt), which adds a third and final fatty acid to the now available amino residue of cysteine via an amide bond. Interestingly, most Gram-positive bacteria lack Lnt and their lipoproteins are usually diacylated rather than triacylated (Kovacs-Simon et al. 2011). Perhaps Gram-negative bacteria triacylate their lipoproteins to strengthen the connection between the OM lipid bilayer and lipoproteins involved cell wall anchoring.

Experimental verification of lipidation is important when examining how lipoproteins interact with leptospiral membranes and the host innate immune system. Several methods are available. A commonly used method is to add radiolabeled palmitate to growth medium to demonstrate incorporation of label into the protein, which can be purified by immunoprecipitation. [^{14}C]palmitate labeled at each of its carbons is the preferred form of palmitate because the higher specific activity results in a much shorter time to identification of bands by autoradiography. It should be noted that spirochetes, including leptospires, can digest fatty acids to two-carbon fragments which are incorporated into amino acid biosynthetic pathways. In this way, [^{14}C]palmitate could potentially label any protein. For this reason, it is desirable to take advantage of the acid-labile linkage of the palmitate to the lipoprotein by demonstrating that the label can be removed from the lipoprotein by treatment of the electrophoresis gel containing the protein with acetic acid: immunoblots would remain positive, while the autoradiogram would become negative. Historically, globomycin has been used to inhibit lipidation of lipoproteins. However, it should be noted that globomycin selectively inhibits lipoprotein signal peptidase, the second enzyme in the series, so proteins could still become acylated through the previous step mediated by Lgt. Indirect evidence for lipidation can be obtained by Triton X-114 detergent fractionation. This detergent is similar to Triton X-100 except that Triton X-114 has a shorter polyethylene side chain, giving Triton X-114 a much lower cloud point. As a result, Triton X-114 solutions that occur in a single phase at 4 °C partition into two phases upon warming to 37 °C: a heavier, detergent-rich "hydrophobic" phase and a lighter, detergent-poor "hydrophilic" phase. Lipoproteins extracted by treatment of bacteria with Triton X-114 on ice should partition into the hydrophobic phase. The combination of sequence analysis plus behavior in Triton X-114 is an argument, albeit indirect, for lipidation.

Significant progress has been made in predicting which leptospiral genes encode lipoproteins. Lipoprotein signal peptides differ from other signal peptides in that they contain a "lipobox" sequence near the carboxy-terminal region of the signal peptide. In *E. coli*, the lipobox sequence is typically Leu-Leu-X-Y-Cys. There is relatively little variation in *E. coli* lipobox sequences and substitutions that do occur are with conservative amino acids: X is typically Ala, but can also be Thr or Ser, while Y is typically Gly, but can also be Ala. Based on sequences from experimentally verified lipoproteins, spirochete lipobox sequences are much more variable than those of *E. coli*. As a consequence, the Psort lipoprotein prediction program, based on lipoprotein sequences of *E. coli* and related bacteria has low (17–33 %) sensitivity for spirochetal lipoproteins. A later algorithm, LipoP, that utilized hidden Markov model statistical methods had significantly greater (50–81 %) sensitivity, but also higher (8–30 %) false positivity. To address these problems, we developed a spirochete-specific lipoprotein algorithm called "SpLip" based on sequences from 28 experimentally verified spirochetal lipoproteins. The SpLip algorithm is a hybrid approach of supplementing weight matrix scoring with rules including exclusion of charged amino acids from the lipobox (Setubal et al. 2006).

The inclusion in SpLip of rules based on sequences of experimentally verified lipoproteins reduces false positive hits, but these rules require further validation. For example, one of the SpLip rules is that the only allowed amino acids at the −1 position are Ala, Gly, Ser, Thr, Asn, Gln, or Cys. Now that a large number of leptospiral genomes have been sequenced, researchers at the J. Craig Venter Institute have discovered that newly sequenced homologs of known lipoproteins may have additional amino acids at the −1 position (Daniel Haft, personal communication). This genome sequence analysis will provide much greater confidence regarding the plasticity of amino acids at positions within the lipobox. It is unclear why spirochetal lipobox sequences are so much more variable than those of *E. coli*. One possible explanation for this difference is that *E. coli* growth rates are so much faster than spirochete growth rates. As a result, *E. coli* enzymes, including those involved in lipoprotein processing, must have much higher rates of catalysis than spirochetal enzymes. Higher catalytic rates may require higher substrate fidelity to maintain enzymatic efficiency.

After lipidation occurs, lipoproteins either remain in the outer leaflet of the inner membrane (IM) or undergo trafficking to one or more of four other possible destinations. From inside to outside these are: the inner leaflet of the OM, the outer leaflet of the OM, as a peripheral OM protein, and secretion beyond the cell. In *E coli*, lipoproteins destined for the OM are recognized by the IM ABC transporter-like sortase complex LolCDE (Yakushi et al. 2000) and then presented to periplasmic lipoprotein-binding chaperone LolA (Yokota et al. 1999) for transport to the OM lipoprotein receptor LolB (Yokota et al. 1999). The *L. interrogans* serovar Copenhageni genome appears to contain multiple homologs of a LolADE subset (LolA-1 and -2, LolD-1 and -2 and LolE-1, -2, and -3) (Fig. 4) (Nascimento et al. 2004). A LolC homolog is missing, as is LolB. LolB homologs so far have only been detected in β- and γ-Proteobacteria, and LolC function might be provided by one of the LolE homologs. While it remains to be determined which of the spirochetal genes are indeed functional Lol orthologs or functionally diverse paralogs, it appears likely that the Lol pathway is involved in shuttling lipoproteins from the IM to the OM.

Even less is known about how lipoproteins travel to the leptospiral surface and beyond. However, it would not be surprising if leptospiral lipoproteins follow the model established for *B. burgdorferi* lipoprotein secretion. In this model, the targeting information of surface lipoproteins was found to be located in the intrinsically disordered N-terminal tether peptides, with sorting signals differing from those in other well-characterized diderm model systems (Kumru et al. 2010, 2011; Schulze and Zückert 2006; Schulze et al. 2010). A surface lipoprotein's periplasmic conformation (or lack thereof) was found to determine its ability to cross the OM, and crossing could be initiated by a disordered C-terminus after insertion of the protein to the periplasmic leaflet of the OM (Chen and Zückert 2011; Schulze et al. 2010). Shown in the context of cell envelope biogenesis (Fig. 4), our evolving working model of the leptospiral lipoprotein transport pathway consists of LolCDE and LolA orthologs being mainly involved in periplasmic sorting, while surface lipoproteins use two additional, so far uncharacterized modules to facilitate

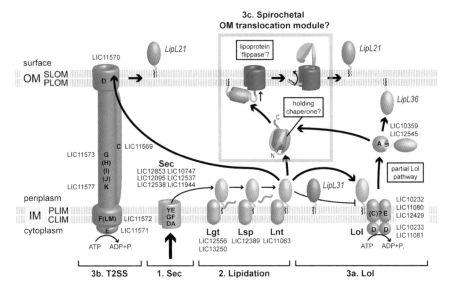

Fig. 4 Leptospiral lipoprotein export. Lipoproteins are exported via the Sec pathway (Step 1) from the cytoplasm to the periplasmic leaflet of the inner membrane *PLIM* where they are lipidated (Step 2). After lipidation, export to the periplasmic leaflet of the outer membrane *PLOM* occurs via the Lol pathway (Step 3a). Export to the surface leaflet of the outer membrane *SLOM* could occur either by the Type II Secretion System (*T2SS*, Step 3b) or by a lipoprotein flippase

translocation, or "flipping," of surface lipoproteins through the OM: (i) a peri-plasmic surface lipoprotein "holding" chaperone functioning like the chaperones guiding transmembrane proteins (TMPs) to the OM (Bos et al. 2007), and (ii) an OM lipoprotein translocase complex functioning similarly to lipid flippases (Pomorski and Menon 2006) (Fig. 4).

Alternative routes to the leptospiral surface are possible. Sec-dependent or -independent bacterial protein secretion pathways in *Leptospira* are limited to a type 2 secretion system, which might be involved in lipoprotein secretion tracking the *Klebsiella* model (d'Enfert et al. 1987; Sauvonnet and Pugsley 1996) (Fig. 4), a twin-arginine translocation (Tat) system, which may provide for export of folded proteins from the cytoplasm to the periplasm (Lee et al. 2006), and a type I secretion system (discussed in Sect. 2.14).

2.4 LipL32, the Major Outer Membrane Lipoprotein

As is strikingly apparent in protein stains of whole bacteria fractionated by SDS-PAGE, LipL32 is the most abundant protein in pathogenic *Leptospira* spp. Localization of LipL32 to the OM was demonstrated by Triton X-114 fractionation (Haake et al. 2000) and isolation of leptospiral OM vesicles by sucrose density gradient ultracentrifugation (Haake and Matsunaga 2002; Nally et al. 2005b). One of the early challenges encountered in these studies was that solubilization with Triton X-114 in the presence of EDTA results in degradation of LipL32 and other leptospiral membrane proteins by endogenous protease(s) when the detergent extract is warmed from 4 to 37 °C. This challenge was overcome by Zuerner et al. (1991) who found that addition of calcium prior to warming the extract prevented LipL32 degradation. The relationship between LipL32 and calcium was further elucidated by the LipL32 crystal structure, which revealed an acidic pocket formed in part by an extraordinary region of the LipL32 sequence in which seven out of eight amino acids are aspartates (Vivian et al. 2009). Co-crystalization of LipL32 with calcium showed that two of these aspartates are involved in calcium ion coordination (Hauk et al. 2009). When the aspartates in the calcium-binding pocket were mutated to alanines, denaturation of LipL32 in response to heat was similar with or without calcium. This elegant study used circular dichroism and tryptophan fluorescence to show that calcium helps LipL32 resist thermal denaturation (Hauk et al. 2012).

The abundance of LipL32 contributed greatly to its unfortunate misidentification as a surface lipoprotein. The first studies to claim LipL32 surface localization involved surface biotinylation experiments (Cullen et al. 2003, 2005). This technique involves addition of the biotinylation reagent sulfo-NHS-LC-biotin, which is considered to be "membrane impermeable" if membranes are intact but is a small enough molecule to penetrate through damaged membranes. This issue is problematic for spirochetes for which the OM is fragile and subject to disruption if organisms are not handled carefully. In this context, it is worth noting that in the second of these biotinylation studies, the cytoplasmic protein GroEL and the periplasmic protein FlaB1 were also found to be biotinylated (Cullen et al. 2005). Surface immunoelectron microscopy studies with LipL32 antibodies showed increased labeling of leptospiral cells compared to control antibodies. However, the number of gold particles (10.8 particles per cell) was far below what would have been expected for such an abundant protein. Seemingly confirmatory whole cell ELISA studies added to the confusion. The LipL32 surface protein dogma was recently overturned when more careful surface immunofluorescence studies were performed, including a number of controls including antisera to positive and negative control antigens and comparisons of intact and methanol fixed organisms (Pinne and Haake 2013). Studies were performed in parallel on intact and fixed organisms and fluorescence microscopy images were obtained using identical exposure times to ensure that they were truly comparable. LipL32 immunofluorescence of intact organisms was mostly negative, but occasionally showed irregular staining patterns, particularly if organisms were disrupted by shear force. However, the homogeneous staining observed with methanol fixed organisms did not occur with intact organisms. These immunofluorescence studies were supplemented with surface proteolysis studies showing that treatment with Proteinase K could digest LipL32 only if organisms were disrupted. Treatment of organisms with Proteinase K had previously been shown to be a reliable method for identifying surface proteins (Pinne and Haake 2009). In conclusion, LipL32 appears to be located in the periplasmic leaflet of the OM, a location shared by LipL36 (Shang et al. 1996). Based on Triton X-114 fractionation, other subsurface lipoproteins including LipL31 (Haake and Matsunaga 2002) and LruB (Verma et al. 2005) appear to be restricted to the periplasmic leaflet of the inner membrane. Interestingly, despite its location, LruA (also known as LipL71) modulates interactions with mammalian apolipoprotein A-I (Zhang et al. 2013).

If LipL32 is not on the leptospiral surface to any significant extent, what is its function? This is an important question given that pathogenic leptospires devote such a large amount of their protein-synthetic resources to expression of LipL32. Based on the Triton X-114 and OM vesicle evidence that LipL32 is an OM protein, it would be logical to conclude that the protein is located in the inner leaflet of the OM. Considering the known size of a LipL32 molecule (29 Å × 50 Å) as determined crystallographically (Vivian et al. 2009), the average length (10 μM) and diameter (0.1 μM) of leptospiral cells, and the quantitation of 38,000 copies of LipL32 molecules per cell (Malmström et al. 2009), it can be estimated that LipL32 occupies an extraordinary 20 % of the leptospiral OM inner surface. Perhaps LipL32 serves some structural role, for example, in OM stabilization? One possible function is as a calcium sink. Calcium is well-known to be important for membrane integrity generally and chelation of divalent cations with EDTA is essential for release of the OM from leptospiral cells (Haake et al. 1991; Haake and Matsunaga 2002; Nally et al. 2005b). However, LipL32 does not appear to be essential for OM integrity, given that a Himar transposon mutant of *L. interrogans* serovar Manilae lacking LipL32 had normal morphology and growth rate compared to the wild type (Murray et al. 2009b).

Aside from serving as a large calcium sink for leptospiral cells, the function of LipL32 is not understood. There is strong evidence that LipL32 is expressed during infection, given that there is intense staining by immunohistochemistry for LipL32 in the kidneys of infected animals (Haake et al. 2000) and that LipL32 is one of the most dominant seroreactive antigens recognized during acute and convalescent leptospirosis (Lessa-Aquino et al. 2013). On the other hand, LipL32 is not essential for infection given that the *lipL32* transposon mutant was able to cause acute, lethal infections in hamsters and chronic infections in rats that were indistinguishable from those caused by the wild-type organism (Murray et al. 2009b). Nevertheless, given the large amount of LipL32 expressed by pathogenic leptospires, this protein has the potential to play a critical role in stimulating the host inflammatory response during infection. Purified, native (and therefore lipidated) LipL32 stimulates an innate immune response through TLR 2 (Werts et al. 2001). Inflammation in the kidney, a major target organ during leptospirosis, is manifested by interstitial nephritis. LipL32 induces interstitial nephritis in kidney proximal tubule cells (Yang et al. 2002) and the inflammation induced by LipL32 is mediated by TLR 2 (Yang et al. 2006). For reasons that remain obscure, LipL32 is one of the most highly conserved leptospiral OMPs among pathogenic leptospires, suggesting that it might be a favorable vaccine target for induction of cross-protective immunity. However, results obtained by immunization with a large variety of different LipL32 constructs remain largely negative or at best indeterminate, which may be related in part to its subsurface location. Readers interested in more information on this subject and other aspects of LipL32 are referred to the excellent, recent review by Murray (2013).

2.5 Loa22 and Other OmpA-Like Proteins

The second most abundant OM protein is Loa22 (Malmström et al. 2009). While there remains some uncertainty as to whether Loa22 is a lipoprotein, it is covered here because of experimental evidence of lipidation: Expression of Loa22 in *E. coli* resulted in labeling with [^{3}H]palmitate (Koizumi and Watanabe 2003). This result is somewhat surprising because of the unusual Loa22 lipobox: SFTLC. As mentioned above, virtually all amino acids found in the −1 position relative to cysteine have been relatively small amino acids, and we are unaware of any documentned examples of a large hydrophobic amino acid like leucine in that location. For this reason, Loa22 is not predicted to be a lipoprotein by the SpLip algorithm. However, it is predicted to be a lipoprotein by the LipoP algorithm. While the [^{3}H]palmitate-labeling data should be considered more convincing than the bioinformatic data, they would have been more conclusive if the experiment also had been performed in *L. interrogans* and if the label had been shown to be acid labile.

Lipoprotein or not, Loa22 represents a conundrum because it is both surface exposed and binds peptidoglycan via a carboxy-terminal OmpA domain. OmpA domains are peptidoglycan binding domains found in proteins that, like OmpA, link membranes to the cell wall situated beneath the OM. In the case of Loa22, the OmpA domain begins at amino acid 111 and occupies more than half the protein. There are strong immunofluorescence data showing that Loa22 is surface exposed (Ristow et al. 2007). One possible explanation for these data is that Loa22, like *E. coli* murein lipoprotein, exists in both peptidoglycan-bound and -free forms. The peptidoglycan-free form of murein lipoprotein has been found to be surface exposed (Cowles et al. 2011). The second explanation is that in the 90 amino acid segment between the signal peptide and the OmpA domain, Loa22 crosses the OM at least once. This 90 amino acid segment is hydrophilic and lacks the amphipathic beta sheets typically found in transmembrane OM proteins. Instead, as shown in Fig. 5a, there is an alpha-helical stretch with a strongly hydrophobic region on one face of the helix. This suggests that Loa22 is similar to the *E. coli* OM lipoprotein Wza, which forms large channels for export of the high molecular weight capsular polysaccharides. Wza forms octamers (Fig. 5b) in which the hydrophobic faces of the Wza monomers interact with the hydrophobic interior of the OM, while the hydrophilic faces form the walls of the channel (Dong et al. 2006). Although the role of Loa22 in the OM remains uncertain, that role appears to be essential for virulence; a *Himar* transposon mutant lacking Loa22 expression was unable to cause lethal infections in hamsters and guinea pigs, although it was able to cause bacteremia and renal colonization (Ristow et al. 2007). It is interesting to note that a homolog of the *loa22* gene with 56 % sequence identity is present in *L. biflexa*,

(a) **(b)**

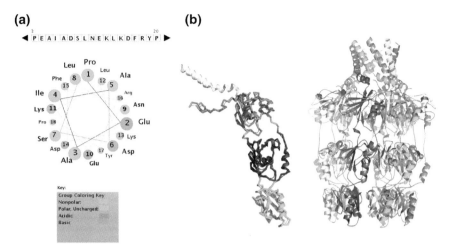

Fig. 5 Loa22 as an alpha-helical transmembrane OM protein. Panel **a** shows a helical wheel for the putative alpha-helical transmembrane domain of Loa22. The collection of nonpolar residues on one face indicates that the transmembrane helix could be amphipathic. Panel **b** shows the monomeric and octameric forms of Wza, which serves as a model for how Loa22 crosses the OM. Reproduced from Dong et al. (2006)

indicating that just because a gene is present or not in leptospiral saprophytes does not predict whether it is likely to be required for virulence in leptospiral pathogens.

Loa22 belongs to a family of seven leptospiral OmpA-like proteins. The other members of the family differ from Loa22 in multiple ways. They do not appear to be lipoproteins, they tend to be much larger proteins, and appear to be more typical transmembrane OM proteins along the lines of the *E. coli* version of OmpA. For example, LIC10050 has a signal peptidase 1 cleavage site and is predicted to be a 78-kD protein with 22 beta-sheet transmembrane segments. However, in all cases, leptospiral OmpA-like proteins are probably important in linking the OM to the peptidoglycan cell wall.

2.6 Outer Membrane Lipoprotein LipL41

LipL41 is the third most abundant OM lipoprotein (Malmström et al. 2009). Levels of *lipL41* transcript (Matsui et al. 2012) and LipL41 protein (Cullen et al. 2002; Nally et al. 2001b) are remarkably unaffected by temperature, osmolarity, and other environmental factors. The stability of LipL41 expression is useful as a control when studying the effects of growth conditions on the expression of other genes and proteins. For example, LipL41 antiserum is frequently included in immunoblots to compare the loading of bacteria per lane (Matsunaga et al. 2013). Although it is treated as one, it would be incorrect to call *lipL41* a "housekeeping gene" until more is known about its function. Although too preliminary to be conclusive, a clue to the function of LipL41 is that it was identified as a potential hemin-binding protein in hemin-agarose affinity chromatography (Asuthkar et al. 2007). King et al. (2013) were unable to confirm hemin-binding activity. However, a subsequent study documented a submicromolar hemin-LipL41 dissociation constant and identified amino acids involved in hemin binding (Lin et al. 2013). Interestingly, the same study found that LipL41 forms a supramolecular assembly consisting of 36 molecules (Lin et al. 2013).

The *lipL41* gene is located immediately upstream of a smaller gene, with which it is co-transcribed. For this reason, the smaller gene has been designated *lep* for *lip*L41 *e*xpression *p*artner (King et al. 2013). Even though *lipL41* transcript levels were unaffected in a lep transposon mutant, LipL41 levels were greatly reduced. Because Lep expression appeared to be required for stable expression of LipL41, perhaps by acting as a chaperone, researchers examined whether Lep bound to LipL41. Lep molecules were found to bind to LipL41 molecules at a molar ratio of 2:1 (King et al. 2013). Neither a *lipL41* nor a *lep* mutant was attenuated for virulence in hamsters. Interestingly, Lep was not detected by whole organism MALDI-TOF (Malmström et al. 2009), indicating that Lep is only required in small amounts transiently during export of LipL41 to the OM.

2.7 The Lig Family of OM Lipoproteins

The Lig family of OM lipoproteins was discovered by screening *L. kirschneri* and *L. interrogans* expression libraries with convalescent human leptospirosis sera. This approach identified GroEL, and DnaK, and LipL41, and three novel genes encoding a series of bacterial immunoglobulin (Ig)-like domains. The proteins encoded by these novel genes were designated as **L**eptospiral **Ig**-like proteins LigA, LigB, and LigC (Matsunaga et al. 2003). The Lig proteins consist of a lipoprotein signal peptide followed by a series of 12–13 Ig-like domains and, in the case of LigB and LigC, a large carboxy-terminal domain. The region upstream of *ligA* and *ligB*, as well as the first six Ig-like domains of LigA and LigB, are virtually identical, indicating that the *ligA* gene resulted from a partial gene duplication event. This event likely occurred relatively late in leptospiral evolution, as *ligA* is found only found in stains of *L. kirschneri* and *L. interrogans* (McBride et al. 2009). In contrast, LigB is found in all pathogenic *Leptospira* species. LigC is also widely distributed but is a pseudogene or absent in some strains. Sequence comparison revealed a surprising degree of mosaicism, indicating genetic rearrangements involving *ligB* gene fragments of *L. interrogans* and *L. kirschneri* (McBride et al. 2009). OMP mosaicism can confer a survival advantage in the face of antigenic pressure.

Temperature and osmolarity are key environmental signals that control the expression of the Lig proteins. In the process of examining the interaction of leptospires with cells in tissue culture, Matsunaga et al. (2005) observed that the addition of EMEM tissue culture medium to leptospiral culture medium induced

LigA and LigB expression and caused a substantial increase in released LigA. Sodium chloride was primarily responsible for these effects. All other EMEM components, including iron, bicarbonate, and oxygen concentrations, had no effect on Lig expression. As shown in Fig. 6, addition of sodium chloride, potassium chloride, or sodium sulfate to leptospiral medium (EMJH) to the level of osmolarity found in the mammalian host (~ 300 mOsm/L) induced expression of both cell-associated LigA and LigB, and release of LigA into the culture supernatant. Osmolarity affects both *lig* transcript and Lig protein levels (Matsunaga et al. 2007b). In addition to its effects on Lig protein expression, osmolarity increases the transcription of the leptospiral sphingomyelinase, Sph2 (Matsunaga et al. 2007b), the putative adhesin, LipL53 (Oliveira et al. 2010), and a number leptospiral lipo-proteins and OMPs (Matsunaga et al. 2007a). These results suggest that leptospires upregulate a defined set of OMPs when they encounter mammalian host tissues and sense an increase in osmolarity. The sensory transduction proteins involved in osmoregulation have not yet been defined.

More recently, it was discovered that expression of the *lig* genes is also regulated by temperature. The long 175 nucleotide 5′ untranslated region is predicted to contain secondary structure that includes and obscures the ribosome binding site and start codon, preventing binding to the ribosome and initiation of translation (Fig. 7). Toeprint experiments showed binding of ribosomes to the *lig* transcript was poor unless most of the left stem of predicted structure 2 (Fig. 7) was removed. In *E. coli*, a *lig′-′bgaB* translational fusion transcribed from a heterologous promoter was regulated by temperature, demonstrating the ability of the *lig* sequences to exert

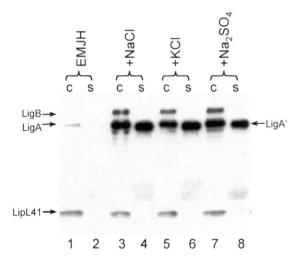

Fig. 6 Induction of Lig expression by osmolarity. Expression of LigA and LigB is strongly induced by addition of salt to Ellinghausen-McCullough-Johnson-Harris *EMJH* medium. LigA is found in both the cellular *c* and supernatant *s* fractions. A variety of salts are effective, indicating that induction of Lig expression is mediated by osmolarity rather than any particular salt component

Fig. 7 Secondary structure of the 5′ untranslated region of the *lig* genes. The mRNA of the lig genes has an unusually long 5′ untranslated region which is predicted to form two stem-loop structures. Structure 2 obscures the ribosome binding site (SD) and start codon and must be unfolded for translation to occur

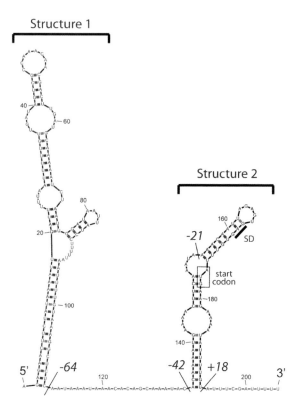

posttranscriptional control by temperature. Mutations on the left or right stem of structure 2 partially relieved inhibition of β-galactosidase expression; inhibition was regained when the mutations were combined to restore base pairing, providing evidence that base-paired RNA is a component of the inhibitory element. These results are consistent with a model in which structure 2 functions as a thermolabile "thermometer," transacting factors may also have a dominant role in melting the inhibitory stem.

The upregulation of LigA and LigB by osmolarity and temperature suggests that these proteins are expressed early during mammalian host infection and may be involved in critical bacterial-host interactions. Various lines of evidence support these conclusions. Patients with leptospirosis have a strong antibody response to the Lig Ig-like repeat domains, suggesting that recombinant Lig repeats would be useful serodiagnostic antigens, confirming that Lig proteins are expressed during infection (Croda et al. 2007). Lig proteins are expressed on the leptospiral surface based on immunoelectron microscopy (Matsunaga et al. 2003) and LigA is released from leptospiral cells (Matsunaga et al. 2005). Osmotic induction of Lig expression resulted in *L. interrogans* becoming more "sticky," with increased adherence to several different extracellular matrix proteins, including fibronectin, fibrinogen, and collagens I and IV (Choy et al. 2007). Heterologous expression of LigA and LigB in *L. biflexa* increased adherence to eukaryotic cells and fibronectin (Figueira et al. 2011). We advocate this "gain of function" approach when studying potential leptospiral adhesins as a way to evaluate the significance of protein-protein interaction assays. LigB binds more avidly to fibronectin and fibrinogen than LigA and the LigB binding activity was localized to 3 of the 12 LigB Ig-like domains; domains 9–11 were both necessary and sufficient to reproduce the binding activity of LigB (Choy et al. 2011). A remarkable aspect of these studies is the range of different proteins to which LigB is able to bind with high avidity. LigB not only binds to complement components and the complement regulatory protein, Factor H, but also inhibits complement activity (Castiblanco-Valencia et al. 2012; Choy 2012). These results suggest that a role of LigB is to coat the leptospiral surface with a variety of circulating host proteins and protect leptospires from host defense mechanisms.

Leptospiral vaccines are discussed in Chapter by Ben Adler, this volume, while their use in humans and animals is described in Chapters by D.A. Haake and P.N. Levett and by W.A. Ellis, this volume. Nevertheless, it should be mentioned in this context that when *L. interrogans* sv Copenhageni is the challenge strain, immunization of hamsters with LigA converts a lethal infection into sublethal kidney colonization. The initial studies showed that the unique part of LigA (Ig-like domains 7–13) was most effective as a vaccine (Silva et al. 2007). Subsequent studies localized the Ig-like domains involved in immunoprotection (Coutinho et al. 2011). There was an absolute requirement for LigA domains 11 and 12. However, these two domains were not sufficient for immunoprotection; a third, flanking domain (either domain 10 or 13) was needed. This requirement for three contiguous Ig-like domains near the carboxy-terminal end of the molecule is highly reminiscent of the finding that LigB domains 9–11 are required for binding activity (see previous paragraph). LigA immunization is effective not only when injected subcutaneously as a purified, recombinant protein, but also when expressed in a lipidated form in *E. coli* that is administered orally (Lourdault et al. 2014). Some important caveats are in order. LigA does not provide sterilizing immunity and because the immunoprotective region of the LigA molecule is subject to variation (McBride et al. 2009), cross-protective immunity may be limited. Additionally, no homologous protection was elicited following immunization of hamsters with LigA from *L. interrogans* serovars Manilae (Deveson Lucas et al. 2011) or Canicola (N. Bomchil, personal communication). An important goal of future studies is to understand why LigA appears to protect against challenge by some serovars but not others.

2.8 More Outer Membrane Lipoproteins

As summarized in Table 1, quantitative MALDI-TOF data reveal that after LipL32, Loa22, and LipL41, the next most abundant OM lipoproteins are LipL36, LipL21, and LipL46 (Malmström et al. 2009). Although LipL36 is an OM protein, it is not surface exposed, being restricted to the inner leaflet of the OM (Haake et al. 1998).

Table 1 Candidate and known leptospiral OM proteins

Name	Locus tag[a]	Type[b]	Size (kd)[c]	Copy number[d]	Knockout virulent?	L. biflexa % identity[e]	Putative function(s), comment[f]
LipL21	10,011	Lip	21	8,830	–	46	–
OmpA	10,050	TM	78*	216*	–	44	Contains OmpA domain
Loa22	10,191	Lip	22	30,329	No	56	Binds peptidoglycan
OmpA	10,258	TM	68*	75*	–	28	Binds peptidoglycan
LigB	10,464	Lip	200	914*	Yes	–	Binds fn, fg, cI, cIV, elst, Ca^{2+}*
LigA	10,465	Lip	130	553*	–	–	Binds fn, fg, col-I, col-IV*
OmpA	10,592	TM	52	118*		39	Also known as Omp52
FecA	10,714	TM	92.5*	529	–	49	TonB DR for Fe^{3+}-dicitrate*
CirA	10,964	TM	86.6*	ND		31	Siderophore uptake receptor
OmpL1	10,973	TM	33	5,441	–	–	Porin*
LipL32	11,352	Lip	32	38,050	Yes	–	Binds Ca^{2+}, lam, cIV, fn*
OstA	11,458	TM	113.5*	145	–	49	LPS assembly
GspD	11,570	TM	66.5*	658	–	62	T2SS channel
BamA	11,623	TM	113*	37	–	64	OMP biogenesis
CirA	11,694	TM	92*	ND		60	Siderophore uptake receptor
LipL46	11,885	Lip	46	5,276	–	54	–
Omp85	12,254	TM	60*	136*	–	–	–
OmpL37	12,263	TM	37	924	–	47	Binds elst*
TolC	12,307	TM	56*	21*	–	48	Export channel
FadL	12,524	TM	52	61*	–	51	Long-chain fatty acid transporter
TolC	12,575	TM	60*	1,064		53	Export channel
TolC	12,693	TM	63.5*	377		50	Export channel
LenA	12,906	Lip	30	ND		–	Binds Factor H, fn, lam
LipL41	12,966	Lip	41	10,531	Yes	–	Binds hemin*

(continued)

Table 1 (continued)

Name	Locus tag[a]	Type[b]	Size (kd)[c]	Copy number[d]	Knockout virulent?	L. biflexa % identity[e]	Putative function(s), comment[f]
OmpL47	13,050	TM	47	5,022	Yes	50	–
LipL36	13,060	Lip	36	14,100		–	Not expressed during infection
TlyC	13,143	TM	50.4*	8*	–	58	Binds fn, lam, cIV*
OmpL54	13,491	TM	54	491	–	44	–
HbpA	20,151	TM	80	14*	Yes[g]	58	TonB DR for hemin*
FecA	20,214	TM	100*	ND	Yes	52	TonB DR for Fe^{3+}-dicitrate

[a] Locus tag for *Leptospira* interrogans serovar Copenhageni, strain L1-130

[b] Type: Lip (lipoprotein), TM (transmembraneOmp), PM (peripheral membrane Omp)

[c] Size (kd): Observed or predicted*

[d] Copy number: Estimated by MS or spectral* methods (Malmström et al. 2009). *ND* None detected

[e] Percent identity with *L. biflexa* homologue

[f] Putative function: T2SS (type 2 secretion system), TonB DR (TonB-dependent receptor), LPS (lipopolysaccharide). Host ligands: fn (fibronectin), fg (fibrinogen), cI (collagen I), cIV (collagen IV), lam (laminin), and elst (elastin). Based on experimental evidence*

[g] Virulent in hamsters but renal colonization deficient in mice

Based on serological evidence (Haake et al. 1998), immunohistochemistry data (Barnett et al. 1999) and downregulation of LipL36 expression at physiologic osmolarity (Matsunaga et al. 2007a, b), LipL36 appears to be expressed only when leptospires are outside the mammalian host. In contrast to LipL36, LipL21 and LipL46 are both surface-exposed and expressed during infection (Cullen et al. 2003, Matsunaga et al. 2006). While not quite as abundant as originally thought, LipL21 is highly expressed during infection based on immunoblot analysis of organisms harvested from infected guinea pigs (Nally et al. 2007) and immuno-histochemistry of liver from infected hamsters (Eshghi et al. 2009). LipL46 can also be detected immunohistochemically in a variety of organs during infection (Matsunaga et al. 2006).

A fundamental difference between leptospiral saprophytes and pathogens is that saprophytes are serum sensitive while pathogens are serum resistant. A common serum resistance mechanism shared by many bacterial pathogens is binding the complement regulators factor H and factor H protein-1. Using a ligand blot approach, *L. interrogans* was found to have two factor H-binding proteins with molecular masses of 25- and 50-kDa. The 25-kDa factor H-binding protein was initialy referred to as LfhA (leptospiral factor H-binding protein) (Verma et al. 2006). A subsequent study identified the same protein as a laminin binding adhesin and applied the des-ignation Lsa24 (leptospiral surface adhesin 24-kD) (Barbosa et al. 2006). Structural analysis revealed that LfhA/Lsa24 was a member of a family of six leptospiral adhesins that share structural similarities with endostatin (Stevenson et al. 2007). For this reason, LfhA/Lsa24 was renamed LenA. In addition to binding Factor H, LenA was subsequently found to bind plasminogen (Verma et al. 2010). Binding of LenA to plasminogen facilitated conversion to plasmin, which in turn degraded fibrinogen, suggesting a role for LenA in penetration through, and/or escape from, fibrin clots. Several other leptospiral OMPs have also been implicated in plasminogen binding and activation (Fernandes et al. 2012; Vieira et al. 2012).

2.9 Transmembrane Outer Membrane Proteins

Transmembrane OMPs are defined as integral OM proteins that contain strands that traverse the lipid bilayer of the OM. Such proteins can be visualized by freeze-fracture electron microscopy (FFEM), a technique that separates the two leaflets of membranes, exposing transmembrane OMPs as studs in a sea of lipid. When applied to spirochetes, FFEM revealed that pathogenic spirochetes, including leptospires, have transmembrane OMPs in far fewer numbers than typical Gram-negative bac-teria (Haake et al. 1991; Radolf et al. 1989; Walker et al. 1991). Transmembrane OMPs are essential for OM-containing bacteria because of their unique ability to form pores or channels that allow bacteria to acquire nutrients and to export toxins and waste products. For researchers interested in bacterial surface antigens, trans-membrane OMPs are of great interest because their surface-exposed loops represent potential targets of a protective immune response.

Transmembrane OMPs have an amino-terminal signal peptide, which facilitates their secretion across the inner membrane to the periplasm by the Sec translocase complex. After removal of the signal peptide by signal peptidase I, transmembrane OMPs are shuttled across the periplasm to the OM by the chaperone SurA (Sklar et al. 2007). LIC12922 of *L. interrogans* serovar Copenhageni has been identified by X-ray crystallography to have both the parvulin and peptide-binding domains of SurA (Giuseppe et al. 2011). The peptide-binding domain allows SurA to keep transmembrane OMPs in an unfolded form until they are delivered to the OMP assembly complex, which consists of the transmembrane OMP, BamA, and several accessory lipoproteins. *L. interrogans* has a BamA homologue with four POTRA domains that are involved in the folding, assembly and insertion of transmembrane OMPs in the OM (Tommassen 2007).

2.10 Discovery of the Porin OmpL1

OmpL1 was one of the first porins to be described in a spirochete, preceded only by the 36.5 kD porin of *Spirochaeta aurantia* (Kropinski et al. 1987). The discovery of OmpL1 resulted from experiments aimed at identifying surface-exposed OMPs. Using a technique called "surface immunoprecipitation," antibodies raised to whole *L. kirschneri* bacteria were added to intact bacteria followed by gentle washing to remove unbound antibodies. The antibody-antigen complexes were solubilized using Triton X-100 detergent and then purified using Protein A beads. In addition to LPS, the surface immunoprecipitate was found to contain three proteins with molecular masses of 33-, 41-, and 44-kD (Haake et al. 1991). The amount of the 33-kD protein was increased in a highly passaged strain of *L. kirchneri*, correlating with the density of transmembrane particles visualized by FFEM. Isolation of the gene encoding the 33-kD protein revealed a series of porin-like transmembrane segments (see next section), and henceforth the protein was called OmpL1 (Haake et al. 1993). The other two proteins were subsequently identified as LipL41 and LipL46. Confirming its role in the leptospiral OM, OmpL1 was later found to have several other properties typical of porins, including: 1. Heat-modifiable electrophoretic mobility; 2. Cross-linkable trimers; and 3. The ability to form channels in lipid bilayers (Shang et al. 1995).

Bacterial porins are of great interest because of their surface exposure and potential to serve as targets of a protective immune response. Like most porins, OmpL1 is hydrophobic and requires detergent for solubilization. Recombinant OmpL1 expressed in *E. coli* with a His6 tag can be purified by nickel chromatography under denaturing conditions. Unfortunately, this denatured form of OmpL1 proved to be ineffective as a vaccine (unpublished results). However, when hamsters were immunized with OmpL1 expressed in *E. coli* as a membrane protein, this resulted in partial protection from lethal and sublethal infection, particularly when combined with a lipidated form of LipL41 (Haake et al. 1999). The *ompL1* gene is present and moderately well conserved (~90 % deduced amino acid sequence identity) across a broad range of pathogenic *Leptospira* species. Interestingly, comparison of sequences from a number of *Leptospira* strains revealed that 20 % of strains carried mosaic *ompL1* genes composed of segments with multiple leptospiral ancestries arising from horizontal DNA transfer and genetic recombination (Haake et al. 2004). These sequence variations, of course, could limit cross-protection from an OmpL1-based vaccine. Other leptospiral genes that have been found to undergo mosaicism include *ligA* and *ligB* (McBride et al. 2009).

2.11 Beta-Barrel Structure of Transmembrane OMPs

As mentioned in the previous section, OmpL1 has a series of transmembrane segments characteristic of channel-forming porins. The transmembrane segments of a number of OMPs from a variety of Gram-negative bacteria have been determined by X-ray crystallography to have a beta-sheet conformation, such that the orientation of amino acid side chains is 180° opposite of those of adjacent amino acids. This allows the side chains of alternating amino acids to interface with the lipid bilayer or with the aqueous pore of the channel. As these transmembrane segments thread their way back and forth across the lipid bilayer, they form the walls of a cylinder or barrel, and such proteins are called "beta barrels." The beta-sheet conformation in these transmembrane strands is the basis for transmembrane OMP prediction programs such as TMBB-PRED (Bagos et al. 2004) and TMBETA-NET (Gromiha and Suwa 2005).

Screening of the *L. interrogans* serovar Copenhageni genome for OMPs by querying the TMBB-PRED webserver revealed 84 genes that met the relatively stringent cutoff score of ≤2.965. As a positive control, the TMBB-PRED algorithm gave OmpL1 a score of 2.900, the sixth best score of any leptospiral protein. A useful feature of TMBB-PRED is that the output includes a plot of the probability of transmembrane membrane beta-strands. As shown in Fig. 8, the TonB-dependent receptor, HbpA received a score of 2.939 and was predicted to have 22 transmembrane beta strands. Using homology-based annotation and sequence-based criteria (signal peptide + ≤3 alpha helices + ≥6 transmembrane beta strands) a list of 184 possible transmembrane OMPs was derived (Pinne et al. 2012). These putative transmembrane OMPs and 177 predicted lipoproteins were expressed by in vitro transcription/translation to construct an OMP proteome array to screen for adherence to fibronectin. 14 novel leptospiral fibronectin-binding proteins were identified, including Lsa66, a previously identified OmpA-like adhesin (Oliveira et al. 2011). Adherence function was confirmed by expression of proteins in *L. biflexa*, conferring dramatically increased fibronectin-binding activity on this surrogate host.

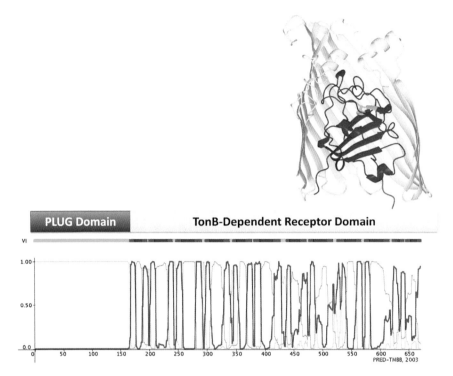

Fig. 8 Topology of TonB-dependent receptor HbpA. Hemin-binding protein A (HbpA, LIC20151) is predicted to have a PLUG domain and a TonB-Dependent Receptor *TBDR* domain. The PLUG domain sits inside the beta-barrel formed by the TBDR domain, reproduced from Oke et al. (2004). The beta-barrel structure is predicted using the TMBB-PRED algorithm

2.12 Experimental Validation of Transmembrane OMPs

A new paradigm has emerged for experimental confirmation of transmembrane OMPs. Originally, Triton X-114 detergent extraction and phase partitioning was thought to be a more or less definitive test for localization of leptospiral proteins (Haake et al. 1991). OMPs were expected to be found, in whole or in part, in the Triton X-114 detergent phase, while cytoplasmic and inner membrane proteins remained in the protoplasmic cylinder fraction and periplasmic proteins fractionated to the aqueous phase. Although many OM components, including LPS and many OMPs, were found in the Triton X-114 detergent phase, it is now clear that a number of transmembrane OMPs do not behave as expected in this detergent (Pinne and Haake 2009).

We now advocate a multistep strategy for defining transmembrane OMPs. The first step is sequence analysis. The sequence of transmembrane OMPs should begin with a signal peptide and signal peptidase I cleavage site but lack a lipobox. The sequence of the mature protein should contain multiple beta-sheet transmembrane segments (predicted using an algorithm such as TMBB-PRED) and should not contain a hydrophobic, membrane-spanning alpha helix. Of course, OMPs such as Loa22 with alpha-helical transmembrane domains are an exception to this rule. The second step is to test whether the protein is an integral membrane protein by treating total leptospiral membranes with reagents, such as high salt, urea, or sodium bicarbonate, that remove membrane-associated proteins (Matsunaga et al. 2002; Pinne and Haake 2009). The third step is to test for surface exposure. Conclusions should not be based on a single method. Several complementary methods are available: surface immunofluorescence, surface proteolysis, and surface biotinylation. In each of these methods, it is essential to include controls. In the case of surface immunofluorescence, control experiments with preimmune sera to show that antibody binding to the leptospiral surface is a result of immunization with the protein of interest must be included. In negative control experiments, it is important to counterstain the slide with DAPI (4′,6-diamidino-2-phenylindole) to show that organisms are present. OmpL1 as a positive control for surface exposure and the endoflagellar protein FlaA1 as a subsurface control must be included. Relatively abundant periplasmic proteins such as FlaA1 are preferred as subsurface controls because these would more readily become surface exposed as a result of OM disruption than cytoplasmic proteins such as GroEL. Information about obtaining antisera for surface and subsurface control antigens is available on our website: http://id-ucla.org/sharing.php.

Using this strategy, four novel leptospiral transmembrane OMPs were defined: OmpL36, OmpL37, OmpL47, and OmpL54 (Pinne and Haake 2009). Each of these four proteins was found to have a signal peptide and signal peptidase I cleavage site and at least 6 membrane-spanning beta-strands. Although OmpL36 and OmpL37 were partially removed from total membrane fractions by sodium bicarbonate, none was removed by high salt or urea. All four proteins were found to be surface exposed by surface immunofluorescence, surface proteolysis, and surface biotinylation except for OmpL36, which was not digested by the highest concentration of proteinase K. It should be noted that OmpL47 (also known as Q8F8Q0) had previously been identified by surface biotinylation as a component of the leptospiral "surfaceome" (Cullen et al. 2005) and is annotated as a glycosyl hydrolase. The behavior of these proteins in Triton X-114 cell fractionation experiments was surprising in that only OmpL54 was found in the Triton X-114 detergent phase. OmpL36 was not extractable with Triton X-114 and was found entirely in the protoplasmic cylinder fraction, which is consistent with the subsequent finding that this protein is a flagellar component (Wunder et al. 2013). While OmpL37 and OmpL47 were partially or completely extracted with Triton X-114, these proteins fractionated into the aqueous phase rather than the detergent phase. These results suggest that localization by Triton X-114 fractionation alone may be unreliable for some types of proteins, especially transmembrane OMPs.

2.13 OMPs Involved in Import Pathways

Pathogenic and saprophytic leptospires appear to have a full complement of TonB-dependent receptors (TB-DRs). TB-DRs are beta-barrel OMPs that function as high affinity receptors and channels for uptake of substrates such as vitamin B_{12} (cobalamin), iron, and other heavy metals. Uptake is energy- dependent and requires interactions between TB-DRs in the OM and TonB in the IM. *L. interrogans* has 12 genes encoding TB-DRs and 3 genes encoding TonB. Thanks to the elegant work of Picardeau and colleagues on TB-DRs of *L. biflexa*, the function of several leptospiral TB-DRs is now known (Louvel et al. 2006). For example, the *L. biflexa* mutant lacking gene LEPBIa2760 was unable to grow on the siderophore desferrioxamine as a source of iron, thereby indicating that this gene encodes the siderophore uptake receptor CirA. Because many TB-DRs are highly conserved across leptospiral species, this information is relevant to pathogenic leptospires. The amino acid sequence of LEPBIa2760 is 77 % identical with that of LIC11694. Likewise, LEPBIa1883 and LIC10714 encode the Fe^{3+}-dicitrate receptor FecA. As shown in Fig. 9, both LIC11694 (CirA) and LIC10714 (FecA) have paralogs that presumably perform similar, if not redundant, functions. LIC20151 has been shown

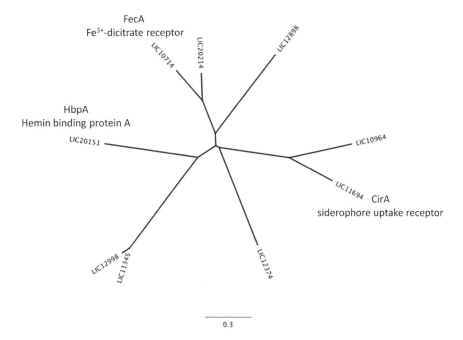

Fig. 9 Relatedness tree for leptospiral TonB-dependent receptors *TBDRs*. The *L. interrogans* serovar Copenhageni strain L1-130 genome is predicted to contain 9 TBDR genes involved in uptake of vitamin B12, iron and other metals. The functions of the three TBDR genes that have been elucidated are shown

to bind hemin, and represents a third TB-DR class. Three additional TB-DR classes remain to be characterized, but presumably are involved in uptake of vitamin B12, copper, or nickel (Schauer et al. 2008). Leptospires also have OM proteins involved in TonB-independent import pathways, such as FadL (LIC12524), the long-chain fatty acid transporter.

2.14 OMPs Involved in Export Pathways (TolC and GspD)

Leptospires have at least two different OMP-mediated export pathways: Type 1 secretion involving TolC and Type 2 secretion involving GspD. Type 1 secretion is Sec-independent, meaning that substrates can be exported directly from the cytoplasm. In the case of proteins (e.g., hemolysins), this means that a signal peptide is not required. Type I secretion can also be involved in efflux of drugs or toxins, such as heavy metals. TolC is the OMP component of the Type 1 secretory apparatus and forms a beta barrel channel in the OM and spans the periplasm to the IM where it engages with a translocase to form a contiguous passage from the cytoplasm to the exterior of the cell. *L. interrogans* encodes seven TolC homologs, presumably to accommodate different types of translocases and substrates. One of these TolC proteins, LIC12575, is expressed at high levels in cultivated cells. Type 2 secretion is Sec-dependent, meaning that proteins exported via this pathway must have a signal peptide and be secreted first to the periplasm before exiting the cell. As discussed above, Type 2 secretion represents a potential pathway for lipoprotein export in *Leptospira* species, as has been demonstrated in *Klebsiella* (d'Enfert et al. 1987; Sauvonnet and Pugsley 1996). Possible substrates include potential lipoproteins LigA and Sph2, which are released from *L. interrogans* in response to elevated osmolarity and/or temperature (Matsunaga et al. 2005, 2007b).

2.15 LipL45 and Related Peripheral Membrane Proteins

LipL45 was first identified as a protein, designated Qlp42, whose expression was upregulated when *L. interrogans* cultures were shifted from 30° to 37 °C (Nally et al. 2001a). Subsequent studies revealed that Qlp42 was initially expressed as a 45-kD lipoprotein, the carboxy-terminal portion of which was removed to become a 31-kD peripheral membrane protein, designated $P31_{LipL45}$ (Matsunaga et al. 2002). Peripheral membrane proteins are membrane-associated proteins that are not integrated into the lipid bilayer and can be removed by treating membranes with a variety of reagents such as high salt, urea, or sodium bicarbonate. The latter two reagents removed $P31_{LipL45}$ from *L. interrogans* membranes, but had no effect on LipL41. Interestingly, in addition to upregulation of expression at higher temperatures, $P31_{LipL45}$ was dramatically increased in stationary phase cultures of *L. interrogans*. The function, membrane location(s), and surface exposure of $P31_{LipL45}$ remain to be determined. Genome sequencing has revealed that LipL45 belongs to a large family of leptospiral proteins; *L. interrogans* has 11 LipL45-related genes, most of which are predicted to be lipoproteins. Although LipL45 itself is the most highly expressed member of the family in cultivated cells (Malmström et al. 2009), two other family members are expressed at comparable levels, which probably explains why $P31_{LipL45}$ appears as a doublet in many strains of pathogenic leptospires (Matsunaga et al. 2002).

Acknowledgments The authors are extremely grateful to Dr. James Matsunaga for his helpful comments on regulation of Lig expression. Current work in Dr. Haake's laboratory is supported by NIH Grant R01 AI034431 and a VA Merit Award. Current work in Dr. Zückert's laboratory is supported by NIH Grant P30 GM103326 and a University of Kansas Medical Center Research Institute Lied Basic Science Pilot Grant.

References

Asuthkar S, Velineni S, Stadimann J, Altmann F, Sritharan M (2007) Expression and characterization of an iron-regulated hemin-binding protein, HbpA, from *Leptospira interrogans* serovar Lai. Infect Immun 75:4582–4591

Bagos PG, Liakopoulos TD, Spyropoulos IC, Hamodrakas SJ (2004) PRED-TMBB: a web server for predicting the topology of beta-barrel outer membrane proteins. Nucleic Acids Res 32: W400–W404

Barbosa AS, Abreu PA, Neves FO, Atzingen MV, Watanabe MM, Vieira ML, Morais ZM, Vasconcellos SA, Nascimento AL (2006) A newly identified leptospiral adhesin mediates attachment to laminin. Infect Immun 74:6356–6364

Barnett JK, Barnett D, Bolin CA, Summers TA, Wagar EA, Cheville NF, Hartskeerl RA, Haake DA (1999) Expression and distribution of leptospiral outer membrane components during renal infection of hamsters. Infect Immun 67:853–861

Bos MP, Robert V, Tommassen J (2007) Biogenesis of the gram-negative bacterial outer membrane. Annu Rev Microbiol 61:191–214

Cao XJ, Dai J, Xu H, Nie S, Chang X, Hu BY, Sheng QH, Wang LS, Ning ZB, Li YX, Guo XK, Zhao GP, Zeng R (2010) High-coverage proteome analysis reveals the first insight of protein modification systems in the pathogenic spirochete *Leptospira interrogans*. Cell Res 20:197–210

Castiblanco-Valencia MM, Fraga TR, Silva LB, Monaris D, Abreu PA, Strobel S, Jozsi M, Isaac L, Barbosa AS (2012) Leptospiral immunoglobulin-like proteins interact with human complement regulators factor H, FHL-1, FHR-1, and C4BP. J Infect Dis 205:995–1004

Chen S, Zückert WR (2011) Probing the *Borrelia burgdorferi* surface lipoprotein secretion pathway using a conditionally folding protein domain. J Bacteriol 193:6724–6732

Choy HA (2012) Multiple activities of LigB potentiate virulence of *Leptospira interrogans*: inhibition of alternative and classical pathways of complement. PLoS ONE 7:e41566

Choy HA, Kelley MM, Chen TL, Moller AK, Matsunaga J, Haake DA (2007) Physiological osmotic induction of *Leptospira interrogans* adhesion: LigA and LigB bind extracellular matrix proteins and fibrinogen. Infect Immun 75:2441–2450

Choy HA, Kelley MM, Croda J, Matsunaga J, Babbitt JT, Ko AI, Picardeau M, Haake DA (2011) The multifunctional LigB adhesin binds homeostatic proteins with potential roles in cutaneous infection by pathogenic *Leptospira interrogans*. PLoS ONE 6:e16879

Coutinho ML, Choy HA, Haake D (2011) A LigA three-domain region protects hamsters from lethal infection by *Leptospira interrogans*. PLoS Neg Trop Dis 5:e1422

Cowles CE, Li Y, Semmelhack MF, Cristea IM, Silhavy TJ (2011) The free and bound forms of Lpp occupy distinct subcellular locations in Escherichia coli. Mol Microbiol 79:1168–1181

Croda J, Ramos JG, Matsunaga J, Queiroz A, Homma A, Riley LW, Haake DA, Reis MG, Ko AI (2007) *Leptospira* immunoglobulin-like proteins as a serodiagnostic marker for acute leptospirosis. J Clin Microbiol 45:1528–1534

Cullen PA, Cordwell SJ, Bulach DM, Haake DA, Adler B (2002) Global analysis of outer membrane proteins from *Leptospira interrogans* serovar Lai. Infect Immun 70:2311–2318

Cullen PA, Haake DA, Bulach DM, Zuerner RL, Adler B (2003) LipL21 is a novel surface-exposed lipoprotein of pathogenic *Leptospira* species. Infect Immun 71:2414–2421

Cullen PA, Xu X, Matsunaga J, Sanchez Y, Ko AI, Haake DA, Adler B (2005) Surfaceome of *Leptospira* spp. Infect Immun 73:4853–4863

d'Enfert C, Ryter A, Pugsley AP (1987) Cloning and expression in *Escherichia coli* of the *Klebsiella pneumoniae* genes for production, surface localization and secretion of the lipoprotein pullulanase. EMBO J 6:3531–3538

Deveson Lucas DS, Cullen PA, Lo M, Srikram A, Sermswan RW, Adler B (2011) Recombinant LipL32 and LigA from *Leptospira* are unable to stimulate protective immunity against leptospirosis in the hamster model. Vaccine 29:3413–3418

Dong C, Beis K, Nesper J, Brunkan-LaMontagne AL, Clarke BR, Whitfield C, Naismith JH (2006) Wza the translocon for *E. coli* capsular polysaccharides defines a new class of membrane protein. Nature 444:226–229

Eshghi A, Cullen PA, Cowen L, Zuerner RL, Cameron CE (2009) Global proteome analysis of Leptospira interrogans. J Proteome Res 8:4564–4578

Eshghi A, Pinne M, Haake DA, Zuerner RL, Frank A, Cameron CE (2012) Methylation and *in vivo* expression of the surface-exposed *Leptospira interrogans* outer membrane protein OmpL32. Microbiol 158:622–635

Farrelly HE, Adler B, Faine S (1987) Opsonic monoclonal antibodies against lipopolysaccharide antigens of *Leptospira interrogans* serovar hardjo. J Med Microbiol 23:1–7

Fernandes LG, Vieira ML, Kirchgatter K, Alves IJ, de Morais ZM, Vasconcellos SA, Romero EC, Nascimento AL (2012) OmpL1 is an extracellular matrix- and plasminogen-interacting protein of *Leptospira* spp. Infect Immun 80:3679–3692

Figueira CP, Croda J, Choy HA, Haake DA, Reis MG, Ko AI, Picardeau M (2011) Heterologous expression of pathogen-specific genes ligA and ligB in the saprophyte *Leptospira biflexa* confers enhanced adhesion to cultured cells and extracellular matrix components. BMC Microbiol 11:129

Giuseppe PO, Von Atzingen M, Nascimento AL, Zanchin NI, Guimaraes BG (2011) The crystal structure of the leptospiral hypothetical protein LIC12922 reveals homology with the periplasmic chaperone SurA. J Struct Biol 173:312–322

Gromiha MM, Suwa M (2005) A simple statistical method for discriminating outer membrane proteins with better accuracy. Bioinformatics 21:961–968

Haake DA (2000) Spirochaetal lipoproteins and pathogenesis. Microbiol 146:1491–1504

Haake DA, Matsunaga J (2002) Characterization of the leptospiral outer membrane and description of three novel leptospiral membrane proteins. Infect Immun 70:4936–4945

Haake DA, Walker EM, Blanco DR, Bolin CA, Miller MN, Lovett MA (1991) Changes in the surface of *Leptospira interrogans* serovar grippotyphosa during in vitro cultivation. Infect Immun 59:1131–1140

Haake DA, Champion CI, Martinich C, Shang ES, Blanco DR, Miller JN, Lovett MA (1993) Molecular cloning and sequence analysis of the gene encoding OmpL1, a transmembrane outer membrane protein of pathogenic *Leptospira* spp. J Bacteriol 175:4225–4234

Haake DA, Martinich C, Summers TA, Shang ES, Pruetz JD, McCoy AM, Mazel MK, Bolin CA (1998) Characterization of leptospiral outer membrane lipoprotein LipL36: downregulation associated with late-log-phase growth and mammalian infection. Infect Immun 66:1579–1587

Haake DA, Mazel MK, McCoy AM, Milward F, Chao G, Matsunaga J, Wagar EA (1999) Leptospiral outer membrane proteins OmpL1 and LipL41 exhibit synergistic immunoprotection. Infect Immun 67:6572–6582

Haake DA, Chao G, Zuerner RL, Barnett JK, Barnett D, Mazel M, Matsunaga J, Levett PN, Bolin CA (2000) The leptospiral major outer membrane protein LipL32 is a lipoprotein expressed during mammalian infection. Infect Immun 68:2276–2285

Haake DA, Suchard MA, Kelley MM, Dundoo M, Alt DP, Zuerner RL (2004) Molecular evolution and mosaicism of leptospiral outer membrane proteins involves horizontal DNA transfer. J Bacteriol 186:2818–2828

Hauk P, Guzzo CR, Roman Ramos H, Ho PL, Farah CS (2009) Structure and calcium-binding activity of LipL32, the major surface antigen of pathogenic *Leptospira* sp. J Mol Biol 390:722–736

Hauk P, Barbosa AS, Ho PL, Farah CS (2012) Calcium binding to leptospira outer membrane antigen LipL32 is not necessary for its interaction with plasma fibronectin, collagen type IV, and plasminogen. J Biol Chem 287:4826–4834

Jost BH, Adler B, Faine S (1989) Experimental immunisation of hamsters with lipopolysaccharide antigens of *Leptospira interrogans*. J Med Microbiol 29:115–120

King AM, Bartpho T, Sermswan RW, Bulach DM, Eshghi A, Picardeau M, Adler B, Murray GL (2013) Leptospiral outer membrane protein LipL41 is not essential for acute leptospirosis but requires a small chaperone protein, Lep, for stable expression. Infect Immun 81:2768–2776

Koizumi N, Watanabe H (2003) Molecular cloning and characterization of a novel leptospiral lipoprotein with OmpA domain. FEMS Microbiol Lett 226:215–219

Kovacs-Simon A, Titball RW, Michell SL (2011) Lipoproteins of bacterial pathogens. Infect Immun 79:548–561

Kropinski AM, Parr TR Jr, Angus BL, Hancock RE, Ghiorse WC, Greenberg EP (1987) Isolation of the outer membrane and characterization of the major outer membrane protein from *Spirochaeta aurantia*. J Bacteriol 169:172–179

Kumru OS, Schulze RJ, Slusser JG, Zückert WR (2010) Development and validation of a FACS-based lipoprotein localization screen in the Lyme disease spirochete *Borrelia burgdorferi*. BMC Microbiol 10:277

Kumru OS, Schulze RJ, Rodnin MV, Ladokhin AS, Zuckert WR (2011) Surface localization determinants of *Borrelia* OspC/Vsp family lipoproteins. J Bacteriol 193:2814–2825

Lee PA, Tullman-Ercek D, Georgiou G (2006) The bacterial twin-arginine translocation pathway. Annu Rev Microbiol 60:373–395

Lessa-Aquino C, Borges Rodrigues C, Pablo J, Sasaki R, Jasinskas A, Liang L, Wunder EA Jr, Ribeiro GS, Vigil A, Galler R, Molina D, Liang X, Reis MG, Ko AI, Medeiros MA, Felgner PL (2013) Identification of seroreactive proteins of *Leptospira interrogans* serovar Copenhageni using a high-density protein microarray approach. PLoS Negl Trop Dis 7:e2499

Lin MH, Chang YC, Hsiao CD, Huang SH, Wang MS, Ko YC, Yang CW, Sun YJ (2013) LipL41, a hemin binding protein from *Leptospira santarosai* serovar Shermani. PLoS ONE 8:e83246

Lo M, Bulach DM, Powell DR, Haake DA, Matsunaga J, Paustian ML, Zuerner RL, Adler B (2006) Effects of temperature on gene expression patterns in *Leptospira interrogans* serovar Lai as assessed by whole-genome microarrays. Infect Immun 74:5848–5859

Lo M, Cordwell SJ, Bulach DM, Adler B (2009) Comparative transcriptional and translational analysis of leptospiral outer membrane protein expression in response to temperature. PLoS Negl Trop Dis 3:e560

Lo M, Murray GL, Khoo CA, Haake DA, Zuerner RL, Adler B (2010) Transcriptional response of *Leptospira interrogans* to iron limitation and characterization of a PerR homolog. Infect Immun 78:4850–4859

Lourdault K, Wang LC, Vieira A, Matsunaga J, Melo R, Lewis MS, Haake DA, Gomes-Solecki M (2014) Oral immunization with *E. coli* expressing a lipidated form of LigA protects hamsters against challenge with *Leptospira interrogans* serovar Copenhageni. Infect Immun doi:10.1128/IAI.01533-13

Louvel H, Bommezzadri S, Zidane N, Boursaux-Eude C, Creno S, Magnier A, Rouy Z, Médigue C, Saint Girons I, Bouchier C, Picardeau M (2006) Comparative and functional genomic analyses of iron transport and regulation in *Leptospira* spp. J Bacteriol 188:7893–7904

Malmström J, Beck M, Schmidt A, Lange V, Deutsch EW, Aebersold R (2009) Proteome-wide cellular protein concentrations of the human pathogen *Leptospira interrogans*. Nature 460:762–766

Matsui M, Soupé ME, Becam J, Goarant C (2012) Differential in vivo gene expression of major *Leptospira* proteins in resistant or susceptible animal models. Appl Environ Microbiol 78:6372–6376

Matsunaga J, Young TA, Barnet JK, Barnett D, Bolin CA, Haake DA (2002) Novel 45-kilodalton leptospiral protein that is processed to a 31-kilodalton growth-phase-regulated peripheral membrane protein. Infect Immun 70:323–334

Matsunaga J, Barocchi MA, Croda J, Young TA, Sanchez Y, Siqueira I, Bolin CA, Reis MG, Riley LW, Haake DA, Ko AI (2003) Pathogenic *Leptospira* species express surface-exposed proteins belonging to the bacterial immunoglobulin superfamily. Mol Microbiol 49:929–945

Matsunaga J, Sanchez Y, Xu X, Haake DA (2005) Osmolarity, a key environmental signal controlling expression of leptospiral proteins LigA and LigB and the extracellular release of LigA. Infect Immun 73:70–78

Matsunaga J, Wernied K, Zuerner R, Frank A, Haake, DA (2006) LipL46 is a novel, surface-exposed lipoprotein expressed during leptospiral dissemination in the mammalian host. Microbiol 152, 3777–3786

Matsunaga J, Lo M, Bulach DM, Zuerner RL, Adler B, Haake DA (2007a) Response of *Leptospira interrogans* to physiologic osmolarity: relevance in signaling the environment-to-host transition. Infect Immun 75:2864–2874

Matsunaga J, Medeiros MA, Sanchez Y, Werneid KF, Ko AI (2007b) Osmotic regulation of expression of two extracellular matrix-binding proteins and a haemolysin of *Leptospira interrogans*: differential effects on LigA and Sph2 extracellular release. Microbiol 153:3390–3398

Matsunaga J, Schlax PJ, Haake DA (2013) Role for cis-acting RNA sequences in the temperature-dependent expression of the multiadhesive Lig proteins in *Leptospira interrogans*. J Bacteriol 195:5092–5101

McBride AJ, Cerqueira GM, Suchard MA, Moreira AN, Zuerner RL, Reis MG, Haake DA, Ko AI, Dellagostin OA (2009) Genetic diversity of the leptospiral immunoglobulin-like (Lig) genes in pathogenic *Leptospira* spp. Infect Genet Evol 9:196–205

Midwinter AC, Vinh T, Faine S, Adler B (1994) Characterization of an antigenic oligosaccharide from *Leptospira interrogans* serovar pomona and its role in immunity. Infect Immun 62:5477–5482

Murray GL (2013) The lipoprotein LipL32, an enigma of leptospiral biology. Vet Microbiol 162:305–314

Murray GL, Morel V, Cerqueira GM, Croda J, Srikram A, Henry R, Ko AI, Dellagostin OA, Bulach DM, Sermswan RW, Adler B, Picardeau M (2009a) Genome-wide transposon mutagenesis in pathogenic *Leptospira* species. Infect Immun 77:810–816

Murray GL, Srikram A, Hoke DE, Wunder EA Jr, Henry R, Lo M, Zhang K, Sermswan RW, Ko AI, Adler B (2009b) Major surface protein LipL32 is not required for either acute or chronic infection with *Leptospira interrogans*. Infect Immun 77:952–958

Murray GL, Srikram A, Henry R, Hartskeerl RA, Sermswan RW, Adler B (2010) Mutations affecting *Leptospira interrogans* lipopolysaccharide attenuate virulence. Mol Microbiol 78:701–709

Nahori MA, Fournie-Amazouz E, Que-Gewirth NS, Balloy V, Chignard M, Raetz CR, Saint Girons I, Werts C (2005) Differential TLR recognition of leptospiral lipid A and lipopolysaccharide in murine and human cells. J Immunol 175:6022–6031

Nally JE, Artiushin S, Timoney JF (2001a) Molecular characterization of thermoinduced immunogenic proteins Q1p42 and Hsp15 of *Leptospira interrogans*. Infect Immun 69:7616–7624

Nally JE, Timoney JF, Stevenson B (2001b) Temperature-regulated protein synthesis by *Leptospira interrogans*. Infect Immun 69:400–404

Nally JE, Chow E, Fishbein MC, Blanco DR, Lovett MA (2005a) Changes in lipopolysaccharide O antigen distinguish acute versus chronic *Leptospira interrogans* infections. Infect Immun 73:3251–3260

Nally JE, Whitelegge JP, Aguilera R, Pereira MM, Blanco DR, Lovett MA (2005b) Purification and proteomic analysis of outer membrane vesicles from a clinical isolate of *Leptospira interrogans* serovar Copenhageni. Proteomics 5:144–152

Nally JE, Whitelegge JP, Bassilian S, Blanco DR, Lovett MA (2007) Characterization of the outer membrane proteome of *Leptospira interrogans* expressed during acute lethal infection. Infect Immun 75:766–773

Nascimento AL, Ko AI, Martins EA, Monteiro-Vitorello CB, Ho PL, Haake DA, Verjovski-Almeida S, Hartskeerl RA, Marques MV, Oliveira MC, Menck CF, Leite LC, Carrer H, Coutinho LL, Degrave WM, Dellagostin OA, El-Dorry H, Ferro ES, Ferro MI, Furlan LR, Gamberini M, Giglioti EA, Góes-Neto A, Goldman GH, Goldman MH, Harakava R, Jerônimo SM, Junqueira-de-Azevedo IL, Kimura ET, Kuramae EE, Lemos EG, Lemos MV, Marino CL, Nunes LR, de Oliveira RC, Pereira GG, Reis MS, Schriefer A, Siqueira WJ, Sommer P, Tsai SM, Simpson AJ, Ferro JA, Camargo LE, Kitajima JP, Setubal JC, Van Sluys MA (2004) Comparative genomics of two *Leptospira interrogans* serovars reveals novel insights into physiology and pathogenesis. J Bacteriol 186:2164–2172

Oke M, Sarra R, Ghirlando R, Farnaud S, Gorringe AR, Evans RW, Buchanan SK (2004) The plug domain of a neisserial TonB-dependent transporter retains structural integrity in the absence of its transmembrane beta-barrel. FEBS lett 564:294–300

Oliveira TR, Longhi MT, Goncales AP, de Morais ZM, Vasconcellos SA, Nascimento AL (2010) LipL53, a temperature regulated protein from *Leptospira interrogans* that binds to extracellular matrix molecules. Microbes Infect 12:207–217

Oliveira R, de Morais ZM, Goncales AP, Romero EC, Vasconcellos SA, Nascimento AL (2011) Characterization of novel OmpA-like protein of *Leptospira interrogans* that binds extracellular matrix molecules and plasminogen. PLoS ONE 6:e21962

Patarakul K, Lo M, Adler B (2010) Global transcriptomic response of *Leptospira interrogans* serovar Copenhageni upon exposure to serum. BMC Microbiol 10:31

Pinne M, Haake DA (2009) A comprehensive approach to identification of surface-exposed, outer membrane-spanning proteins of *Leptospira interrogans*. PLoS ONE 4:e6071

Pinne M, Haake DA (2011) Detection of leptospiral surface-exposed proteins via immunofluorescence. J Vis Exp 53:2805

Pinne M, Haake DA (2013) LipL32 is a subsurface lipoprotein of *Leptospira interrogans*: presentation of new data and reevaluation of previous studies. PLoS ONE 8:e51025

Pinne M, Matsunaga J, Haake DA (2012) A novel approach to identification of leptospiral ligand-binding proteins: an outer-membrane protein microarray. J Bacteriol 194:6074–6087

Pomorski T, Menon AK (2006) Lipid flippases and their biological functions. Cell Mol Life Sci 63:2908–2921

Que-Gewirth NS, Riberio AA, Kalb SR, Cotter RJ, Bulach DM, Adler B, Saint Girons I, Werts C, Raetz CR (2004) A methylated phosphate group and four amide-linked acyl chains in *Leptospira interrogans* Lipid A. J Biol Chem 279:25420–25429

Raddi G, Morado DR, Yan J, Haake DA, Yang XF, Liu J (2012) Three-dimensional structures of pathogenic and saprophytic *Leptospira* species revealed by cryo-electron tomography. J Bacteriol 194:1299–1306

Radolf JD, Norgard MV, Schulz WW (1989) Outer membrane ultrastructure explains the limited antigenicity of virulent *Treponema pallidum*. Proc Natl Acad Sci USA 86:2051–2055

Ren SX, Fu G, Jiang XG, Zeng R, Miao YG, Xu H, Zhang YX, Xiong H, Lu G, Lu LF, Jiang HQ, Jia J, Tu YF, Jiang JX, Gu WY, Zhang YQ, Cai Z, Sheng HH, Yin HF, Zhang Y, Zhu GF, Wan M, Huang HL, Qian Z, Wang SY, Ma W, Yao ZJ, Shen Y, Qiang BQ, Xia QC, Guo XK, Danchin A, Saint Girons I, Somerville RL, Wen YM, Shi MH, Chen Z, Xu JG, Zhao GP (2003) Unique physiological and pathogenic features of *Leptospira interrogans* revealed by whole-genome sequencing. Nature 422:888–893

Ristow P, Bourhy P, da Cruz McBride FW, Figueira CP, Huerre M, Ave P, Saint Girons I, Ko AI, Picardeau M (2007) The OmpA-like protein Loa22 is essential for leptospiral virulence. PLoS Pathog 3:e97

Ruiz N, Kahne D, Silhavy TJ (2009) Transport of lipopolysaccharide across the cell envelope: the long road of discovery. Nat Rev Microbiol 7:677–683

Sauvonnet N, Pugsley AP (1996) Identification of two regions of *Klebsiella oxytoca* pullulanase that together are capable of promoting beta-lactamase secretion by the general secretory pathway. Mol Microbiol 22:1–7

Schauer K, Rodionov DA, de Reuse H (2008) New substrates for TonB-dependent transport: do we only see the 'tip of the iceberg'? Trends Biochem Sci 33:330–338

Schulze RJ, Zuckert WR (2006) *Borrelia burgdorferi* lipoproteins are secreted to the outer surface by default. Mol Microbiol 59:1473–1484

Schulze RJ, Chen S, Kumru OS, Zückert WR (2010) Translocation of *Borrelia burgdorferi* surface lipoprotein OspA through the outer membrane requires an unfolded conformation and can initiate at the C-terminus. Mol Microbiol 76:1266–1278

Setubal JC, Reis M, Matsunaga J, Haake DA (2006) Lipoprotein computational prediction in spirochaetal genomes. Microbiol 152:113–121

Shang ES, Exner MM, Summers TA, Martinich C, Champion CI, Hancock RE, Haake DA (1995) The rare outer membrane protein, OmpL1, of pathogenic *Leptospira* species is a heat-modifiable porin. Infect Immun 63:3174–3181

Shang ES, Summers TA, Haake DA (1996) Molecular cloning and sequence analysis of the gene encoding LipL41, a surface-exposed lipoprotein of pathogenic *Leptospira* species. Infect Immun 64:2322–2330

Silva EF, Medeiros MA, McBride AJ, Matsunaga J, Esteves GS, Ramos JG, Santos CS, Croda J, Homma A, Dellagostin OA, Haake DA, Reis MG, Ko AI (2007) The terminal portion of leptospiral immunoglobulin-like protein LigA confers protective immunity against lethal infection in the hamster model of leptospirosis. Vaccine 25:6277–6286

Sklar JG, Wu T, Kahne D, Silhavy TJ (2007) Defining the roles of the periplasmic chaperones SurA, Skp, and DegP in *Escherichia coli*. Genes Develop 21:2473–2484

Sperandeo P, Deho G, Polissi A (2009) The lipopolysaccharide transport system of Gram-negative bacteria. Biochim Biophys Acta 1791:594–602

Srikram A, Zhang K, Bartpho T, Lo M, Hoke DE, Sermswan RW, Adler B, Murray GL (2011) Cross-protective immunity against leptospirosis elicited by a live, attenuated lipopolysaccharide mutant. J Infect Dis 203:870–879

Stevenson B, Choy HA, Pinne M, Rotondi ML, Miller MC, Demoll E, Kraiczy P, Cooley AE, Creamer TP, Suchard MA, Brissette CA, Verma A, Haake DA (2007) *Leptospira interrogans* endostatin-like outer membrane proteins bind host fibronectin, laminin and regulators of complement. PLoS ONE 2:e1188

Tommassen J (2007) Getting into and through the outer membrane. Science 317:903–904

Verma A, Artiushin S, Matsunaga J, Haake DA, Timoney JF (2005) LruA and LruB, novel lipoproteins of pathogenic *Leptospira interrogans* associated with equine recurrent uveitis. Infect Immun 73:7259–7266

Verma A, Hellwage J, Artiushin S, Zipfel PF, Kraiczy P, Timoney JF, Stevenson B (2006) LfhA, a novel factor H-binding protein of *Leptospira interrogans*. Infect Immun 74:2659–2666

Verma A, Brissette CA, Bowman AA, Shah ST, Zipfel PF, Stevenson B (2010) Leptospiral endostatin-like protein A (LenA) is a bacterial cell-surface receptor for human plasminogen. Infect Immun 78:2053–2059

Vieira ML, Atzingen MV, Oliveira R, Mendes RS, Domingos RF, Vasconcellos S, Nascimento AL (2012) Plasminogen binding proteins and plasmin generation on the surface of *Leptospira* spp.: the contribution to the bacteria-host interactions. J Biomed Biotechnol 2012:758513

Viriyakosol S, Matthias MA, Swancutt MA, Kirkland TN, Vinetz JM (2006) Toll-like receptor 4 protects against lethal *Leptospira interrogans* serovar icterohaemorrhagiae infection and contributes to in vivo control of leptospiral burden. Infect Immun 74:887–895

Vivian JP, Beddoe T, McAlister AD, Wilce MC, Zaker-Tabrizi L, Troy S, Byres E, Hoke DE, Cullen PA, Lo M, Murray GL, Adler B, Rossjohn J (2009) Crystal structure of LipL32, the most abundant surface protein of pathogenic *Leptospira* spp. J Mol Biol 387:1229–1238

Walker EM, Borenstein LA, Blanco DR, Miller JN, Lovett MA (1991) Analysis of outer membrane ultrastructure of pathogenic *Treponema* and *Borrelia* species by freeze-fracture electron microscopy. J Bacteriol 173:5585–5588

Werts C (2010) Leptospirosis: a Toll road from B lymphocytes. Chang Gung Med J 3:591–601

Werts C, Tapping RI, Mathison JC, Chuang TH, Kravchenko V, Saint Girons I, Haake DA, Godowski PJ, Hayashi F, Ozinsky A, Underhill DM, Kirschning CJ, Wagner H, Aderem A, Tobias PS, Ulevitch RJ (2001) Leptospiral endotoxin activates cells via a TLR2-dependent mechanism. Nature Immunol 2:346–352

Wunder EA Jr, Figueira CP, Benaroudj N, Hu B, Tong BA, Trajtenberg F, Liu J, Reis MG, Charon N, Buschiazzo A, Picardeau M, Ko AI (2013) *Leptospira* Fcp1 is a key protein in determining the coiled morphology of purified flagella and conferring translational motility and virulence for the spirochete. In: 8th Scientific Meeting of the International Leptospirosis Society, Fukuoka, Japan

Xue F, Dong H, Wu J, Wu Z, Hu W, Sun A, Troxell B, Yang XF, Yan J (2010) Transcriptional responses of *Leptospira interrogans* to host innate immunity: significant changes in metabolism, oxygen tolerance, and outer membrane. PLoS Negl Trop Dis 4:e857

Yakushi T, Masuda K, Narita S, Matsuyama S, Tokuda H (2000) A new ABC transporter mediating the detachment of lipid-modified proteins from membranes. Nat Cell Biol 2:212–218

Yang CW, Wu MS, Pan MJ, Hsieh WJ, Vandewalle A, Huang CC (2002) The *Leptospira* outer membrane protein LipL32 induces tubulointerstitial nephritis-mediated gene expression in mouse proximal tubule cells. J Am Soc Nephrol 13:2037–2045

Yang CW, Hung CC, Wu MS, Tian YC, Chang CT, Pan MJ, Vandewalle A (2006) Toll-like receptor 2 mediates early inflammation by leptospiral outer membrane proteins in proximal tubule cells. Kidney Int 69:815–822

Yokota N, Kuroda T, Matsuyama S, Tokuda H (1999) Characterization of the LolA-LolB system as the general lipoprotein localization mechanism of *Escherichia coli*. J Biol Chem 274:30995–30999

Zhang K, Murray GL, Seemann T, Srikram A, Bartpho T, Sermswan RW, Adler B, Hoke DE (2013) Leptospiral LruA is required for virulence and modulates an interaction with mammalian apolipoprotein AI. Infect Immun 81:3872–3879

Zuerner RL, Knudtson W, Bolin CA, Trueba G (1991) Characterization of outer membrane and secreted proteins of *Leptospira interrogans* serovar pomona. Microb Pathog 10:311–322

Host Response to *Leptospira* Infection

Richard L. Zuerner

Abstract Pathogenic *Leptospira* has the capacity to infect a broad range of mammalian hosts. Leptospirosis may appear as an acute, potentially fatal infection in accidental hosts, or progress into a chronic, largely asymptomatic infection in natural maintenance hosts. The course that *Leptospira* infection follows is dependent upon poorly understood factors, but is heavily influenced by both the host species and bacterial serovar involved in infection. Recognition of pathogen-associated molecular patterns (PAMPs) by a variety of host pattern recognition receptors (PRRs) activates the host immune system. The outcome of this response may result in bacterial clearance, limited bacterial colonization of a few target organs, principally the kidney, or induction of sepsis as the host succumbs to infection and dies. This chapter describes current knowledge of how the host recognizes *Leptospira* and responds to infection using innate and acquired immune responses. Aspects of immune-mediated pathology and pathogen strategies to evade the host immune response are also addressed.

Contents

R.L. Zuerner (✉)
Department of Biomedical Sciences and Veterinary Public Health, Swedish University for Agricultural Sciences, 75007 Uppsala, Sweden
e-mail: Richard.Zuerner@gmail.com

© Springer-Verlag Berlin Heidelberg 2015   223
B. Adler (ed.), *Leptospira and Leptospirosis*, Current Topics in Microbiology and Immunology 387, DOI 10.1007/978-3-662-45059-8_9

1 Introduction

Leptospira can cause two distinctly different disease manifestations depending on the mammalian host and infecting serovar. Infection leads to either a chronic, nearly asymptomatic infection or an acute, potentially life-threatening disease. The most severe form, classic Weil's disease, or acute leptospirosis, occurs most commonly in accidental hosts, including humans, with a wide range of disease manifestations (Faine et al. 1999). In contrast, infection of a normal maintenance host will typically result in a chronic infection with little outward sign of infection (Faine et al. 1999). Maintenance hosts most commonly show evidence of infection during pregnancy, manifested by the appearance of reproductive failure (infertility, abortions, still-births, or birth of weak offspring). It is important to note that the same bacterial strain can often cause both acute and chronic infections, depending largely on the mammalian species that is infected. Development of chronic or acute infection is dependent upon poorly understood factors that pair specific mammalian host species with selected *Leptospira* serovars. Presumably, the interplay between the host immune system and infecting strain of bacteria is critical in directing the outcome of *Leptospira* infection.

Keeping in mind the dual nature of *Leptospira* is key to understanding the disease and how the immune system responds to infection. Early work by Adler, Faine, and coworkers clearly established the importance of antibody in providing immune protection in leptospirosis, at least for some host species (Adler and Faine 1977). However, these studies do not tell the full story. Components of both innate and acquired immune systems have been identified that respond to *Leptospira* infection. Both humoral and cell-mediated immunity (CMI) are needed for immune protection against *Leptospira*, yet at the same time immunological processes may also contribute to tissue damage during infection. Infected hosts are challenged by a number of bacterial properties that alter the host response or that contribute to immune evasion and persistent infection.

Although *Leptospira* can infect a wide range of mammalian species, most experimental infection studies have been conducted in golden Syrian hamsters, a species particularly susceptible to acute infection (Morton 1942). However, lack of well characterized immunological reagents for use with hamster tissues has limited our understanding of many aspects of the immune response to *Leptospira* infection. Although a wide variety of reagents are available for characterization of the mouse immune response, most mouse strains are refractory to infection by pathogenic strains of *Leptospira* after about 1 month of age (Packchanian 1940). This situation has slowed analysis of many aspects of the host immune response during leptospirosis. Studies involving experimental infection of other mammalian hosts, notably cattle, have helped to establish a prominent role for components of the cellular immune response in development of protective immunity, especially in maintenance hosts. Thus, the overall view of the immune response during leptospirosis draws on knowledge gained from the host responses in widely divergent mammalian genera infected with diverse species of *Leptospira*.

From the perspective of the host, pathogenic spirochetes, including *Leptospira*, are difficult adversaries to remove. Pathogenic spirochetes express few proteins on the outer membrane surface (Haake et al. 1991, see the chapter by D.A. Haake and W.R. Zückert, this volume), and may vary expression of surface proteins in response to environmental factors such as iron, temperature, and osmolarity (Lo et al. 2006; Matsunaga et al. 2005, 2007). Limited expression of antigenic surface proteins presents few targets for pathogen recognition and development of a protective immune response by the host. Additionally, spirochete outer membranes are loosely attached to the peptidoglycan layer and are easily removed by mild detergent (Haake et al. 1991; Zuerner et al. 1991). Lateral movement of outer membrane antigens through the lipid bilayer with little or no impediment enables the bacteria freedom of movement when bound by antibody (Charon et al. 1981). Thus, attachment of antibody to surface proteins does not impede motility, often a key factor in tissue penetration. Although leptospiral LPS is less pyrogenic than typical Gram-negative LPS, it stimulates a strong immune response that may, or may not, be important for immunoprotection, depending on the nature of the host–serovar interaction.

This chapter reviews historic and recent findings related to the immune response of the host to *Leptospira* infection, the bacterial targets of the immune response, and possible role of the immune response in contributing to disease manifestations. Complicating our ability to develop an understanding of how hosts resist *Leptospira* infection is the variability associated with past experimentation, which has often used different *Leptospira* species, serovars, and strains, and different mammalian host species. Additionally, a critical flaw in some studies has been the use of strains that had undergone many in vitro passages in bacteriological media without first assessing infectivity (ID_{50}) or lethality (LD_{50}) before animal experimentation. Consequently, findings from different laboratories may appear contradictory, yet could simply represent differences between mammalian hosts or the species, serovar, or strain used in experimentation. Recent development of genetic tools has facilitated construction of defined leptospiral mutants, and this is allowing us to discern the importance of specific bacterial genes in virulence (see the chapter by M. Picardeau, this volume). Likewise, recent development of highly inbred or genetic knockout strains of mice with known genetic deficiencies is now leading to a limited, but growing, understanding of the genetic basis of host susceptibility to infection. It is therefore important to bear in mind that most of the studies described in this chapter are drawn from experiments conducted with widely variable use of hosts and pathogens. Continued development and use of highly infectious (i.e., strains with low ID_{50}) knockout mutants should help to resolve the relative importance of specific genes in host selection and virulence.

2 Animal Models

A wide variety of animal species have been used as hosts for experimental lepto-spirosis. Early studies used guinea pigs as a preferred animal model host to study acute infection (Noguchi 1918). In the mid-twentieth century, it was discovered that hamsters were particularly susceptible to *Leptospira* infection (Morton 1942). Owing to their general good health, rapid growth, and lower cost, hamsters are now routinely used as the primary model for acute leptospirosis (Haake 2006). Hamsters retain susceptibility to acute infection with increasing age more than many other animal species and mimic acute infections that share some similarities to clinical disease in humans. Hamsters have been used extensively to test bacterial strain infectivity and virulence, and as a model for testing vaccine efficacy. Indeed, the hamster model of infection is so predictable that many government and international organizations use the hamster model for testing vaccine efficacy.

Common laboratory mice (*Mus musculus*) and rats (*Rattus novegicus*) are generally unsuitable as hosts for acute leptospirosis; these species are only susceptible to developing acute leptospirosis within a very short window of time after birth (Packchanian 1940), unless they have specific genetic deficiencies. Infection of mice or rats older than a few weeks of age will more likely lead to development of chronic infections limited to colonization of kidney. However, as will be described in more detail below, infection of cyclophosphamide-treated mice (Adler and Faine 1976) or mice with toll-like receptor (TLR) deficiencies (Pereira et al. 1998) can result in lethal infection. Use of well-defined genetic knockout (KO) mouse strains in leptospirosis research is becoming more common. Rats are also being used as experimental hosts to study chronic leptospirosis (Athanazio et al. 2008; Monahan et al. 2008; Tucunduva de Faria et al. 2007). Use of rats and mice allows access to well-defined tools and the availability of genetically defined strains is leading to new knowledge on components of the immune system that are important for protective immunity.

Although experimental studies using livestock are quite expensive, cattle, goats, and pigs have been used as experimental hosts for infection and vaccination studies for leptospirosis. This is due in large part on the concern for zoonotic transmission between livestock and humans, the impact of leptospirosis on livestock production costs, and the need for effective vaccines in production animals. Research on leptospirosis in cattle has provided new information on the role of CMI in controlling leptospirosis.

Experimental small animals are most often inoculated with *Leptospira* by intraperitoneal (IP) injection (Haake 2006). Although an unnatural method of disease transmission, IP injection is an efficient, reproducible method for inoculation of small animals such as hamsters and leads to rapid dissemination in the animal. Two alternative methods of experimental inoculation of *Leptospira* thought to mimic natural routes of infection include conjunctival instillation (Thiermann and Handsaker 1985) and subcutaneous injection (Truccolo et al. 2002).

Virulent leptospires injected into the peritoneum establish a transient peritonitis and can be detected in and around blood vessels within 2 days (Zuerner et al. 2012). In acute leptospirosis, the bacteria may first migrate to the pancreas and potentially reduce insulin production, as seen in some human infections (Spichler et al. 2007). Within 3–4 days enough bacteria can be detected in the kidney to be visualized by microscopic examination of stained sections. If the infection does not progress to fulminant leptospirosis, the bacteria often remain in the kidney with occasional migration to other tissue (including brain and pancreas) (Zuerner et al. 2012). However, in hamsters, many *Leptospira* strains produce acute infections and the bacteria can be detected in nearly all tissue in the body, including freely swimming in blood. The interval between injection of virulent *Leptospira* and onset of clinical signs of infection varies, and is dependent upon the strain used, number of in vitro passages, and infectious dose. Standardized tests for vaccine potency or virulence checks for strains are limited to 28 days, by which time most animals should have shown clinical signs of infection.

Many *Leptospira* infection studies have used death as an endpoint, a practice that has been replaced with use of alternative criteria such as onset of clinical signs of infection, at which point animals are euthanized to avoid pain and distress. This approach leads to calculation of a modified LD_{50}. Determination of ID_{50} is often more difficult, due to the requirement to detect *Leptospira* by culture or through direct examination of tissue. There is considerable variation in LD_{50} values for different strains. Critical points for consideration when planning experimental infections are the age and number of in vitro passes of the culture. Older cultures, or cultures that have been propagated in vitro for several passages, tend to lose virulence. Using hamster virulence as a guide, LD_{50} values for *Leptospira* strains may vary from <10 to >10^8 (Haake 2006).

3 Host Detection of Pathogens

3.1 Pattern Recognition Receptors

How does the immune system detect the presence of microbial pathogens? Mammalian cells display a variety of receptors on the cell surface with the design and purpose to recognize molecular signatures that are characteristic for microbial pathogens; these signatures are referred to as pathogen-associated molecular patterns (PAMPs) (Akira et al. 2006; Iwasaki and Medzhitov 2010). PAMPs include a wide variety of molecules such as bacterial LPS, lipoproteins, peptidoglycan, and flagella proteins. The host receptors, referred to as pattern recognition receptors (PRRs), interact with PAMPs, initiating a series of intracellular signals that trigger the host response to infection. Host receptors that recognize PAMPs include toll-like receptors (TLRs) and C-type lectin receptors (CLRs) (Akira et al. 2006; Iwasaki and Medzhitov 2010). A related group of receptors that recognize damage associated molecular patterns (DAMPs), which develop during infection, include receptors for advanced glycosylation end products (RAGE) (Williams et al. 2010). Nucleotide-binding oligomerization domain (NOD)-like receptors (NLRs) recognize both PAMPs and DAMPs. Interaction of PAMPs and DAMPs with appropriate receptors leads to intracellular signaling cascades that trigger the innate immune response and help direct acquired immune responses (Iwasaki and Medzhitov 2010; Williams et al. 2010). Therefore, understanding these receptors and the responses they initiate are essential in developing an understanding of how the host responds to infection.

3.1.1 Toll-like Receptors

Toll-like receptors are the most thoroughly studied PRRs and in many cases initiate the first part of the host response to infection (Aderem and Ulevitch 2000). Most of the published research on recognition of *Leptospira* by PRRs has focused on TLRs, and therefore this section will focus on TLR detection of PAMPs and subsequent cellular responses. TLRs are a group of related transmembrane proteins with an extracellular pattern recognition domain and a cytoplasmic domain responsible for transmitting the signal generated from the extracellular domain to the host response network (Napetschnig and Wu 2013). The cytoplasmic portions of TLRs share a protein domain with the interleukin 1 receptor (IL-1R). This intracellular toll/inter-leukin 1 receptor (TIR) domain interacts with cytoplasmic proteins to initiate a signaling cascade that triggers the host cell to respond to the threat of infection.

LPS has been used extensively to study the intricacies of TLR signaling and the host response to LPS will be used here to provide an overview of the TLR signaling pathway (Fig. 1 summarizes this process) and to highlight some unusual attributes of the response to *Leptospira*. Detection of LPS from most Gram-negative bacterial genera involves TLR4, myeloid differentiation protein 2 (MD-2), and CD14. CD14 binds LPS and transfers the molecule to MD-2 (Kawai and Akira 2010). When MD-2 binds the lipid A portion of a LPS molecule, it undergoes a structural change and forms a protein pocket that interacts with TLR4 (Park et al. 2009). This interaction initiates the intracellular TIR domains to come together and form a site where adaptor proteins assemble into oligomeric structures and initiate the intra-cellular signaling cascade. The TIR domains of most TLRs interact with MyD88, a protein that forms an oligomeric structure called a Myddosome with IRAK4, IRAK1, and IRAK2 (Napetschnig and Wu 2013). MyD88 forms the top of the structure with IRAK4 forming a layer between MyD88 and IRAK1/IRAK2. MyD88, IRAK1, IRAK2, and IRAK4 are phosphokinases, and one proposed model suggests MyD88 promotes phosphorylation of IRAK4, with subsequent down-stream phosphorylation from IRAK4 to IRAK1 and IRAK2 (Napetschnig and Wu 2013). Phosphorylation by the myddosome complex to additional kinases (including p38 MAP kinase) ensues, thereby activating transcriptional regulatory proteins, including nuclear factor kB (NFkB), AP1, and Sp-1 (Napetschnig and Wu 2013), described in more detail below.

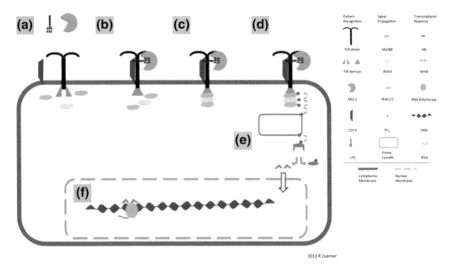

Fig. 1 Pattern recognition and host response. **a** Before PAMP (shown here as LPS) interaction with MD-2, the two TIR domains of the TLR1/TLR2 heterodimer or TLR2/TLR2 homodimer are disassociated from each other, and CD14 is not tightly associated with the TLRs. **b** The MD-2/LPS complex binds the TLR dimer, and CD14 joins the complex; this process leads to structural changes in the TLRs that bring the TIR domains together. **c** MyD88 binds the TIR domain and forms the myddosome consisting of MyD88 (*top*), IRAK4 (*middle*), and IRAK1/2 (*bottom*). **d** Phosphorylation from MyD88 through the myddosome is passed to one of several cytoplasmic kinases. **e** The phosphorylation cycle is propagated through a new cascade, ultimately leading to phosphorylation of IκB. Phosphorylated IκB undergoes ubiquitination, releasing NFκB. **f** NFκB migrates to the nucleus and activates transcription of immune response genes resulting in induction of the immune response

Although most of the TLR research on *Leptospira* has focused on TLR2 and 4 (see below), studies on other spirochetes, particularly *Borrelia burgdorferi*, have shown that TLR5 (Bernardino et al. 2008; Cabral et al. 2006), TLR8 (Cervantes et al. 2011), and TLR7 and TLR9 (Petzke et al. 2009) also play a role in recognizing spirochetes. TLR1, TLR2 and TLR6 are structurally similar and can form heterodimers that are involved in lipoprotein detection, TLR5 detects the presence of flagellin, TLR7 and TLR8 recognize single stranded RNA and imidazoquinoline compounds, and TLR9 recognizes unmethylated CpG motifs in DNA (Akira et al. 2006).

TLRs use a variety of accessory proteins during PAMP recognition and some of these proteins, e.g., MD-2, appear to have multiple functions. For example, LPS-bound MD-2 is also phosphorylated, possibly during endocytosis of the LPS-TLR4-MD-2 complex (Gray et al. 2011). In addition, TLR complexes can also function from within intracellular compartments. TLR4-MD-2 appears to be capable of sensing the presence of LPS; LPS binding through this pathway induces a distinct set of LPS inducible genes (Shibata et al. 2011). While the Myddosomes connect most TLRs to the intracellular signaling network, TIR-domain-containing adapter-inducing interferon-β (TRIF), a protein recognized by TLR3 for signal propagation, is also used for this purpose (Napetschnig and Wu 2013; Petnicki-Ocwieja et al. 2013).

Myddosome-mediated signals primarily result in induction of inflammatory cytokine and chemokine expression, whereas TRIF-mediated signals induce type I interferons (Kawai and Akira 2010). TLR2-TRIF mediated signaling was recently demonstrated in response to *B. burgdorferi* infection in mice (Miller et al. 2010), and may have a role in detecting other spirochetes, including *Leptospira*. These studies highlight the complexity of signal transduction in recognition of microbial pathogens and rapid growth in our understanding of how host cells sense the presence of microbial pathogens.

3.1.2 Other Pattern Recognition Receptors

NLRs are large oligomeric cytoplasmic proteins that contain the NOD domain, which in NLRs is referred to as NACHT (Leemans et al. 2011). The NOD domain is centrally located, and NLRs also have a carboxy-terminal leucine-rich repeat (LRR) motif. Interaction of NLRs with the appropriate PAMP or DAMP leads to formation of multiprotein structures called inflammasomes. Once formed, inflammasomes activate caspase-1, which in turn activates proinflammatory cytokines IL-1β and IL-8 (Leemans et al. 2011). If the inflammasome is not properly regulated, then a pro-inflammatory cycle ensues leading to host directed tissue damage (Leemans et al. 2011), for example, during acute lung injury (ALI). Currently, the NLRP3 inflammasome is the best characterized, and is often associated with a variety of inflammatory disorders including chronic kidney disease (Anders and Muruve 2011).

Other PRRs include the mannose receptor, a member of the CLR family. The mannose receptor has been associated with binding of *B. burgdorferi* to monocyte/macrophages (Cinco et al. 2002). *B. burgdorferi* interaction with $\alpha_3\beta_1$ integrin also induces proinflammatory cytokine production, independent of TLRs or MyD88 (Behera et al. 2006). The binding to the $\alpha_3\beta_1$ integrin sends a signal to the c-Jun NH(2)-terminal kinase (JNK) pathway and leading to induction of a proinflammatory response (Behera et al. 2006). The roles of these other PRRs in *Leptospira* infection have not been well defined.

3.1.3 PRR-Mediated Transcription Response

The signaling cascade triggered by interaction of PAMPs with the appropriate receptor results in activation of several transcription factors, most notably NFkB (Napetschnig and Wu 2013). Nonactivated NFkB is located in the cytosol and bound by the inhibitor IkB. A portion of the signaling cascade leads to phosphorylation of IkB kinase (IKK), which in turn phosphorylates IkB. Phosphorylated IkB is recruited to proteosomes and degraded, thereby releasing NFkB (Napetschnig and Wu 2013). IkB-free NFkB migrates to the nucleus where it binds chromosomal DNA at specific sites with the assistance of accessory transcription factors, e.g., activator protein-1 (AP-1), that are also activated by phosphorylation (Napetschnig and Wu 2013). These events lead to transcriptional activation of response genes enabling the activated cells to respond to infection. NFkB can be activated by a variety of molecular signals and pathways, including TNF-α, and IL-1 via TRAF6. This process initiates the innate response to infection, induces the expression of inflammatory cytokines and chemokines, and helps direct development of the acquired immune response.

4 Innate Immunity

4.1 TLR Recognition and Response

The vast majority of research on pattern recognition of *Leptospira* has focused on the role of TLRs. Although leptospiral LPS has low endotoxicity, it stimulates a strong antibody response during infection (Chapman et al. 1988), or as a result of vaccination with whole-killed cell bacterins (Bolin et al. 1989). As noted above, LPS from most bacteria is predominantly detected using TLR4. However, LPS from *Leptospira* spp. is primarily recognized in humans by TLR2/TLR1 (Werts et al. 2001). Leptospiral LPS is recognized primarily by TLR2, but TLR4 also contributes to activation of murine cells (Nahori et al. 2005). Information regarding TLR recognition of leptospiral LPS is not available for other mammalian species.

The C3H/HeJ mouse strain lacks functional TLR4. Infection of C3H/HeJ mice with *Leptospira interrogans* serovar Icterohaemorrhagiae leads to acute leptospirosis and death (Pereira et al. 1998). Subsequent studies have shown that C3H/HeJ mice are also susceptible to infection with *L. interrogans* serovars Copenhageni and Manilae (Viriyakosol et al. 2006; Koizumi 2003; Nally et al. 2005) indicating that this is not a serovar-specific property. These studies suggest that TLR4 is of critical importance in controlling *Leptospira* infection in mice. The respective roles of TLR2 and TLR4 were studied using mice with genetically defined mutations in TLR2 and TLR4 (Chassin et al. 2009), and results from this and related studies have helped to define links between innate and adaptive immunity and control of *Leptospira* infection. In these studies, C57BL/6 J wild type (WT) mice were used as a control group and bred with TLR2$^{-/-}$, TLR4$^{-/-}$, and double TLR2/TLR4 knockout (DKO) mice, followed by backcrossing to insure that the TLR mutations were studied in a uniform C57BL/6 J genetic background. The resulting mutant strains and WT were inoculated with *L. interrogans* serovar Icterohaemorrhagiae and the outcome of infection assessed. Consistent with previous results using TLR4 deficient C3H/HeJ mice as hosts for *Leptospira*, infection of C57BL/6 J TLR4$^{-/-}$ mice also resulted in lethal infections, as did infections in DKO mice (Chassin et al. 2009). TLR4$^{-/-}$ mice survived longer than DKO mice, a finding that suggests loss of TLR2 increases susceptibility to lethal infection over the TLR4 deficiency alone. The bacterial loads in liver, lung, and kidney were assessed, and compared to WT C57BL/6 J mice in which bacteria were cleared. DKO strains had high bacterial loads in all three organs, but TLR2$^{-/-}$ or TLR4$^{-/-}$ knockout mice had significantly lower bacterial loads in kidney and lung, as compared to DKO mice, and in these two organs resembled WT mice. Infected $TLR4^{-/-}$ mice had high bacterial loads in the liver, whereas $TLR2^{-/-}$ mice resembled WT mice with little or no bacteria detected (Chassin et al. 2009). These studies led to a model where TLR2 and TLR4 have overlapping functions in kidney, but functional TLR4 receptors are needed for bacterial clearance in liver (Chassin et al. 2009). Removal of leptospires from liver in $TLR2^{-/-}$ mice is consistent with the finding that cytokine expression in mouse macrophages involves LPS interaction with TLR4 (Chassin et al. 2009; Viriyakosol et al. 2006). In addition, there is also evidence for TLR-independent induced inflammation (Chassin et al. 2009).

4.1.1 NLR Mediated Response

Detection of PAMP and DAMP signals by NLRs also occurs during leptospirosis. The NLRP3 inflammasome is primed by TLR2/4 interaction with LPS and activated by a depression of the Na/K-ATPase pump by leptospiral glycolipoprotein (Burth et al. 1997; Lacroix-Lamande et al. 2012). Leptospiral glycoliporotein is a suspected cytotoxic component of the *Leptospira* outer membrane (Vinh et al. 1986), and has previously been shown to activate peripheral blood mononuclear cells (Diament et al. 2002). Chronic inflammasome activation may be one pathway leading to the development of tissue lesions, especially in kidney; the NLRP3 inflammasome can be triggered by either sterile or infectious stimuli (Anders and Muruve 2011; Vilaysane et al. 2010). Inflammasome activation has been implicated in a variety of chronic kidney diseases (Anders and Muruve 2011), and specific activation of the NLRP3 inflammasome and induction of IL-1β and IL-18 secretion has been associated with the development of chronic kidney disease in a noninfectious mouse model (Vilaysane et al. 2010).

4.1.2 CLR Mediated Response

DC-SIGN and mannose-binding protein are two CLRs that have been identified as having possible roles in *Leptospira* recognition. The mannose-binding lectin (MBL) is elevated in serum during leptospirosis, with higher serum levels being detected in human patients during an outbreak of more classical Weil's disease than in an outbreak of more moderate disease manifestations (Miranda et al. 2009). This finding suggests that MBL may be useful as a marker for severe leptospirosis (Miranda et al. 2009). *Leptospira* detection by human monocyte-derived dendritic cells via DC-SIGN induced secretion of the proinflammatory cytokine TNF-α and IL-12 (which enhances the cytotoxicity of NK and $CD8^+$ T cells) (Gaudart et al. 2008). However, DC-SIGN induced limited secretion of the anti-inflammatory cytokine IL-10 (Gaudart et al. 2008). Low passage, virulent serovar Pyrogenes strain 2317 induced greater TNF-α and IL-12 secretion than a high passage avirulent derivative of strain 2317 (Gaudart et al. 2008). These results are consistent with studies that show high serum TNF-α correlates with a poor prognosis in human leptospirosis patients (Tajiki and Salomão 1996; Kyriakidis et al. 2011; Wagenaar et al. 2009a). Serum IL-10 levels are also elevated during acute leptospirosis, but this may be in response to high levels of inflammatory cytokines; IL-10 functions to restrain the inflammatory response. The inability of high serum levels of IL-10 to control the inflammation response may lead to immune pathology (see Sect. 6). IL-10 is important for limiting *Borrelia turicatae* growth in mice, showing a commonality in the need for a balanced immune response to survive infections caused by these spirochetes (Londoño et al. 2008).

4.1.3 Cytokine Induction

The role of inflammatory cytokines in C57BL/6 J mice and assorted mutants was also examined (Chassin et al. 2009). Levels of inflammatory cytokines were highest in DKO mice in kidney and liver as compared to WT, TLR2$^{-/-}$, or TLR4$^{-/-}$ mice. This result may be due in part to the higher bacterial load in liver and kidney because DKO mutants were unable to clear bacteria during infection, and the observed induction of inflammatory cytokines was by a non-TLR based pathway (Chassin et al. 2009). MyD88$^{-/-}$ mice have approximately the same levels of inflammatory cytokines as TLR2-TLR4 DKO mice, leading to the conclusion that TLRs other than TLR2 and TLR4 do not play a significant role in detecting *Leptospira,* or for inducing production of IL-1β, IL-6, and chemokines There is no evidence that TLR3, which uses a MyD88-independent signaling pathway, has a significant role in recognition of *Leptospira* antigens. TNF-α-induced CCL5 (also known as RANTES), CXCL1 (also known as KC) and CXCL2 (also known as MIP-2) (Chassin et al. 2009). This conclusion is inconsistent with another report concluding that TNF-α production is largely TLR5-dependent in human leukocytes (Goris et al. 2011). These differences may indicate either a difference in the relative importance of TLRs in different tissues or the ability of leukocytes from different host species to use different TLRs for pathogen detection. However, a general program of robust production of inflammatory cytokines is consistent across diverse mammalian hosts; the findings cited above are similar to studies conducted in hamsters that also have high inflammatory cytokine production during the acute phase of infection (Lowanitchapat et al. 2010; Marinho et al. 2009; Matsui et al. 2011; Vernel-Pauillac and Merien 2006; Vernel-Pauillac and Goarant 2010).

The array of circulating cytokines and chemokines induced at significant levels in both humans and mice during leptospirosis includes IL1-β, IL-6, IL-10, MCP-1, and TNF-α (Wang et al. 2012). In humans, GM-CSF (granulocyte macrophage colony-stimulating factor) and CCL2 (also known as macrophage chemotactic protein 1, MCP-1) were also found at increased levels in sera (Wang et al. 2012); these two compounds promote granulocyte and monocyte production and recruit leukocytes to sites of inflammation, respectively. Human patients also had elevated IL-11; IL-11 contributes to platelet replenishment due to thrombobocytopenia (a frequent complication of leptospirosis) and induction of acute phase proteins (Wang et al. 2012). There is also in vitro evidence of locally produced cytokine and chemokine production; CXCL1/KC, iNOS, and CCL2/MCP-1, are produced by cultured renal cells using a TLR1/2 driven pathway via MyD88 and a MAP38 kinase pathway (Hung et al. 2006a, b; Yang et al. 2006). The result of CXCL1/KC synthesis in the kidney may help recruit neutrophils to the site of infection. However, another consequence of chemokine/cytokine synthesis in the kidney may be accumulation of fibrous tissue and decreased kidney function (see Sect. 6).

4.2 Cellular Response

Monocytes/macrophages utilize PRR-mediated activation to provide innate immune protection of the host, especially during the early stages of infection. Leptospiral LPS and hemolysins stimulate macrophages to produce IL-1β, IL-6, IFN, and TNF-α (Isogai et al. 1990; Wang et al. 2012). In addition, macrophages treated with leptospiral LPS have enhanced phagocytic activity (Isogai et al. 1990). The role of macrophages in protection against *Leptospira* infection was suggested in a study where mice were treated with silica to inhibit macrophage function, and it was found that treated mice were impaired in bacterial clearance and had increased susceptibility to infection (Isogai et al. 1986). The role of antibody appears to be important for macrophage-mediated killing of *Leptospira*; several independent studies have shown that phagocytosis leading to decreased bacterial viability requires opsonization with homologous antibody (Banfi et al. 1982; Cinco et al. 1981; Vinh et al. 1982). Opsonization may overcome an inherent immune evasion mechanism of *Leptospira* that impairs macrophage function; freshly isolated virulent strains can induce macrophage apoptosis (Merien et al. 1997; Jin et al. 2009) or limit lysosomal fusion with bacteria-laden phagosomes (Toma et al. 2011).

Polymorphonuclear leukocytes (PMNs) include granulocytes, eosinophils, and neutrophils, and these cells comprise important components of the innate immune response, but their role in protection against *Leptospira* infection is unclear. Two antibacterial peptides produced by bovine neutrophils, Bac5 (also known as cathelicidin-2) and Bac7 (cathelicidin-7), can kill *Leptospira* (Scocchi et al. 1993). Intact *Leptospira,* leptospiral peptidoglycan or LPS induce PMN adherence to endothelial cells (Isogai et al. 1989a; Dobrina et al. 1995). However, resistance to PMN phagocytosis has been suggested as a potential virulence factor for *Leptospira* (Wang et al. 1984). Acute infection with a hamster lethal strain of *Leptospira borgpetersenii* serovar Hardjo resulted in the in vivo formation in blood of large bacterial–neutrophil aggregates without bacterial clearance (Zuerner et al. 2012). Much like the findings described above noting that macrophages depend on antibody for phagocytosis, PMNs also require assistance from the humoral response to provide immune sera for phagocytosis of *Leptospira* (McGrath et al. 1984; Wang et al. 1984). These results are similar to those reported for *B. burgdorferi*, which appears to be more susceptible to PMN attack in the presence, rather than absence, of antibody (Lusitani et al. 2002).

Although platelets have traditionally been associated with hemostasis, recent studies have shown these cells are important components of the innate immune response (Yeaman 2009). Platelets utilize TLRs to detect PAMPs, and produce antimicrobial peptides and cytokines (Cognasse et al. 2008). Activated platelets contribute to the activation of neutrophils and neutrophil extracellular formation (Yeaman 2009). Leptospiral LPS induces platelet aggregation (Isogai et al. 1989b), and thrombocytopenia often occurs in about half of human leptospirosis patients (Edwards et al. 1986). By contributing to platelet removal, *Leptospira* may be able to subvert part of the innate immune system during the early stages of infection.

5 Acquired Immunity

5.1 Humoral Response

Antibodies against *Leptospira* have a key role in providing immune protection against lethal infection in many potential host species. Adler and Faine concluded that antibody to *Leptospira* is essential for protective immunity with the discovery that mice treated with cyclophosphamide, which preferentially kills B cells, were susceptible to lethal *Leptospira* infection (Adler and Faine 1976, 1977). Nude mice, which lack a thymus, and therefore cannot produce T cells, were resistant to infection (Adler and Faine 1977). Mice lacking a functional Rag gene are unable to produce functional B and T cells due to an inability to undergo V(D)J recombination in immunoglobulin and T cell receptor genes. Likewise, SCID mice lack an enzyme responsible for DNA recombination needed for maturation of antigen specific B and T cells. μMT mice lack functional B cells. Infection with *L. interrogans* of Rag$^{-/-}$, SCID mice, μMT, or nude mice treated with cyclophosphamide results in lethal infection (Adler and Faine 1977; Bandeira et al. 2011; Chassin et al. 2009; Nally et al. 2005). Adler and Faine (1977) clearly demonstrated the importance antibody (and therefore B cells) by injecting cyclophosphamide-treated nude mice with antibody to *Leptospira* resulting in protection against lethal *Leptospira* infection. Chassin et al. (2009) reported similar results: μMT mice were protected from lethal challenge using passive transfer of immune sera collected from infected WT mice at 20-days PI. These studies are consistent with an earlier study that showed transfer of maternal antibodies protected mice from becoming chronic carriers of *Leptospira* (Birnbaum et al. 1972). In contrast, T cells do not appear to have an important role in providing protection from lethal challenge in the mouse model; CD3$^{-/-}$ (T cell deficient) mice are resistant to lethal challenge (Chassin et al. 2009).

A key *Leptospira* antigen that is important for the development of immune protection in many host species is LPS. Immunization with *Leptospira* LPS protects hamsters against homologous challenge (Jost et al. 1989). Passive transfer of antibody to LPS has also been used successfully to protect mice, guinea pigs, monkeys, and dogs before lethal infectious challenge (Jost et al. 1986; Challa et al.

2011; Schoone et al. 1989). Indeed, development of antibody to the LPS component of whole cell bacterins is thought to be key for immune protection against lethal infection with several *Leptospira* serovars in many animal species. Development of agglutinating antibodies, predominantly IgM (Adler and Faine 1978), is important for serological diagnosis of exposure to *Leptospira* using the microscopic agglutination test (MAT). Antibodies to LPS develop early in infection (Chapman et al. 1991). However, LPS is the serovar-specific antigen in *Leptospira* and therein lies one of the problems with relying on the LPS component in vaccines for developing protective immunity against a broad spectrum of serovars; antibodies against LPS provide limited cross-protection against other serovars and may provide short duration of immunity. Development of antibody to leptospiral proteins has greater likelihood of cross-protection (Sonrier et al. 2000; Srikram et al. 2011; see the chapters by D.A. Haake and W.R. Zückert and by B. Adler, this volume). The major outer membrane protein of pathogenic *Leptospira,* LipL32, stimulates a significant early and sustained antibody response during infection (Haake et al. 1991, 2000; Zuerner et al. 1991). LipL32 is proteolytically cleaved in vitro (Haake et al. 2000; Zuerner et al. 1991; Cullen et al. 2002) and the protein is post-translationally modified (Witchell et al. 2014), processes that may limit exposure of antigenic epitopes of this protein on the cell surface (Pinne and Haake 2013). While antibodies to LipL32 are good indicators of infection, development of antibody to this protein does not appear to be protective (Lucas et al. 2011), and LipL32 is not needed for successful infection (Murray et al. 2009). Differential methylation of OmpL32 glutamic residues is another method by which Leptospira may alter exposure of antigenic epitopes during infection (Eshghi et al. 2012b). A more complete review of vaccine development is presented in the chapter by B. Adler, this volume, but, on the whole, the most successful *Leptospira* vaccines produced to date are composed of whole, killed bacteria (Bey and Johnson 1982), suggesting that a complex mixture of antigens may be required for protection.

5.2 Cell-Mediated Immunity

Although the data described above show the critical importance of a Th2, or B cell-mediated protective immunity, both B and T lymphocytes have important roles in promoting an immune response to *Leptospira* infection. Rag$^{-/-}$ mice do not produce significant levels of IFN-γ in liver or kidney, indicating either B or T cells, or both classes of lymphocytes, are required for IFN-γ production during infection (Chassin et al. 2009). B cells appear to be primarily responsible for IFN-γ production and bacterial clearance in the liver, whereas T cells are responsible for these roles in the kidney (Chassin et al. 2009). Furthermore, histological evidence of kidney tissue damage is greater in CD3$^{-/-}$ animals lacking functional T cells, as compared to WT or µMT (B cell deficient) mice. Histological examination of infected kidneys showed evidence of interstitial inflammation and development of nodular infiltrates in T cell deficient mice that were absent from kidneys of infected

WT or B cell deficient mice (Chassin et al. 2009). Finally, serological markers of renal damage were elevated in infected T cell deficient mice, but not infected WT or B cell deficient mice. Combined, these data provide a compelling argument that the Th1, or CMI, response involving T cells is an important component of the immune response as it relates to *Leptospira* infection.

The studies above focused on protection against lethal *Leptospira* challenge. There is less information on what components of the immune response are critical to prevent against development of chronic infection by *Leptospira*. Elimination of chronic leptospirosis, especially in maintenance hosts, is important to reduce the likelihood of disease transmission to accidental hosts. Vaccination and challenge studies using serovar Hardjo infections of cattle have led to a better understanding of the immune response in regard to *Leptospira* infection of its natural maintenance host. In contrast to the animal studies described above that show antibody to LPS to be protective against lethal leptospirosis, similar studies in cattle have shown that high titers of antibody to LPS fail to protect cattle from infection with serovar Hardjo, the most common serovar associated with chronic bovine leptospirosis (Bolin et al. 1989). Vaccines in this class fail to induce a Th1, or CMI, response in cattle (Naiman et al. 2001b, 2002; Zuerner et al. 2011). Refined whole cell monovalent serovar Hardjo vaccines that protect against significant renal colonization stimulate antibody production, but also induce CMI (Bolin et al. 2000; Bolin and Alt 2001; Ellis et al. 2000). These vaccines stimulate $CD4^+$ and $\gamma\delta$ T cells to proliferate and produce IFN-γ in a recall response when exposed to serovar Hardjo antigens (Blumerman et al. 2007a; Naiman et al. 2001b, 2002). In short-term vaccine efficacy studies, where cattle were challenged approximately 4 months after vaccination, these vaccines either prevented renal colonization and urinary shedding of bacteria (Bolin et al. 2000; Bolin and Alt 2001; Ellis et al. 2000) or eliminated urinary shedding within a few weeks after challenge (Zuerner et al. 2011). However, duration of protective immunity remains a problem. Some animals may develop renal colonization with lesion formation if infected 1 year after vaccination (Zuerner et al. 2011). Nevertheless, the general success of these vaccines in limiting renal colonization provides a model to understand the role of CMI in controlling *Leptospira* infection in cattle, and perhaps other species.

Analysis of how bovine peripheral blood mononuclear cells (PBMCs) respond to vaccination and subsequent infectious challenge has revealed several characteristics of a protective Th1 response to *Leptospira* infection. Analysis of how cattle respond to *L. borgpetersenii* serovar Hardjo has played a key role in characterizing bovine $\gamma\delta$ T cells because this class of lymphocytes replicate in response to vaccination with a monovalent serovar Hardjo and demonstrate a strong recall response to leptospiral antigens (Baldwin et al. 2002; Naiman et al. 2001a, b; Zuerner et al. 2011). $\gamma\delta$ T cells are a unique class of $CD4^-$ $CD8^-$ T cells that comprise approximately 30 % of the normal adult ruminant PBMC population (Hein and Mackay 1991). This unique class of T cells comprises a smaller percentage of PBMCs in nonruminant species, and is not as well characterized as $CD4^+$ and $CD8^+$ $\alpha\beta$ T cells. Most bovine $\gamma\delta$ T cells possess the WC1 scavenger receptor on the cell surface (Baldwin et al. 2000). WC1 is one of several members of the scavenger receptor cysteine-rich (SRCR) family (Wang et al. 2011), a group of surface proteins that bind a variety of PAMPs including lipoproteins, lipoteichoic acid, and leucine-rich repeat proteins (Loimaranta et al. 2009). A protective monovalent serovar Hardjo vaccine induces a positive recall response to leptospiral antigens in CD4$^+$ αβ- and γδ-T cells, but the response of CD8$^+$ cells has varied between studies (Baldwin et al. 2002; Naiman et al. 2001b, 2002; Zuerner et al. 2011). Several studies have shown that the phenotype of *Leptospira* antigen-stimulated WC1$^+$ γδ T cells is consistent with Th1 polarized cells: (1) they express the transcription factors T-bet and GATA-3, as well as IL-12Rβ2 which encodes the high affinity IL-12 receptor (Rogers et al. 2005a, b); (2) they are activated by treatment with IL-12; (3) γδ T cells have elevated transcription of genes associated with cytotoxic activity (Blumerman et al. 2007b); and (4) cells have elevated expression of B-cell activating factor (BAFF, also referred to as BLysS, for B lymphocyte stimulator), and NDFIP2 (Blumerman et al. 2007b), a gene that promotes IFN-γ production in Th1 polarized lymphocytes (Lund et al. 2007). One of the characteristics of CD4$^+$ T cells stimulated with *Leptospira* antigens is increased transcription of genes encoding cytotoxic functions and CXCL6 (granulocyte chemotactic protein), a chemokine that attracts neutrophils (Blumerman et al. 2007b).

Several studies on human patients have shown that exposure to *Leptospira* antigens induces a proliferative response in PBMCs. In particular, there is preferential expansion of γδ T cells in leptospirosis patient blood samples stimulated with *Leptospira* antigens (Barry et al. 2006; Klimpel et al. 2003). However, Tuero et al. (2010) did not detect the presence of a T cell memory response in patient blood following infection. The presence of inflammatory cytokines (de Fost et al. 2003) showed that *Leptospira* induced significant increases in human PBMC expression of IFN-γ, TNF-α, and IL-12 receptor, consistent with a strong Th1 response to infection. In addition, patients with, or suspected of having, leptospirosis had elevated concentrations of T- and NK-cell derived cytotoxic compounds or chemokines (De Fost et al. 2007).

NK cells are a group of cytotoxic lymphocytes often considered part of the innate immune response. However, recent reports have shown that NK cells have the capacity to mount a recall response to antigens (Cooper et al. 2009; Sun et al. 2009). NK cells, defined as CD335$^+$ (i.e., containing the natural cytotoxicity receptor, NKp46) from cattle vaccinated with a monovalent serovar Hardjo vaccine demonstrated a recall response by expressing IFN-γ when exposed to *Leptospira* antigens (Zuerner et al. 2011). Surprisingly, NK cells from sham vaccinated cattle also demonstrated an antigen recall response, that by 6 weeks post challenge, was indistinguishable from cells obtained from vaccinated animals (Zuerner et al. 2011). A key difference in the response of lymphocytes from vaccinates versus sham vaccinates may be the ability of the vaccine to induce sustained lymphocyte proliferation with IFN-γ expression following infectious challenge (Naiman et al. 2001b, 2002; Zuerner et al. 2011). The presence of immune cells in vaccinated animals at initiation of infection may limit the initial tissue colonization by *Leptospira*, and allow the host to eventually resolve the infection. In contrast, infection of nonimmune animals likely allows substantial colonization of host tissue that cannot be removed by the host without additional forms of intervention, e.g., antibiotic treatment.

6 Immune Pathology

Some of the manifestations of acute leptospirosis may be the result of unrestrained activation of the host immune response. Several lines of evidence suggest that robust activation of inflammasomes may contribute to tissue damage, particularly lung and kidney. The two triggers (e.g., LPS and potassium efflux) needed to obtain high-level activation of inflammasomes resulting in robust production of IL-1β (Mariathasan and Monack 2007) are present during acute leptospirosis. LPS is an outer membrane component and potassium efflux is induced by the leptospiral glycolipoprotein (Lacroix-Lamande et al. 2012). Overstimulation of the inflammasome can contribute to tissue damage to lung (Xiang et al. 2011) and kidney (Vilaysane et al. 2010; Anders and Muruve 2011). Consistent with this hypothesis, evidence for "massive overexpression" of proinflammatory cytokines in hamsters experiencing severe leptospirosis has been presented (Matsui et al. 2011). Other studies have found high inflammatory cytokine levels associated with lethal infection of hamsters (Marinho et al. 2009; Vernel-Pauillac and Goarant 2010). Human patients suffering from acute leptospirosis also have evidence of overexpression of inflammatory cytokines, and soluble ST2 and long pentraxin PTX3 have been indicated as possible markers for acute infection (Wagenaar et al. 2009a, b). Elevated expression of neutrophil che-mokines CXCL1 (Hung et al. 2006a, b) and CXCL6 (Blumerman et al. 2007b) may promote PMN migration, cell activation, and inflammation, all of which are asso-ciated with acute lung injury (Li et al. 2009). The presence of neutrophil–bacterial aggregates during acute infection (Zuerner et al. 2011), coupled with extracellular net formation can result in release of neutrophil granules and tissue damage (Abraham 2003; Lee and Downey 2001). Several immune receptors were upregu-lated in lung tissue from human patients that had died from acute leptospirosis and experienced pulmonary involvement (Del Carlo Bernardi et al. 2012).

Pathogenic *Leptospira* binds to chondroitin sulfate B, a proteoglycan of host cells (Breiner et al. 2009). Interaction of pathogenic *Leptospira* with endothelial cells induces cellular changes that are consistent with disruption of endothelial barriers, thereby aiding bacterial invasion (Martinez-Lopez et al. 2010). Interest-ingly, this process, at least in vitro, can be blocked using the ACE inhibitor lys-inopril, suggesting that pharmaceutical treatments that supplement antibiotic therapy may be useful in limiting tissue damage (Martinez-Lopez et al. 2010). Tissue from infected animals often shows evidence of tubulointerstitial nephritis, an accumulation of extracellular matrix (ECM) proteins in the kidney (Araujo et al. 2010), a process that can be replicated with mouse proximal tubule cells treated with *Leptospira* OMP preparation, which may well contain LPS (Yang et al. 2000). Evidence for a TLR2-driven signaling cascade stimulating ECM production in response to exposure to *Leptospira* outer membrane proteins, especially LipL32, was recently shown using immortalized human kidney cells (Hsu et al. 2010; Tian et al. 2011). Production of CXCL1/KC attracts neutrophils and monocytes (Hsu et al. 2010), and production TGF-B1 likely drives synthesis of type I and type IV collagen (Tian 2006), leading to fibrosis. In situ expression of inflammatory cytokines has been suggested as contributing to tissue damage in acute lung injury and pulmonary fibrosis (Kolb et al. 2001), and a similar mechanism of tissue damage and errant repair may also occur in renal tissue following infection with *Leptospira* and contribute to the development of tubulointerstitial nephritis.

iNOS expression may present a double-edged sword with respect to protecting the host and damaging tissue. Production of iNOS is important for host survival (Prêtre et al. 2011), but two studies have suggested that iNOS activity may contribute to damage observed during *Leptospira*-induced pulmonary hemorrhage (Chen et al. 2007; Yang and Hsu 2005).

Leptospirosis induced autoimmunity may contribute to the development of uveitis and loss of eyesight in horses (Faber et al. 2000; Verma and Stevenson 2012) and humans (Chu et al. 1998; Mancel et al. 1999). Antibodies from uveitis horses recognize two *Leptospira* proteins, LruA and LruB that share antigenic cross reactivity with eye proteins in horses (Verma et al. 2005). Sera from human uveitis patients also recognize LruA and LruB (Verma et al. 2008). Development of antibodies to other host proteins in leptospirosis patients has been reported, for example antibodies to host cardiolipin following infection (Rugman et al. 1991), but this has not been associated with development of autoimmune disease.

Autoimmunity, in the form of Goodpasture's syndrome, has also been suggested as contributing to the development of pulmonary hemorrhage in a guinea pig model (Nally et al. 2004). In that model it was proposed that autoantibodies to connective tissue triggered by *Leptospira* infection were the cause of pulmonary damage. This hypothesis has since been disproven (Craig et al. 2009).

7 Immune Evasion

Leptospira has several proteins that have the capacity to bind components of the complement system, including factor H (fH) and factor H-like (fHl) proteins. By binding components of the complement system, *Leptospira* avoids complement activation and cell damage. Among the leptospiral proteins capable of binding components of the complement system are two endostatin-like proteins LenA (LfhA) and LenB (Stevenson et al. 2007; Verma et al. 2010), LigA and LigB (Castiblanco-Valencia et al. 2012), and LIC11834, and LIC12253 (Domingos et al. 2012). Some of these proteins, as well as many other *Leptospira* proteins including other members of the endostatin-like proteins (Stevenson et al. 2007) and LipL32 (Choy et al. 2011), bind a variety of host proteins, thereby masking bacterial antigens and contributing to evasion from the host immune system.

The major outer membrane protein of pathogenic *Leptospira*, LipL32, induces a strong antibody response and is a TLR2 agonist (Hsu et al. 2010). However, mutants in LipL32 are still infectious, and LipL32 monovalent vaccines are not protective (Lucas et al. 2011), findings consistent with a recent report that challenges the long-held belief that LipL32 is exposed on the bacterial surface (Pinne and Haake 2013). If the subsurface localization of this protein is confirmed, then perhaps the robust antigenic activity of LipL32 serves to divert the immune response away from effective targets for immune clearance and instead direct the immune response to antigens for which antibodies do not impair in vivo bacterial survival.

Leptospira may also mask antigenic sites on outer membrane proteins. Amino acids in OmpL32 are methylated, and the pattern of methylation changes depending on various environmental factors (Eshghi et al. 2012b). This process likely alters antibody access to this protein, thereby interfering with opsonization. As noted above, LipL32 is also post-translationally modified in a way that may alter antibody binding to antigenic domains on the major outer membrane protein (Witchell et al. 2014).

Leptospira is also able to penetrate host cells, including macrophages, and induce apoptosis (Merien et al. 1997, 1998; Jin et al. 2009). This function likely abrogates the normal role of macrophages in innate immunity and bacterial clearance. Expression of catalase may contribute to intracellular survival of *Leptospira* (Eshghi et al. 2012a).

8 Conclusions

We are gaining new insight into the complexities involved as mammalian hosts respond to *Leptospira* infection. The infection is a perpetual battle between host and bacterium, each with its own arsenal of weapons to attack the other. On the host side, an array of inflammatory cytokines and chemokines is used to stimulate cells to resist infection and kill the bacteria. The bacteria present an array of molecules to the host immune system that may initiate a destructive immune response leading to sepsis and death, or in a more limited setting, chronic tissue damage as the bacteria establishes a persistent infection. Information is needed on how to avoid over induction of a proinflammatory response and instead develop a measured response that limits host tissue damage while contributing to bacterial death. Identification of bacterial evasion strategies and key bacterial antigens is needed to enable development of safe, effective vaccines that promote clearance of bacteria from the host. These findings provide a basis for future study on the immune response to *Leptospira* infection. Future work may involve genetic determinants of susceptibility; several genetic polymorphisms that may predispose humans to severe infection have been identified (Fialho et al. 2009), and may be important for anticipating treatment strategies, especially in areas where humans are chronic carriers of endemic strains of *Leptospira.*

References

Abraham E (2003) Neutrophils and acute lung injury. Crit Care Med 31:S195–S199
Aderem A, Ulevitch RJ (2000) Toll-like receptors in the induction of the innate immune response. Nature 406:782–787
Adler B, Faine S (1976) Susceptibility of mice treated with cyclophosphamide to lethal infection with *Leptospira interrogans* Serovar Pomona. Infect Immun 14:703–708

Adler B, Faine S (1977) Host immunological mechanisms in the resistance of mice to leptospiral infections. Infect Immun 17:67–72

Adler B, Faine S (1978) The antibodies involved in the human immune response to leptospiral infection. J Med Microbiol 11:387–400

Akira S, Uematsu S, Takeuchi O (2006) Pathogen recognition and innate immunity. Cell 124:783–802

Anders H-J, Muruve DA (2011) The inflammasomes in kidney disease. J Am Soc Nephrol 22:1007–1018

Araujo ER, Seguro AC, Spichler A, Magaldi AJ, Volpini RA, De Brito T (2010) Acute kidney injury in human leptospirosis: an immunohistochemical study with pathophysiological correlation. Virchows Arch 456:367–375

Athanazio DA, Santos CS, Santos AC, McBride FWC, Reis MG (2008) Experimental infection in tumor necrosis factor alpha receptor, interferon gamma and interleukin 4 deficient mice by pathogenic *Leptospira interrogans*. Acta Trop 105:95–98

Baldwin CL, Sathiyaseelan T, Rocchi M, McKeever D (2000) Rapid changes occur in the percentage of circulating bovine WC1(+)gamma delta Th1 cells. Res Vet Sci 69:175–180

Baldwin CL, Sathiyaseelan T, Naiman B, White AM, Brown R, Blumerman S, Rogers A, Black SJ (2002) Activation of bovine peripheral blood gammadelta T cells for cell division and IFN-gamma production. Vet Immunol Immunopathol 87:251–259

Bandeira M, Santos CS, de Azevedo EC, Soares LM, Macedo JO, Marchi S, da Silva CLR, Chagas-Junior AD, McBride AJA, McBride FWC, Reis MG, Athanazio DA (2011) Attenuated nephritis in inducible nitric oxide synthase knockout C57BL/6 mice and pulmonary hemorrhage in CB17 SCID and aecombination activating gene 1 knockout C57BL/6 mice infected with *Leptospira interrogans*. Infect Immun 79:2936–2940

Banfi E, Cinco M, Bellini M, Soranzo MR (1982) The role of antibodies and serum complement in the interaction between macrophages and leptospires. Microbiol 128:813–816

Barry M, Wisnewski AV, Matthias MA, Inouye SK, Vinetz JM (2006) Suburban leptospirosis: atypical lymphocytosis and γ-δ T cell response. Clin Infect Dis 43:1304–1307

Behera AK, Hildebrand E, Uematsu S, Akira S, Coburn J, Hu LT (2006) Identification of a TLR-independent pathway for *Borrelia burgdorferi*-induced expression of matrix metalloproteinases and inflammatory mediators through binding to integrin alpha 3 beta 1. J Immunol 177:657–664

Bernardino ALF, Myers TA, Alvarez X, Hasegawa A, Philipp MT (2008) Toll-like receptors: insights into their possible role in the pathogenesis of lyme neuroborreliosis. Infect Immun 76:4385–4395

Bey RF, Johnson RC (1982) Immunogenicity and humoral and cell-mediated immune responses to leptospiral whole cell, outer envelope, and protoplasmic cylinder vaccines in hamsters and dogs. Am J Vet Res 43:835–840

Birnbaum S, Shenberg E, Torten M (1972) The influence of maternal antibodies on the epidemiology of leptospiral carrier state in mice. Am J Epidemiol 96:313–317

Blumerman SL, Herzig CTA, Baldwin CL (2007a) WC1+ gammadelta T cell memory population is induced by killed bacterial vaccine. Eur J Immunol 37:1204–1216

Blumerman SL, Herzig CTA, Wang F, Coussens PM, Baldwin CL (2007b) Comparison of gene expression by co-cultured WC1+ gammadelta and CD4+ alphabeta T cells exhibiting a recall response to bacterial antigen. Mol Immunol 44:2023–2035

Bolin CA, Zuerner RL, Trueba G (1989) Effect of vaccination with a pentavalent leptospiral vaccine containing *Leptospira interrogans* serovar Hardjo type hardjo-bovis on type hardjo-bovis infection of cattle. Am J Vet Res 50:2004–2008

Bolin CA, Alt DP, Zuerner RL (2000) Protection of cattle from renal and genital tract colonization with *Leptospira borgpetersenii* serovar Hardjo. In: Proceedings of the 21st world buiatrics congress, Punte del Este, Uruguay

Bolin CA, Alt DP (2001) Use of a monovalent leptospiral vaccine to prevent renal colonization and urinary shedding in cattle exposed to *Leptospira borgpetersenii* serovar Hardjo. Am J Vet Res 62:996–1000

Breiner DD, Fahey M, Salvador R, Novakova J, Coburn J (2009) *Leptospira interrogans* binds to human cell surface receptors including proteoglycans. Infect Immun 77:5528–5536

Burth P, Younes-Ibrahim M, Gonçalez FH, Costa ER, Faria MV (1997) Purification and characterization of a Na+, K+ ATPase inhibitor found in an endotoxin of *Leptospira interrogans*. Infect Immun 65:1557–1560

Cabral ES, Gelderblom H, Hornung RL, Munson PJ, Martin R, Marques AR (2006) *Borrelia burgdorferi* lipoprotein-mediated TLR2 stimulation causes the down-regulation of TLR5 in human monocytes. J Infect Dis 193:849–859

Castiblanco-Valencia MM, Fraga TR, Silva LBd, Monaris D, Abreu PAE, Strobel S, Józsi M, Isaac L, Barbosa AS (2012) Leptospiral immunoglobulin-like proteins interact with human complement regulators factor H, FHL-1, FHR-1, and C4BP. J Infect Dis 205:995–1004

Cervantes JL, Dunham-Ems SM, La Vake CJ, Petzke MM, Sahay B, Sellati TJ, Radolf JD, Salazar JC (2011) Phagosomal signaling by *Borrelia burgdorferi* in human monocytes involves Toll-like receptor (TLR) 2 and TLR8 cooperativity and TLR8-mediated induction of IFN-beta. Proc Nat Acad Sci USA 108:3683–3688

Challa S, Nally JE, Jones C, Sheoran AS (2011) Passive immunization with *Leptospira* LPS-specific agglutinating but not non-agglutinating monoclonal antibodies protect guinea pigs from fatal pulmonary hemorrhages induced by serovar Copenhageni challenge. Vaccine 29:4431–4434

Chapman AJ, Adler B, Faine S (1988) Antigens recognised by the human immune response to infection with *Leptospira interrogans* serovar Hardjo. J Med Microbiol 25:269–278

Chapman AJ, Everard CO, Faine S, Adler B (1991) Antigens recognized by the human immune response to severe leptospirosis in Barbados. Epidemiol Infect 107:143–155

Charon N, Lawrence C, O'Brien S (1981) Movement of antibody-coated latex beads attached to the spirochete *Leptospira interrogans*. Proc Natl Acad Sci USA 78:7166

Chassin C, Picardeau M, Goujon J-M, Bourhy P, Quellard N, Darche S, Badell E, d' Andon MF, Winter N, Lacroix-Lamande S, Buzoni-Gatel D, Vandewalle A, Werts C (2009) TLR4- and TLR2-mediated B cell responses control the clearance of the bacterial pathogen, *Leptospira interrogans*. J Immunol 183:2669–2677

Chen HI, Kao SJ, Hsu YH (2007) Pathophysiological mechanism of lung injury in patients with leptospirosis. Pathology 39:339–344

Choy HA, Kelley MM, Croda J, Matsunaga J, Babbitt JT, Ko AI, Picardeau M, Haake DA (2011) The multifunctional LigB adhesin binds homeostatic proteins with potential roles in cutaneous infection by pathogenic *Leptospira interrogans*. PLoS ONE 6:e16879

Chu KM, Rathinam R, Namperumalsamy P, Dean D (1998) Identification of *Leptospira* species in the pathogenesis of uveitis and determination of clinical ocular characteristics in South India. J Infect Dis 177:1314–1321

Cinco M, Banfi E, Soranzo MR (1981) Studies on the interaction between macrophages and leptospires. Microbiol 124:409–413

Cinco M, Cini B, Perticarari S, Presani G (2002) *Leptospira interrogans* binds to the CR3 receptor on mammalian cells. Microb Pathog 33:299–305

Cognasse F, Hamzeh-Cognasse H, Lafarge S, Delezay O, Pozzetto B, McNicol A, Garraud O (2008) Toll-like receptor 4 ligand can differentially modulate the release of cytokines by human platelets. Br J Haematol 141:84–91

Cooper MA, Elliott JM, Keyel PA, Yang L, Carrero JA, Yokoyama WM (2009) Cytokine-induced memory-like natural killer cells. Proc Nat Acad Sci USA 106:1915–1919

Craig SB, Graham GC, Burns M-A, Dohnt MF, Wilson RJ, Smythe LD, Jansen CC, McKay DB (2009) Leptospirosis and Goodpasture's syndrome: testing the aetiological hypothesis. Ann Trop Med Parasitol 103:647–651

Cullen PA, Cordwell SJ, Bulach DM, Haake DA, Adler B (2002) Global analysis of outer membrane proteins from *Leptospira interrogans* serovar Lai. Infect Immun 70:2311–2318

de Fost M, Hartskeerl RA, Groenendijk MR, van der Poll T (2003) Interleukin 12 in part regulates gamma interferon release in human whole blood stimulated with *Leptospira interrogans*. Clin Diagn Lab Immunol 10:332–335 de Fost M, Chierakul W, Limpaiboon R, Dondorp A, White NJ, van der Poll T (2007) Release of granzymes and chemokines in Thai patients with leptospirosis. Clin Microbiol Infect 13:433–436

Del Carlo Bernardi F, Ctenas B, da Silva LFF, Nicodemo AC, Saldiva PHN, Dolhnikoff M, Mauad T (2012) Immune receptors and adhesion molecules in human pulmonary leptospirosis. Hum Pathol 43:1601–1610

Diament D, Brunialti MKC, Romero EC, Kallas EG, Salomão R (2002) Peripheral blood mononuclear cell activation induced by Leptospira interrogans glycolipoprotein. Infect Immun 70:1677–1683

Dobrina A, Nardon E, Vecile E, Cinco M, Patriarca P (1995) Leptospira icterohemorrhagiae and leptospire peptidolgycans induce endothelial cell adhesiveness for polymorphonuclear leukocytes. Infect Immun 63:2995–2999

Domingos RF, Vieira ML, Romero EC, Goncales AP, Morais ZM, Vasconcellos SA, Nascimento AL (2012) Features of two proteins of Leptospira interrogans with potential role in host-pathogen interactions. BMC Microbiol 12:50

Edwards CN, Nicholson GD, Hassell TA, Everard CO, Callender J (1986) Thrombocytopenia in leptospirosis: the absence of evidence for disseminated intravascular coagulation. Am J Trop Med Hyg 35:352–354

Ellis W, McDowell S, Mackie D, Pollock M, Taylor M (2000). Immunity to bovine leptospirosis. In: Proceedings of the 21st world buiatrics congress, Punte del Este, Uruguay

Eshghi A, Lourdault K, Murray GL, Bartpho T, Sermswan RW, Picardeau M, Adler B, Snarr B, Zuerner RL, Cameron CE (2012a) Leptospira interrogans catalase is required for resistance to H_2O_2 and for virulence. Infect Immun 80:3892–3899

Eshghi A, Pinne M, Haake DA, Zuerner RL, Frank A, Cameron CE (2012b) Methylation and in vivo expression of the surface-exposed Leptospira interrogans outer-membrane protein OmpL32. Microbiol 158:622–635

Faber NA, Crawford M, Lefebvre RB, Buyukmihci NC, Madigan JE, Willits NH (2000) Detection of Leptospira spp. in the aqueous humor of horses with naturally acquired recurrent uveitis. J Clin Microbiol 38:2731–2733

Faine S, Adler B, Perolat P, Bolin C (1999) Leptospira and leptospirosis. MediSci, Melbourne

Fialho RN, Martins L, Pinheiro JP, Bettencourt BF, Couto AR, Santos MR, Peixoto MJ, Garrett F, Leal J, Tomás AM, Bruges-Armas J (2009) Role of human leukocyte antigen, killer-cell immunoglobulin-like receptors, and cytokine gene polymorphisms in leptospirosis. Hum Immunol 70:915–920

Gaudart N, Ekpo P, Pattanapanyasat K, van Kooyk Y, Engering A (2008) Leptospira interrogans is recognized through DC-SIGN and induces maturation and cytokine production by human dendritic cells. FEMS Immunol Med Microbiol 53:359–367

Goris MGA, Wagenaar JFP, Hartskeerl RA, van Gorp ECM, Schuller S, Monahan AM, Nally JE, van der Poll T, van 't Veer C (2011) Potent innate immune response to pathogenic Leptospira in human whole blood. PLoS ONE 6:e18279

Gray P, Dagvadorj J, Michelsen KS, Brikos C, Rentsendorj A, Town T, Crother TR, Arditi M (2011) Myeloid Differentiation Factor-2 interacts with lyn kinase and is tyrosine phosphorylated following lipopolysaccharide-induced activation of the TLR4 signaling pathway. J Immunol 187:4331–4337

Haake DA, Walker EM, Blanco DR, Bolin CA, Miller MN, Lovett MA (1991) Changes in the surface of Leptospira interrogans serovar Grippotyphosa during in vitro cultivation. Infect Immun 59:1131–1140

Haake DA, Chao G, Zuerner RL, Barnett JK, Barnett D, Mazel M, Matsunaga J, Levett PN, Bolin CA (2000) The leptospiral major outer membrane protein LipL32 is a lipoprotein expressed during mammalian infection. Infect Immun 68:2276–2285

Haake DA (2006) Hamster model of leptospirosis. Curr Protoc Microbiol 12:Unit 12E

Hein W, Mackay C (1991) Prominence of gamma delta T cells in the ruminant immune system. Immunol Today 12:30–34

Hsu S-H, Lo Y-Y, Tung J-Y, Ko Y-C, Sun Y-J, Hung C-C, Yang CW, Tseng F-G, Fu C-C, Pan R-L (2010) Leptospiral outer membrane lipoprotein LipL32 binding on toll-like receptor 2 of renal cells as determined with an atomic force microscope. Biochemistry 49:5408–5417

Hung C-C, Chang C-T, Chen K-H, Tian Y-C, Wu MS, Pan MJ, Vandewalle A, Yang C-W (2006a) Upregulation of chemokine CXCL1/KC by leptospiral membrane lipoprotein preparation in renal tubule epithelial cells. Kidney Int 69:1814–1822

Hung C-C, Chang C-T, Tian Y-C, Wu MS, Yu C-C, Pan MJ, Vandewalle A, Yang CW (2006b) Leptospiral membrane proteins stimulate pro-inflammatory chemokines secretion by renal tubule epithelial cells through toll-like receptor 2 and p38 mitogen activated protein kinase. Nephrol Dial Transplant 21:898–910

Isogai E, Kitagawa H, Isogai H, Kurebayashi Y, Ito N (1986) Phagocytosis as a defense mechanism against infection with leptospiras Zentralbl Bakteriol Mikrobiol Hyg A 261:65–74

Isogai E, Isogai H, Wakizaka H, Miura H, Kurebayashi Y (1989a) Chemiluminescence and phagocytic responses of rat polymorphonuclear neutrophils to leptospires. Zentralbl Bakteriol 272:36–46

Isogai E, Kitagawa H, Isogai H, Matsuzawa T, Shimizu T, Yanagihara Y, Katami K (1989b) Effects of leptospiral lipopolysaccharide on rabbit platelets. Zentralbl Bakteriol Mikrobiol Hyg A 271:186–196

Isogai E, Isogai H, Fujii N, Oguma K (1990) Macrophage activation by leptospiral lipopolysaccharide. Zentralbl Bakteriol 273:200–208

Iwasaki A, Medzhitov R (2010) Regulation of adaptive immunity by the innate immune system. Science 327:291–295

Jin D, Ojcius DM, Sun D, Dong H, Luo Y, Mao Y, Yan J (2009) *Leptospira interrogans* induces apoptosis in macrophages via caspase-8- and caspase-3-dependent pathways. Infect Immun 77:799–809

Jost BH, Adler B, Vinh T, Faine S (1986) A monoclonal antibody reacting with a determinant on leptospiral lipopolysaccharide protects guinea pigs against leptospirosis. J Med Microbiol 22:269–275

Jost BH, Adler B, Faine S (1989) Experimental immunisation of hamsters with lipopolysaccharide antigens of *Leptospira interrogans*. J Med Microbiol 29:115–120

Kawai T, Akira S (2010) The role of pattern-recognition receptors in innate immunity: update on Toll-like receptors. Nat Immunol 11:373–384

Klimpel GR, Matthias MA, Vinetz JM (2003) *Leptospira interrogans* activation of human peripheral blood mononuclear cells: preferential expansion of TCR gamma delta+ T cells vs TCR alpha beta+ T cells. J Immunol 171:1447–1455

Koizumi N (2003) Identification of a novel antigen of pathogenic *Leptospira spp.* that reacted with convalescent mice sera. J Med Microbiol 52:585–589

Kolb M, Margetts PJ, Anthony DC, Pitossi F, Gauldie J (2001) Transient expression of IL-1β induces acute lung injury and chronic repair leading to pulmonary fibrosis. J Clin Invest 107:1529–1536

Kyriakidis I, Samara P, Papa A (2011) Serum TNF-α, sTNFR1, IL-6, IL-8 and IL-10 levels in Weil's syndrome. Cytokine 54:117–120

Lacroix-Lamande S, d'Andon MF, Michel E, Ratet G, Philpott DJ, Girardin SE, Boneca IG, Vandewalle A, Werts C (2012) Downregulation of the Na/K-ATPase pump by leptospiral glycolipoprotein activates the NLRP3 inflammasome. J Immunol 188:2805–2814

Lee WL, Downey GP (2001) Neutrophil activation and acute lung injury. Curr Opin Crit Care 7:1–7

Leemans JC, Cassel SL, Sutterwala FS (2011) Sensing damage by the NLRP3 inflammasome. Immunol Rev 243:152–162

Li Y, Xiang M, Yuan Y, Xiao G, Zhang J, Jiang Y, Vodovotz Y, Billiar TR, Wilson MA, Fan J (2009) Hemorrhagic shock augments lung endothelial cell activation: role of temporal alterations of TLR4 and TLR2. Am J Physiol Regul Integr Comp Physiol 297:R1670–R1680

Lo M, Bulach DM, Powell DR, Haake DA, Matsunaga J, Paustian ML, Zuerner RL, Adler B (2006) Effects of temperature on gene expression patterns in *Leptospira interrogans* serovar Lai as assessed by whole-genome microarrays. Infect Immun 74:5848–5859

Loimaranta V, Hytönen J, Pulliainen AT, Sharma A, Tenovuo J, Strömberg N, Finne J (2009) Leucine-rich repeats of bacterial surface proteins serve as common pattern recognition motifs of human scavenger receptor gp340. J Biol Chem 284:18614–18623

Londoño D, Marques A, Hornung RL, Cadavid D (2008) IL-10 helps control pathogen load during high-level bacteremia. J Immunol 181:2076–2083

Lowanitchapat A, Payungporn S, Sereemaspun A, Ekpo P, Phulsuksombati D, Poovorawan Y, Chirathaworn C (2010) Expression of TNF-alpha, TGF-beta, IP-10 and IL-10 mRNA in kidneys of hamsters infected with pathogenic *Leptospira*. Comp Immunol Microbiol Infect Dis 33:423–434

Lucas DSD, Cullen PA, Lo M, Srikram A, Sermswan RW, Adler B (2011) Recombinant LipL32 and LigA from *Leptospira* are unable to stimulate protective immunity against leptospirosis in the hamster model. Vaccine 29:3413–3418

Lund RJ, Löytömäki M, Naumanen T, Dixon C, Chen Z, Ahlfors H, Tuomela S, Tahvanainen J, Scheinin J, Henttinen T, Rasool O, Lahesmaa R (2007) Genome-wide identification of novel genes involved in early Th1 and Th2 cell differentiation. J Immunol 178:3648–3660

Lusitani D, Malawista SE, Montgomery RR (2002) *Borrelia burgdorferi* are susceptible to killing by a variety of human polymorphonuclear leukocyte components. J Infect Dis 185:797–804

Mancel E, Merien F, Pesenti L, Salino D, Angibaud G, Perolat P (1999) Clinical aspects of ocular leptospirosis in New Caledonia (South Pacific). Aust N Z J Ophthalmol 27:380–386

Mariathasan S, Monack DM (2007) Inflammasome adaptors and sensors: intracellular regulators of infection and inflammation. Nat Rev Immunol 7:31–40

Marinho M, Oliveira-Júnior IS, Monteiro CMR, Perri SH, Salomão R (2009) Pulmonary disease in hamsters infected with *Leptospira interrogans*: histopathologic findings and cytokine mRNA expressions. Am J Trop Med Hyg 80:832–836

Martinez-Lopez DG, Fahey M, Coburn J (2010) Responses of human endothelial cells to pathogenic and non-pathogenic *Leptospira* species. PLoS Negl Trop Dis 4:e918

Matsui M, Rouleau V, Bruyère-Ostells L, Goarant C (2011) Gene expression profiles of immune mediators and histopathological findings in animal models of leptospirosis: comparison between susceptible hamsters and resistant mice. Infect Immun 79:4480–4492

Matsunaga J, Sanchez Y, Xu X, Haake DA (2005) Osmolarity, a key environmental signal controlling expression of leptospiral proteins LigA and LigB and the extracellular release of LigA. Infect Immun 73:70–78

Matsunaga J, Medeiros MA, Sanchez Y, Werneid KF, Ko AI (2007) Osmotic regulation of expression of two extracellular matrix-binding proteins and a haemolysin of *Leptospira interrogans*: differential effects on LigA and Sph2 extracellular release. Microbiol 153:3390–3398

McGrath H, Adler B, Vinh T, Faine S (1984) Phagocytosis of virulent and avirulent leptospires by guinea-pig and human polymorphonuclear leukocytes in vitro. Pathology 16:243–249

Merien F, Baranton G, Perolat P (1997) Invasion of Vero cells and induction of apoptosis in macrophages by pathogenic Leptospira interrogans are correlated with virulence. Infect Immun 65:729–738

Merien F, Truccolo J, Rougier Y, Baranton G, Perolat P (1998) *In vivo* apoptosis of hepatocytes in guinea pigs infected with *Leptospira interrogans* serovar Icterohaemorrhagiae. FEMS Microbiol Lett 169:95–102

Miller JC, Maylor-Hagen H, Ma Y, Weis JH, Weis JJ (2010) The Lyme disease spirochete *Borrelia burgdorferi* utilizes multiple ligands, including RNA, for interferon regulatory factor 3-dependent induction of type I interferon-responsive genes. Infect Immun 78:3144–3153

Miranda KA, Vasconcelos LRS, Coelho LCBB, Lima Filho JL, Cavalcanti MSM, Moura P (2009) High levels of serum mannose-binding lectin are associated with the severity of clinical signs of leptospirosis. Braz J Med Biol Res 42:353–357

Monahan AM, Callanan JJ, Nally JE (2008) Proteomic analysis of *Leptospira interrogans* shed in urine of chronically infected hosts. Infect Immun 76:4952–4958

Morton HE (1942) Susceptibility of Syrian hamsters to leptospirosis. Proc Soc Exp Biol Med (New York, NY) 49:566–568

Murray GL, Srikram A, Hoke DE, Wunder EA, Henry R, Lo M, Zhang K, Sermswan RW, Ko AI, Adler B (2009) Major surface protein LipL32 is not required for either acute or chronic infection with *Leptospira interrogans*. Infect Immun 77:952–958

Nahori M-A, Fournié-Amazouz E, Que-Gewirth NS, Balloy V, Chignard M, Raetz CRH, Saint Girons I, Werts C (2005) Differential TLR recognition of leptospiral lipid A and lipopolysaccharide in murine and human cells. J Immunol 175:6022–6031

Naiman BM, Alt D, Bolin CA, Zuerner R, Baldwin CL (2001a) Protective killed *Leptospira borgpetersenii* vaccine induces potent Th1 immunity comprising responses by CD4 and γδ T lymphocytes. Infect Immun 69:7550–7558

Naiman BM, Alt DP, Bolin CA, Zuerner RL, Baldwin CL (2001b) Protective killed *Leptospira borgpetersenii* vaccine induces potent Th1 immunity comprising responses by CD4 and γδ T lymphocytes. Infect Immun 69:7550–7558

Naiman BM, Blumerman S, Alt D, Bolin CA, Brown R, Zuerner RL, Baldwin CL (2002) Evaluation of type 1 immune response in naïve and vaccinated animals following challenge with *Leptospira borgpetersenii* serovar Hardjo: involvement of WC1(+) gammadelta and CD4 T cells. Infect Immun 70:6147–6157

Nally JE, Chantranuwat C, Wu X-Y, Fishbein MC, Pereira MM, da Silva JJP, Blanco DR, Lovett MA (2004) Alveolar septal deposition of immunoglobulin and complement parallels pulmonary hemorrhage in a guinea pig model of severe pulmonary leptospirosis. Am J Pathol 164:1115–1127

Nally JE, Fishbein MC, Blanco DR, Lovett MA (2005) Lethal infection of C3H/HeJ and C3H/SCID Mice with an isolate of *Leptospira interrogans* serovar Copenhageni. Infect Immun 73:7014–7017

Napetschnig J, Wu H (2013) Molecular Basis of NF-κB Signaling. Annu Rev Biophys 42:443–468

Noguchi H (1918) A comparative study of experimental prophylactic inoculation against *Leptospira icterohaemorrhagiae*. J Exp Med 28:561–570

Packchanian A (1940) Susceptibility and resistance of certain species of american deer mice, genus *Peromyscus*, and other rodents to *Leptospira icterohaemorrhagiae*. Public Health Rep 55:1389–1402

Park BS, Song DH, Kim HM, Choi BS, Lee H, Lee JO (2009) The structural basis of lipopolysaccharide recognition by the TLR4-MD-2 complex. Nature 458:1191–1195

Pereira MM, Andrade J, Marchevsky RS, Ribeiro dos Santos R (1998) Morphological characterization of lung and kidney lesions inC3H/HeJ mice infected with *Leptospira interrogans* serovar icterohaemorrhagiae: Defect of CD4+ and CD8+ T-cells are prognosticators of the disease progression. Exp Toxicol Pathol 50:191–198

Petnicki-Ocwieja T, Chung E, Acosta DI, T RL, Shin OS, Ghosh S, Kobzik L, Li X, Hu LT (2013) TRIF mediates Toll-Like Receptor 2-dependent inflammatory responses to *Borrelia burgdorferi*. Infect Immun 81:402–410

Petzke MM, Brooks A, Krupna MA, Mordue D, Schwartz I (2009) Recognition of *Borrelia burgdorferi*, the Lyme disease spirochete, by TLR7 and TLR9 induces a type I IFN response by human immune cells. J Immunol 183:5279–5292

Pinne M, Haake DA (2013) LipL32 is a subsurface lipoprotein of *Leptospira interrogans*: presentation of new data and reevaluation of previous studies. PLoS ONE 8:e51025

Prêtre G, Olivera N, Cédola M, Haase S, Alberdi L, Brihuega B, Gómez RM (2011) Role of inducible nitric oxide synthase in the pathogenesis of experimental leptospirosis. Microb Pathog 51:203–208

Rogers AN, VanBuren DG, Hedblom E, Tilahun ME, Telfer JC, Baldwin CL (2005a) Function of ruminant gammadelta T cells is defined by WC1.1 or WC1.2 isoform expression. Vet Immunol Immunopathol 108:211–217

Rogers AN, VanBuren DG, Hedblom EE, Tilahun ME, Telfer JC, Baldwin CL (2005b) Gammadelta T cell function varies with the expressed WC1 coreceptor. J Immunol 174:3386–3393

Rugman FP, Pinn G, Palmer MF, Waite M, Hay CR (1991) Anticardiolipin antibodies in leptospirosis. J Clin Pathol 44:517–519

Schoone GJ, Everard COR, Korver H, Carrington DG, Inniss VA, Baulu J, Terpstra WJ (1989) An immunoprotective monoclonal antibody directed against *Leptospira interrogans* serovar Copenhageni. Microbiol 135:73–78

Scocchi M, Romeo D, Cinco M (1993) Antimicrobial activity of two bactenecins against spirochetes. Infect Immun 61:3081–3083

Shibata T, Motoi Y, Tanimura N, Yamakawa N, Akashi-Takamura S, Miyake K (2011) Intracellular TLR4/MD-2 in macrophages senses Gram-negative bacteria and induces a unique set of LPS-dependent genes. Int Immunol 23:503–510

Sonrier C, Branger C, Michel V, Ruvoën-Clouet N, Ganière JP, André-Fontaine G (2000) Evidence of cross-protection within *Leptospira interrogans* in an experimental model. Vaccine 19:86–94

Spichler A, Spichler E, Moock M, Vinetz JM, Leake JAD (2007) Acute pancreatitis in fatal anicteric leptospirosis. Am J Trop Med Hyg 76:886–887

Srikram A, Zhang K, Bartpho T, Lo M, Hoke DE, Sermswan RW, Adler B, Murray GL (2011) Cross-protective immunity against leptospirosis elicited by a live, attenuated lipopolysaccharide mutant. J Infect Dis 203:870–879

Stevenson B, Choy HA, Pinne M, Rotondi ML, Miller MC, Demoll E, Kraiczy P, Cooley AE, Creamer TP, Suchard MA, Brissette CA, Verma A, Haake DA (2007) *Leptospira interrogans* endostatin-like outer membrane proteins bind host fibronectin, laminin and regulators of complement. PLoS ONE 2:e1188

Sun JC, Beilke JN, Lanier LL (2009) Adaptive immune features of natural killer cells. Nature 457:557–561

Tajiki H, Salomão R (1996) Association of plasma levels of tumor necrosis factor alpha with severity of disease and mortality among patients with leptospirosis. Clin Infect Dis 23:1177–1178

Thiermann AB, Handsaker AL (1985) Experimental infection of calves with *Leptospira interrogans* serovar Hardjo: conjunctival versus intravenous route of exposure. Am J Vet Res 46:329–331

Tian Y-C (2006) Leptospiral outer membrane protein induces extracellular matrix accumulation through a TGF-beta1/smad-dependent pathway. J Am Soc Nephrol 17:2792–2798

Tian Y-C, Hung C-C, Li Y-J, Chen Y-C, Chang M-Y, Yen T-H, Hsu H-H, Wu MS, Phillips A, Yang CW (2011) *Leptospira santorosai* Serovar Shermani detergent extract induces an increase in fibronectin production through a Toll-like receptor 2-mediated pathway. Infect Immun 79:1134–1142

Toma C, Okura N, Takayama C, Suzuki T (2011) Characteristic features of intracellular pathogenic *Leptospira* in infected murine macrophages. Cell Microbiol 13:1783–1792

Truccolo J, Charavay F, Merien F, Perolat P (2002) Quantitative PCR assay to evaluate ampicillin, ofloxacin, and doxycycline for treatment of experimental leptospirosis. Antimicrob Agents Chemother 46:848–853

Tucunduva de Faria M, Athanazio D, Goncalves Ramos E, Silva E, Reis M, Ko A (2007) Morphological alterations in the kidney of rats with natural and experimental *Leptospira* infection. J Comp Pathol 137:231–238

Tuero I, Vinetz JM, Klimpel GR (2010) Lack of demonstrable memory T cell responses in humans who have spontaneously recovered from leptospirosis in the Peruvian Amazon. J Infect Dis 201:420–427

Verma A, Artiushin S, Matsunaga J, Haake DA, Timoney JF (2005) LruA and LruB, novel lipoproteins of pathogenic *Leptospira interrogans* associated with equine recurrent uveitis. Infect Immun 73:7259–7266

Verma A, Rathinam SR, Priya CG, Muthukkaruppan VR, Stevenson B, Timoney JF (2008) LruA and LruB antibodies in sera of humans with leptospiral uveitis. Clin Vacc Immunol 15:1019–1023

Verma A, Brissette CA, Bowman AA, Shah ST, Zipfel PF, Stevenson B (2010) Leptospiral endostatin-like protein a is a bacterial cell surface receptor for human plasminogen. Infect Immun 78:2053–2059

Verma A, Stevenson B (2012) Leptospiral uveitis–there is more to it than meets the eye! Zoonoses Public Health 59:132–141

Vernel-Pauillac F, Merien F (2006) Proinflammatory and immunomodulatory cytokine mRNA time course profiles in hamsters infected with a virulent variant of *Leptospira interrogans*. Infect Immun 74:4172–4179

Vernel-Pauillac F, Goarant C (2010) Differential cytokine gene expression according to outcome in a hamster model of leptospirosis. PLoS Negl Trop Dis 4:e582

Vilaysane A, Chun J, Seamone ME, Wang W, Chin R, Hirota S, Li Y, Clark SA, Tschopp J, Trpkov K, Hemmelgarn BR, Beck PL, Muruve DA (2010) The NLRP3 inflammasome promotes renal inflammation and contributes to CKD. J Am Soc Nephrol 21:1732–1744

Vinh T, Adler B, Faine S (1982) The role of macrophages in the protection of mice against leptospirosis: *in vitro* and *in vivo* studies. Pathology 14:463–468

Vinh T, Adler B, Faine S (1986) Glycolipoprotein cytotoxin from *Leptospira interrogans* serovar Copenhageni. J Gen Microbiol 132:111–123

Viriyakosol S, Matthias MA, Swancutt MA, Kirkland TN, Vinetz JM (2006) Toll-Like Receptor 4 protects against lethal *Leptospira interrogans* serovar icterohaemorrhagiae infection and contributes to *in vivo* control of leptospiral burden. Infect Immun 74:887–895

Wagenaar JFP, Gasem MH, Goris MGA, Leeflang M, Hartskeerl RA, van der Poll T, van 't Veer C, van Gorp ECM (2009a) Soluble ST2 levels are associated with bleeding in patients with severe leptospirosis. PLoS Negl Trop Dis 3:e453

Wagenaar JFP, Goris MGA, Gasem MH, Isbandrio B, Moalli F, Mantovani A, Boer KR, Hartskeerl RA, Garlanda C, van Gorp ECM (2009b) Long pentraxin PTX3 is associated with mortality and disease severity in severe leptospirosis. J Infect 58:425–432

Wang B, Sullivan JA, Sullivan GW, Mandell GL (1984) Role of specific antibody in interaction of leptospires with human monocytes and monocyte-derived macrophages. Infect Immun 46:809–813

Wang F, Herzig CTA, Chen C, Hsu H, Baldwin CL, Telfer JC (2011) Scavenger receptor WC1 contributes to the γδ T cell response to *Leptospira*. Mol Immunol 48:801–809

Wang H, Wu Y, Ojcius DM, Yang XF, Zhang C, Ding S, Lin X, Yan J (2012) Leptospiral hemolysins induce proinflammatory cytokines through Toll-like receptor 2-and 4-mediated JNK and NF-κB signaling pathways. PLoS ONE 7:e42266

Werts C, Tapping RI, Mathison JC, Chuang T-H, Kravchenko V, Saint Girons I, Haake DA, Godowski PJ, Hayashi F, Ozinsky A, Underhill DM, Kirschning CJ, Wagner H, Aderem A, Tobias PS, Ulevitch RJ (2001) Leptospiral lipopolysaccharide activates cells through a TLR2-dependent mechanism. Nat Immunol 2:346–352

Williams A, Flavell RA, Eisenbarth SC (2010) The role of NOD-like receptors in shaping adaptive immunity. Curr Opin Immunol 22:34–40

Witchell TD, Eshghi A, Nally JE, Hof R, Boulanger MJ, Wunder EA, Ko AI, Haake DA, Cameron CE (2014) Post-translational modification of LipL32 during Leptospira interrogans infection. PLoS Negl Trop Dis. Accepted 19 Sept 2014

Xiang M, Shi X, Li Y, Xu J, Yin L, Xiao G, Scott MJ, Billiar TR, Wilson MA, Fan J (2011) Hemorrhagic shock activation of NLRP3 inflammasome in lung endothelial cells. J Immunol 187:4809–4817

Yang C-W, Wu MS, Pan MJ, Hong JJ, Yu CC, Vandewalle A, Huang CC (2000) *Leptospira* outer membrane protein activates NF-kappaB and downstream genes expressed in medullary thick ascending limb cells. J Am Soc Nephrol 11:2017–2026

Yang C-W, Hung C-C, Wu MS, Tian Y-C, Chang C-T, Pan MJ, Vandewalle A (2006) Toll-like receptor 2 mediates early inflammation by leptospiral outer membrane proteins in proximal tubule cells. Kidney Int 69:815–822

Yang G-G, Hsu Y-H (2005) Nitric oxide production and immunoglobulin deposition in leptospiral hemorrhagic respiratory failure. J Formos Med Assoc 104:759–763

Yeaman MR (2009) Platelets in defense against bacterial pathogens. Cell Mol Life Sci 67:525–544

Zuerner RL, Knudtson W, Bolin CA, Trueba G (1991) Characterization of outer membrane and secreted proteins of *Leptospira interrogans* serovar Pomona. Microb Pathog 10:311–322

Zuerner RL, Alt DP, Palmer MV, Thacker TC, Olsen SC (2011) A *Leptospira borgpetersenii* serovar Hardjo vaccine induces a Th1 Response, activates NK cells, and reduces renal colonization. Clin Vacc Immunol 18:684–691

Zuerner RL, Alt DP, Palmer MV (2012) Development of chronic and acute golden Syrian hamster infection models with *Leptospira borgpetersenii* serovar Hardjo. Vet Pathol 49:403–411

Vaccines Against Leptospirosis

Ben Adler

Abstract Vaccines against leptospirosis followed within a year of the first isolation of *Leptospira*, with the first use of a killed whole cell bacterin vaccine in guinea pigs published in 1916. Since then, bacterin vaccines have been used in humans, cattle, swine, and dogs and remain the only vaccines licensed at the present time. The immunity elicited is restricted to serovars with related lipopolysaccharide (LPS) antigen. Likewise, vaccines based on LPS antigens have clearly demonstrated protection in animal models, which is also at best serogroup specific. The advent of leptospiral genome sequences has allowed a reverse vaccinology approach for vaccine development. However, the use of inadequate challenge doses and inappropriate statistical analysis invalidates many of the claims of protection with recombinant proteins.

Contents

B. Adler (✉)
Department of Microbiology, Australian Research Council Centre of Excellence in Structural and Functional Microbial Genomics, Monash University, Clayton, VIC 3800, Australia
e-mail: Ben.Adler@monash.edu

© Springer-Verlag Berlin Heidelberg 2015   251
B. Adler (ed.), *Leptospira and Leptospirosis*, Current Topics in Microbiology and Immunology 387, DOI 10.1007/978-3-662-45059-8_10

1 Bacterin Vaccines

Pathogenic *Leptospira* was first isolated in Japan in 1914. Within a year, Japanese researchers had successfully immunized guinea pigs (Ido et al. 1916). They showed that injection of leptospires inactivated with phenol elicited protective immunity in guinea pigs and that immunity could be transferred with immune serum administered concurrently with the infecting leptospires, demonstrating for the first time the importance of antibodies in immunity to leptospirosis in an animal model. The first large-scale human use took place in Japan, where Wani vaccinated 10,000 coal miners between 1919 and 1921. He also showed passive protection of guinea pigs with human immune serum (Alston and Broom 1958).

In the ensuing years, a variety of methods was used to kill leptospires for use as vaccines, including heat, formalin, phenol, ethanol, freeze-thawing, and irradiation. However, in the past 100 years very little has changed and at the present time the only licensed vaccines remain whole cell, inactivated bacterins. These have been used widely in cattle, swine, and dogs; specific usage for individual animal species is detailed in chapter by W.A. Ellis, this volume. Because of problems with reactogenicity due to components of the leptospires and constituents of the growth media, bacterin vaccines for humans have not gained acceptance to the same degree as for animals. Attempts to overcome these problems have included the development of protein-free growth media (Christopher et al. 1982; Torten et al. 1973). However, yields were generally much poorer than in conventional media containing serum or BSA. Nevertheless, human bacterin vaccines have been used successfully in several regions, including China, Japan, Cuba, and Europe. The use of currently available human vaccines is described in the chapter by D.A. Haake and P.N. Levett, this volume.

Immunity elicited by bacterin vaccines is restricted to serovars with related agglutinating antigens and is generally humorally mediated, with the exception of Hardjo infection in cattle (Naiman et al. 2001). This restriction, therefore, requires a good knowledge of the regional epidemiology, which can be reliably gained only by culture and identification of locally prevalent serovars. Reliance on serological surveys to predict local serovars is not recommended. A second consequence of the limitation of immunity to serologically-related serovars is that in situations where multiple serovars are circulating, multivalent vaccines are required. Accordingly, bacterin vaccines containing up to four serovars are commonly used in many countries, especially in dogs and pigs (see the chapter by W.A. Ellis, this volume). Claims for protection against additional, closely-related serovars are probably valid. In some countries, locally-produced vaccines, especially for use in cattle, may contain up to eight serovars. Efficacy studies to demonstrate protection against all the included serovars have very rarely, if ever, been performed. Any possible antigenic competition effects between such large numbers of serovars are completely unknown. A final drawback of bacterin vaccines arises from the fact that the immunity elicited is directed mainly against the leptospiral lipopolysaccharide

(LPS), a T-independent antigen, and therefore involves IgM antibodies and lack of a memory response. The duration of immunity is therefore relatively short, with annual vaccination recommended in almost all cases.

2 Live Vaccines

The lack of detailed knowledge about leptospiral pathogenesis (see the chapter by G.L. Murray, this volume) and the unavailability of genetic tools for easy manipulation of pathogenic *Leptospira* spp. (see the chapter by M. Picardeau, this volume) have to date precluded any development of rationally-attenuated, live vaccines. Nevertheless, serovar Pomona attenuated by laboratory passage was used as a live vaccine and shown to elicit protective immunity in hamsters, swine, and cattle (Stalheim 1968). Although demonstrated to be safe and to be effective in stimulating a duration of immunity which lasted at least 14 months (Stalheim 1971), the basis for attenuation was unknown; the vaccine has not been developed further and no live vaccines are currently licensed.

More recently, a defined LPS biosynthetic mutant of serovar Manilae was shown to be attenuated in hamsters, which showed no clinical signs of infection, and did not become renal carriers (Srikram et al. 2010). The mutant was also unable to colonize the kidneys of mice (Marcsisin et al. 2013). Immunization with the mutant elicited protective immunity against homologous challenge and also against heterologous challenge with serovars Pomona (Srikram et al. 2010) or Autumnalis (Unpublished results). Killed bacteria stimulated only homologous protection. Significantly, there was no detectable reactivity against either Pomona or Autumnalis LPS, strongly suggesting that immunity was mediated by protein antigens. The identity of the protective antigens is unknown.

3 Lipopolysaccharide Vaccines

Unlike some of the other major spirochete genera *Treponema* and *Borrelia*, the major surface component of *Leptospira* is LPS. Furthermore, leptospiral LPS is a protective antigen. Monoclonal antibodies against LPS can protect against acute lethal infection in guinea pigs and hamsters (Jost et al. 1986; Schoone et al. 1989) and also protected dogs, based on recovery of leptospires from blood (Schoone et al. 1989). The protection shown in early studies with an "outer sheath" preparation (Auran et al. 1972) was almost certainly mediated by LPS; indeed, LPS was shown by silver staining and western blotting to be a major constituent of this preparation (Adler B; unpublished results). Likewise, it is clear that a reported protective "glycolipid" antigen (Masuzawa et al. 1990) was in fact LPS. Immunization with as little as 2.5 µg of purified LPS, or the polysaccharide (PS) component of LPS, was sufficient to elicit the production of agglutinating, protective antibodies in hamsters

(Jost et al. 1989). The immunogenicity of PS could be enhanced by conjugation with a protein carrier, diphtheria toxoid (Midwinter et al. 1990). An oligosaccharide derived from LPS and conjugated to diphtheria toxoid elicited the production of agglutinating, opsonic antibodies (Midwinter et al. 1994), suggesting that the conjugate would be protective, but protection studies were not undertaken. The structure of leptospiral lipid A has been determined (Que-Gewirth et al. 2004), but the structure of the carbohydrate component remains unknown. However, genome sequences have identified LPS biosynthetic loci with close to 100 genes, suggesting that the LPS structure is very complex (Bulach et al. 2006; Nascimento et al. 2004).

An intriguing possibility was raised by the use of LPS derived from saprophytic *Leptospira biflexa* to immunize hamsters against infection with the pathogenic serovar Manilac (Matsuo et al. 2000). However, the claims of protection must be tempered by the fact that all hamsters, including controls, survived challenge, despite the use of a high $>10^6$ challenge dose. Protection was based on clinical and pathological criteria, but the use of small animal groups precludes the drawing of any statistically meaningful results. It is possible that the effects observed were due to activation of the innate immune response by *L. biflexa* LPS. The work has not been reproduced, but significantly, an earlier study in which children were immunized with an inactivated *L. biflexa* vaccine reported no agglutinating antibodies against pathogenic serovars (Rottini et al. 1972). In addition, another study found no protection against challenge with Canicola in gerbils immunized with *L. biflexa* (Sonrier et al. 2000).

The clear capacity of LPS and LPS-derived components to elicit protective immunity held the possibility of development of immunoconjugate vaccines, similar to those developed against pneumococcal and *Haemophilus influenzae* infections. However, this development has not eventuated, most probably because of the large number of leptospiral serovars, the cost involved, and the unknown but complex structure of leptospiral LPS. There is no prospect of LPS-based vaccines in the near future.

4 Cross-Protective Immunity

It seems apparent that heterologous immunity does not usually follow natural infection, at least in humans. The author has experience of two examples where culture confirmed infection with one serovar (Pomona) was followed less than 3 months later by infection, again culture confirmed, with a different serovar (Hardjo). Nevertheless, the stimulation of cross-protective immunity remains an important focus and goal in leptospirosis vaccine research. Several studies have shown that this is feasible.

Some inkling that cross immunity might exist was noticed as early as 1928 (Fletcher 1928) and perhaps even earlier, although these studies were primitive by today's standards. In work now 50 years old, Kemenes (1964) investigated cross immunity in guinea pigs, which recovered from one infection and were then infected with a heterologous serovars. He showed a level of cross immunity between serovars Pomona and Canicola and also between Pomona and Icterohaemorrhagiae. Cross immunity did not extend to serovars Sejroe or Hyos (now Tarassovi). Of course, the nature of the antigens involved was and remains unknown, but interestingly, both of these serovars are now classified in the species *Leptospira borgpetersenii*, while Pomona, Canicola, and Icterohaemorrhagiae belong to *Leptospira interrogans*.

Using a similar approach, Plesko and Lataste-Dorolle (1970) showed limited, but incomplete, cross immunity between several serovars, including Bratislava, Icterohaemorrhagiae and Copenhageni, Pomona, Lora (all *L. interrogans*) and Grippotyphosa (*L. kirschneri*). In a subsequent study, significant, but not complete, interserovar immunity was demonstrated in hamsters between four serovars of *L. borgpetersenii*, viz. Tarassovi, Javanica, Poi and Arborea (Plesko and Hlavata 1971). Again, the responsible antigens remain unknown. However, it is notable that all of these studies used live leptospires, highlighting the possibility that cross-protective antigens may be expressed exclusively in vivo, or at best, expressed at low levels in vitro.

There appears to have been no further work in this area for several decades until Sonrier et al. (2000) investigated the cross-protective capacity of LPS and whole cell extracts, obtained from in vitro-grown bacteria, in gerbils. Not surprisingly, LPS elicited only homologous protection. However, whole cell extracts from Icterohaemorrhagiae ($p = 0.003$) but not from Autumnalis ($p = 0.2$) protected against challenge with Canicola. In a modified reverse experiment, a chloroform-methanol-water extract of the phenol phase (designated as protein in this paper) LPS preparation from Canicola protected against challenge with Icterohaemorrhagiae ($p = 0.002$). However, the claim of protein-mediated cross protection must be tempered by two caveats. The phenol phase can also contain leptospiral LPS (Shinagawa and Yanagawa 1972; Vinh et al. 1989) and there is a well-established MAT cross-reactivity between serovars Canicola and Icterohaemorrhagiae. The possibility that the observed protection was actually mediated by LPS cannot be excluded.

A more recent study examined cross immunity between four serovars, using formalin-inactivated vaccines in hamsters (Rosario et al. 2012). Serovars Canicola and Copenhageni belong to *L. interrogans*, serovar Ballum to *L. borgpetersenii*, while serovar Mozdok may be classified as either *L. borgpetersenii* or *L. kirschneri*, depending on the strain (not specified in this paper). All four vaccines elicited 100 % homologous immunity, as well as varying levels of cross immunity. The Mozdok vaccine elicited only homologous immunity. Immunization with Copenhageni stimulated immunity against challenge with Ballum but not the other two heterologous serovars. The claimed protection against Canicola was not significant ($p = 0.087$). However, vaccination with Ballum or Canicola induced solid heterologous immunity except against Mozdok, with 100 % survival except for the Ballum-Copenhageni combination (70 %; $p = 0.003$).

As described above (Sect. 2), a genetically defined LPS biosynthesis mutant of serovar Manilae was able to stimulate 100 % immunity in hamsters against challenge with Autumnalis (Unpublished results) or Pomona (Srikram et al. 2010).

What conclusions can realistically be drawn from these studies? Although the results have been variable, it seems clear that it is possible to stimulate heterologous immunity and that the antigens involved are probably proteins which may well be expressed poorly or not at all under the standard conditions used to culture leptospires in vitro. Although some progress has been made in recent years, the identity of the antigen(s) involved remains poorly understood.

5 Recombinant Proteins as Vaccines

The development of recombinant DNA techniques and the availability of leptospiral whole genome sequences have resulted in a resurgence of activity to identify protective antigens and to develop defined subunit vaccines. However, much of the vaccination work reported in the literature suffers from the use of inadequate challenge doses, lack of reproducibility, and inappropriate statistical analysis. Accordingly, many of the claims about protection from infection, especially those claiming partial protection, cannot be substantiated.

5.1 The Lipoprotein LipL32

The leptospiral outer membrane lipoprotein LipL32 (Haake et al. 2000) would appear to have all the hallmarks of a virulence factor and/or protective antigen. It is the most abundant protein in the leptospiral cell and the outer membrane and is present exclusively in pathogenic *Leptospira* spp., where it is highly conserved. Surprisingly, therefore, a defined *lipL32* mutant retained virulence for hamsters, whether infected parenterally or conjunctivally, and was unaffected in its ability to colonize the renal tubules of rats (Murray et al. 2009). Originally identified as a major component of the leptospiral surface (Cullen et al. 2005), its surface location has recently been re-evaluated (Pinne and Haake 2013).

LipL32 is the most studied leptospiral protein (Murray 2013). Its ability to elicit protective immunity against acute infection with several different serovars has been reported numerous times using a range of antigen delivery methods and animal models (Table 1). However, a rigorous evaluation reveals major deficiencies in many of these reports, with the most common problems being the use of inadequate challenge dose, small groups of animals, and inappropriate statistical analysis. Accordingly, the majority of publications does not present a credible case for protection when survival is used as the criterion (Table 1).

The original work in gerbils delivered LipL32 either as a recombinant protein or via the *lipL32* gene introduced as plasmid DNA or using an adenovirus vector. Claims of protection must be tempered by the high survival rates in control animals resulting in lack of statistically significant protection (Table 1). Similar problems arise when assessing the results of attempts to immunize hamsters with LipL32

Table 1 Protection studies with LipL32

Origin serovar	Challenge serovar	Antigen	Animal	Delivery	Claimed protection[a]	P value[b]	Notes	References
Autumnalis	Canicola	lipL32 adenovirus	Gerbil	Adenovirus 10^9 pfu	86 %	0.054–0.06	50 % survival in control groups	Branger et al. (2001)
Autumnalis or Copenhageni	Canicola	lipL32 DNA	Gerbil	Plasmid DNA 100 μg	60 %	0.18	35 % survival in control group	Branger et al. (2005)
Autumnalis or Copenhageni	Canicola	LipL32	Gerbil	Protein 50 μg	0–50 %	0.48–0.71	13–60 % survival in control groups	Branger et al. (2005)
Copenhageni	Copenhageni	LipL32	Hamster	BCG 10^6 cfu	16–60 %	0.015–0.72	Highly variable results across three experiments	Seixas et al. (2007)
Icterohaemorrhagiae	Pomona	Anti-LipL32 monoclonal antibody	Hamster	Anti-LipL32 monoclonal antibody	100 %	<0.0001	Low challenge dose $5 \times LD_{50}$. Leptospires isolated from tissues at 21 day necropsy	Maneewatch et al. (2008)
Lai	Lai	LipL32	Guinea pig	Protein 200 μg	50 %	0.01	High challenge dose > 10^8	Luo et al. (2010)
Lai	Ballum	LipL32	Guinea pig	Protein 200 μg	58 %	0.005	High challenge dose > 10^8	Luo et al. (2010)

(continued)

Table 1 (continued)

Origin serovar	Challenge serovar	Antigen	Animal	Delivery	Claimed protection[a]	P value[b]	Notes	References
Pomona	Pomona	LipL32	Hamster	Protein 50 µg	Nil	1.0	No protection based on lung histopathology	Cao et al. (2011)
Manilae or Hardjo	Manilae	LipL32 and fragments	Hamster	Protein 50 µg	Nil	1.0	No survival in control groups. Hamster sera reacted with intact LipL32	Deveson Lucas et al. (2011)
Copenhageni	Copenhageni	LipL32-LTB fusion	Hamster	Protein 43–60 µg	40–100 %	0.44	0–60 % survival in control groups	Grassmann et al.(2012)
Copenhageni	Copenhageni	LipL32 +LTB	Hamster	Protein 43–60 µg	60–100 %	0.17–0.44	0–60 % survival in control groups	Grassmann et al.(2012)

[a] Protection based on survival compared with control animals

[b] Fisher's exact test

expressed in *Mycobacterium bovis* BCG. A proper statistical analysis shows that significance was achieved ($p = 0.022$, Fisher's exact test) in only one of three experiments. Claimed protection of hamsters immunized with LipL32 and LTB, either as a mixture or as a fusion protein, likewise do not withstand proper analysis. Importantly, two additional studies in hamsters showed unequivocal lack of protection following immunization with recombinant entire LipL32 or fragments thereof (Table 1; Cao et al. 2011; Deveson Lucas et al. 2011).

In contrast, partial but significant protection was generated in guinea pigs immunized with LipL32 and challenged with either serovar Lai (homologous) or Ballum (Table 1; Luo et al. 2010). However, even here the conclusion must be tempered by the apparently low virulence of the challenge strains, necessitating the use of a very high challenge dose.

A more compelling case for LipL32 as a protective antigen arises from the clear and highly significant protection conferred to hamsters that received mouse monoclonal antibodies against LipL32 (Table 1; Maneewatch et al. 2008). What then, are we to make of these apparently contradictory findings? Given that the most credible protection has been mediated by antibodies generated in mice or guinea pigs, is it possible that these animal species respond with antibody isotypes that are protective, but hamsters do not? Or do these protective antibodies recognize unique LipL32 epitopes? LipL32 in *Leptospira* is glycosylated (Ricaldi et al. 2012), but recombinant proteins used in vaccination studies would almost certainly not be glycosylated. Any role for LipL32-linked glycans in immunity remains completely unknown.

A further possibility is that cell-mediated immunity plays an as yet undefined role in the variable levels of protection observed. Intriguingly, in cattle where immunity, at least to serovar Hardjo, is not antibody dependent but is correlated with IFN-γ release by T-cells, the antigen which is the major stimulator of IFN-γ release is LipL32 (Deveson Lucas et al. 2014). The possibility thus exists that LipL32 is a protective antigen in some animal species but not in others. In the case of humans at least, there is a compelling argument that LipL32 does not mediate protection. LipL32 is expressed during human infection and is immunogenic; indeed it has been used as a serodiagnostic antigen (Flannery et al. 2001). However, in the face of this antibody response, immunity following human infection is restricted to serovars with related LPS. Whether this restriction is true for other animal species remains equivocal. Another possibility might be that antibodies elicited during natural infection are not directed against as yet undefined protective epitopes. The role of LipL32 in immunity thus remains enigmatic and warrants further investigation.

5.2 The Lig Proteins

The Lig proteins were identified as major components of the leptospiral surface which are not expressed under normal in vitro growth conditions (Matsunaga et al.

2003, 2005). The Lig proteins have been investigated as vaccine candidates against challenge infection with three different serovars (Table 2). As is the case with LipL32 studies, many of the claims of protection must be tempered due to the use of inadequate challenge doses, poor reproducibility, and inappropriate statistical analyses. There are no studies which present a credible case for LigB as a protective antigen (Table 2). Koizumi and Watanabe (2004) reported >90 % protection of C3H/HeJ mice immunized with LigA and/or LigB, but with 40 % survival in the GST-immunized control groups, yielding statistical insignificance. A study with LigA in hamsters claimed efficacy (Table 2; Palaniappan et al. 2006), but control animals showed 75 % survival. A subsequent attempt to immunize hamsters with DNA encoding LigA also claimed protection (Faisal et al. 2008); however, a proper statistical analysis of those data does not support the claim of enhanced survival (Table 2). Nevertheless, several other studies have now shown unequivocal protection of hamsters immunized with the C-terminal portion of LigA, with *ligA* DNA, or with specific domains within the LigA C-terminus (Table 2). An alternative approach was used to deliver lipidated LigA expressed in *E. coli* orally to hamsters. Significant protection was elicited in single experiments against a low intradermal challenge dose, but not against a slightly higher intraperitoneal challenge (Table 2; Lourdault et al. 2014). LigA therefore shows significant promise as a protective protein antigen, at least against some serovars. Potential explanations for the conflicting results include the use of different adjuvants, challenge doses, and challenge serovars. Indeed, one study found no homologous protection in hamsters immunized with Canicola LigA (Table 2; N. Bomchil, Personal communication), whereas Copenhageni LigA elicited 100 % protection against homologous challenge. A similar lack of homologous protection was observed with serovar Manilae (Table 2; Deveson Lucas et al. 2011). The possibility therefore remains that the protective capacity of LigA may not necessarily extrapolate to all species or serovars.

5.3 Other Recombinant Proteins

There has been a range of other recombinant proteins tested for protective capacity. Similar problems arise with the majority of claims, which report a single experiment, or lack of reproducibility and therefore do not withstand proper statistical analysis. These are summarized in Table 3 and will not be discussed further here. Notably, Murray et al. (2013) found no protection elicited by any of the 238 recombinant proteins tested from serovar Hardjo, when colonization of hamster kidneys was used as the criterion for protection. The list of proteins tested contained several for which claims of protection had been made previously.

Two studies report protection elicited by the FlaB flagellar subunit protein (Table 3). The first (Dai et al. 1997) was performed in mice, which were challenged with a very high dose of 2.5×10^{10} leptospires; despite this dose, 40 % of controls survived, but the numbers used yielded significant protection (Table 3). In the

Table 2 Protection studies with Lig proteins

Origin serovar	Challenge serovar	Antigen	Animal	Delivery	Claimed protection[a]	P value[b]	Notes	References
Manilae	Manilae	LigA or LigB C-ter-minus. GST fusions	C3H/ HEJ mouse	Protein 10 µg	90 %	0.077	40 % survival in GST control group. Protec-tion significant only when compared with PBS group	Koizumi and Watanabe (2004)
Manilae	Manilae	LigA C-ter-minus plus LigB C-ter-minus. GST fusion	C3H/ HEJ mouse	Protein 10 µg	100 %	0.167	40 % survival in GST control group. Protec-tion significant when com-pared with PBS group	Koizumi and Watanabe (2004)
Pomona	Pomona	LigA C-ter-minus plus LigA N-ter-minus. GST fusions.	Hamster	Protein 50 µg	100 %	0.077–1.0	57–88 % sur-vival in control groups	Palaniappan et al. (2006)
Copenhageni	Copenhageni	LigA C-ter-minus. His tag	Hamster	Protein 10–80 µg	63–100 %	0.00008–0.026	Better protec-tion with higher protein doses	Silva et al. (2007)
Copenhageni	Copenhageni	LigB C-ter-minus. His tag	Hamster	Protein 10–80 µg	Nil	1.0	No protection	Silva et al. (2007)

(continued)

Table 2 (continued)

Origin serovar	Challenge serovar	Antigen	Animal	Delivery	Claimed protection[a]	P value[b]	Notes	References
Pomona	Pomona	ligA DNA	Hamster	Plasmid DNA 50 μg	100 %	0.077–0.20	50–75 % survival in control groups	Faisal et al. (2008)
Pomona	Pomona	LigB fragments	Hamster	Protein 50 μg	25–87 %	0.01–1.0	Variability across experiments. Significant protection with C-terminus (p = 0.04) or C- plus N-terminal fragments (p = 0.01) obtained in 2 of 3 experiments	Yan et al. (2009)
Pomona	Pomona	LigB fragments	Hamster	Protein 50 μg	33–50 %	0.182–0.455	2 or 3 survivors in groups of 6	Cao et al. (2011)
Pomona	Pomona	LigA C-terminus	Hamster	Liposomes or PLGA microspheres 10/ 20 μg	76–92 %	<10⁻⁷	LigA with alum adjuvant elicited 50 % protection (p = 0.002)	Faisal et al. (2009)
Copenhageni	Copenhageni	LigA C-terminus and sub-fragments. His tag	Hamster	Protein 100 μg	50–100 %	0.01–0.43	Domains 10–13 required for 100 % protection. Use of four animals	Coutinho et al. (2011)

(continued)

Table 2 (continued)

Origin serovar	Challenge serovar	Antigen	Animal	Delivery	Claimed protection[a]	P value[b]	Notes	References
Manilae	Manilae	LigA C-terminus	Hamster	Protein 30 µg	Nil	0.474	per group limits conclusions. Hamster sera reacted with intact LigA in *Leptospira*	Deveson Lucas et al. (2011)
Canicola	Copenhageni	*ligA* or *ligB* DNA	Hamster	Plasmid DNA 100 µg	62*–100 %	0.03 to <10⁻⁶	*One LigB group. remainder all 100 % protection	Forster et al. (2013)
Canicola	Canicola	LigA C-terminus	Hamster	Protein 100 µg	Nil	1.0	No protection. 100 % homologous protection with Copenhageni in the same study	Bomchil. N. (Personal communication)
Copenhageni	Copenhageni	LigA lipidated C-terminal domains 7–13	Hamster	*E. coli* total 37–148 mg. repeat oral immunization	38–63 %	0.026–0.2	Protection against intradermal but not intraperitoneal challenge. Single experiments	Lourdault et al. (2014)

[a] Protection based on survival compared with control animals
[b] Fisher's exact test

Table 3 Protection studies with other recombinant proteins

Origin serovar	Challenge serovar	Antigen	Animal	Delivery	Claimed protection[a]	P value[b]	Notes	References
Lai	Lai	*flaB* DNA	Mouse	*E. coli* 10^7 cfu plus plasmid DNA	78 %	0.02	Challenge dose 2.5 × 10^10 40 % survival in control group which received only plasmid vector without *E. coli*	Dai et al. (1997)
Grippotyphosa	Grippotyphosa	OmpL1 LipL41 and OmpL1	Hamster	Protein 50 µg, in *E. coli* membrane	100 %	0.009	33 % survival in control group. Protection seen in one of three experiments. No protection with His-tagged protein(s)	Haake et al. (1999)
Lai	Lai	*flaB2* DNA	Guinea pig	Plasmid DNA 100 µg	90 %	0.005	Single experiment reported	Dai et al. (2000)
Copenhageni	Pomona	*ompL1* DNA	Hamster	Plasmid DNA 100 µg	33 %	0.455	2/6 survival compared with 0/6 in control group	Maneewatch et al. 2007)
Pomona	Pomona	Lp1454, Lp1118, McelI. GST fusions.	Hamster	Protein 50 µg	71–100 %	0.07–0.59	50 % survival in control groups. No significant protection when all three combined	Chang et al. (2007)
Lai	Lai	*lipL21* DNA	Guinea pig	Plasmid DNA 100 µg	Nil	1.0	All animals survived. Protection claimed on the basis of changes in weight gain	He et al. (2008)

(continued)

Table 3 (continued)

Origin serovar	Challenge serovar	Antigen	Animal	Delivery	Claimed protection[a]	P value[b]	Notes	References
Pomona	Pomona	Lp0607, Lp118, Lp1454 combined	Hamster	Protein trapped in leptospiral or *E. coli* liposomes	75 %	0.0006	No protection with proteins trapped in phosphatidylcholine liposomes ($p = 0.245$). No protection with proteins mixed with any liposomes ($p = 1.0$)	Faisal et al. (2009)
Copenhageni	Copenhageni	Lic12720, Lic10494, Lic12922 His tag	Hamster	Protein 50 µg	30–44 %	0.04*–1.0	*Lic 12720 in one of two experiments	Atzingen et al. (2010)
Pomona	Pomona	Lp0222, Lp3685, Lp4337	Hamster	Protein 50 µg	33–83 %	0.08–1.0	Protection not significant	Yan et al. (2010)
Copenhageni	Copenhageni	Lic10325, Lic13059 His tag	Hamster	Protein 60 µg	33 %	0.455	2/6 survival compared with 0/6 in control group	Felix et al. (2011)
Copenhageni	Copenhageni	Lsa21, Lsa66, Lic11030. His tag	Hamster	Protein 50 µg	20–30 %	0.21–0.48	Claimed protection for any of the proteins was not reproduced in a second experiment	Atzingen et al. (2012)

(continued)

Table 3 (continued)

Origin serovar	Challenge serovar	Antigen	Animal	Delivery	Claimed protection[a]	P value[b]	Notes	References
Copenhageni	Icterohaemorrhagiae	*lemA* DNA and LemA prime boost	Hamster	Protein 100 µg plasmid DNA 100 µg	87 %	0.002	LemA alone (p = 0.8). *lemA* alone (p = 0.03). Survivors culture and lesion positive. Results from single experiment	Hartwig et al. (2013)
Copenhageni	Copenhageni	Leptallo1. His tag	Hamster	Protein 50 µg	30 %	0.211	No significant protection	Hashimoto et al. (2013)
Lai	Lai	GroEL His tag	Hamster	Protein 100–200 µg	50–75 %	0.007–0.077	Single experiment reported. Claim that GroEL antiserum agglutinated multiple serovars	Li et al. (2013)
Hardjo	Hardjo	238 recombinant proteins	Hamster	Protein 25 µg in pools of five	Nil	1.0	Kidney colonization used to assess protection	Murray et al. (2013)

[a] Protection based on survival compared with control animals
[b] Fisher's exact test

second study (Dai et al. 2000), guinea pigs were immunized with plasmid DNA encoding FlaB, and again apparently significant protection was obtained, although only a single experiment was performed. It is difficult to know how to interpret these results. Leptospiral flagellar antigens are not surface exposed and indeed, do not react with specific antibodies unless the leptospiral cells are first permeabilized (Zhang et al. 2013). It is the opinion of this author that the protection claims with flagellar antigens are not credible.

An even stranger claim is that of a recent study which reported significant protection of hamsters with recombinant GroEL (Table 3; Li et al. 2013). The chaperone GroEL is a cytoplasmic protein; indeed, it is used routinely as a cytoplasmic marker in cell fractionation experiments. The report that anti-GroEL antiserum agglutinated all eight leptospiral serovars tested thus borders on bizarre. An independent assessment of specific rabbit anti-GroEL antiserum found no evidence whatsoever of agglutination of whole leptospires (B. Adler, unpublished observations).

Despite these mainly negative or unconvincing findings, there are some credible reports of immunoprophylaxis. One of the earliest reports of protective immunity elicited by defined protein antigens (Haake et al. 1999) involved immunization of hamsters with *E. coli* membrane fractions containing a combination of OmpL1 and LipL41. This preparation induced significant protection against homologous challenge with *Leptospira kirschneri* serovar Grippotyphosa, but only in one of three experiments. These studies have not been repeated.

The hypothetical LemA protein induced partial, but highly significant, protection in hamsters when delivered using a prime boost, DNA plus protein strategy. Surviving animals were culture and lesion positive. Interestingly, LemA alone did not elicit significant immunity, whereas *lemA* alone was marginally protective ($p = 0.03$) despite not eliciting a detectable antibody response (Table 3; Hartwig et al. 2013). Unfortunately, these results were based on a single experiment.

Faisal et al. (2009) reported significant protection in hamsters immunized with a combination of three proteins of unknown function, Lp0607, Lp118 and Lp1454, when delivered trapped in liposomes derived from polar lipids of *L. biflexa* (termed leptosomes). Intriguingly, no protection was observed if the proteins were trapped in phosphatidylcholine liposomes, nor if the proteins were delivered mixed with, rather than trapped in, either of the liposome preparations (Table 3). The leptosomes stimulated significantly higher Th1 and Th2 responses, although it is not clear which of these was involved in mediating protection. However, here again, the protection data were based on a single experiment.

6 Conclusions

On the centennial of the discovery of *Leptospira* as the causative agent of Weil's disease the only vaccines licensed for use in animals and humans are inactivated bacterins not very different from those first used 90 years ago. The post-genomic era has seen a flurry of activity to identify protein components of the leptospiral cell that are able to elicit cross-protective immunity. As outlined in this review, the majority of claims for protection are not credible, based on the data reported. However, this should not be viewed as painting too bleak a picture. It may well be that some of these proteins will be shown to be capable of stimulating immunity when they are tested in repeat experiments, perhaps in combination, and with sufficiently large numbers of animals, proper challenge doses, and with appropriate statistical analysis. This prospect is exemplified by LigA. Despite a number of protection claims which do not withstand proper scrutiny, there is now sufficient evidence that LigA is a protective antigen, at least in some leptospiral species and serovars, and currently represents the most likely candidate vaccine antigen. There is thus a realistic possibility of the development of defined, protein-based vaccines in the next decade.

A final cautionary point should be borne in mind. The experience with Hardjo vaccines in cattle has emphasized the fact that mechanisms of immunity to leptospirosis, and therefore the identity of the antigen(s) mediating that immunity, cannot necessarily be extrapolated from laboratory animals to production or companion animals, to humans, or even among different animal species. The caveat may also hold for different serovars; the assumption should not be made that immunity elicited by an antigen against a particular serovar in a particular animal, can be generalized to other species.

Acknowledgments Original work in the author's laboratory was supported by the National Health and Medical Research Council and the Australian Research Council.

References

Alston JM, Broom JC (1958) Leptospirosis in man and animals. E & S Linvingstone, Edinburgh and London

Atzingen MV, Goncales AP, de Morais ZM, Araujo ER, De Brito T, Vasconcellos SA, Nascimento AL (2010) Characterization of leptospiral proteins that afford partial protection in hamsters against lethal challenge with *Leptospira interrogans*. J Med Microbiol 59:1005–1015

Atzingen MV, Vieira ML, Oliveira R, Domingos RF, Mendes RS, Barros AT, Goncales AP, de Morais ZM, Vasconcellos SA, Nascimento AL (2012) Evaluation of immunoprotective activity of six leptospiral proteins in the hamster model of leptospirosis. Open Microbiol J 6:79–87

Auran NE, Johnson RC, Ritzi DM (1972) Isolation of the outer sheath of *Leptospira* and its immunogenic properties in hamsters. Infect Immun 5:968–975

Branger C, Sonrier C, Chatrenet B, Klonjkowski B, Ruvoen-Clouet N, Aubert A, Andre-Fontaine G, Eloit M (2001) Identification of the hemolysis-associated protein 1 as a cross-protective immunogen of *Leptospira interrogans* by adenovirus-mediated vaccination. Infect Immun 69:6831–6838

Branger C, Chatrenet B, Gauvrit A, Aviat F, Aubert A, Bach JM, Andre-Fontaine G (2005) Protection against *Leptospira interrogans* sensu lato challenge by DNA immunization with the gene encoding hemolysin-associated protein 1. Infect Immun 73:4062–4069

Bulach DM, Zuerner RL, Wilson P, Seemann T, McGrath A, Cullen PA, Davis J, Johnson M, Kuczek E, Alt DP, Peterson-Burch B, Coppel RL, Rood JI, Davies JK, Adler B (2006) Genome reduction in *Leptospira borgpetersenii* reflects limited transmission potential. Proc Natl Acad Sci USA 103:14560–14565

Cao Y, Faisal SM, Yan W, Chang YC, McDonough SP, Zhang N, Akey BL, Chang YF (2011) Evaluation of novel fusion proteins derived from extracellular matrix binding domains of LigB as vaccine candidates against leptospirosis in a hamster model. Vaccine 29:7379–7386

Chang YF, Chen CS, Palaniappan RU, He H, McDonough SP, Barr SC, Yan W, Faisal SM, Pan MJ, Chang CF (2007) Immunogenicity of the recombinant leptospiral putative outer membrane proteins as vaccine candidates. Vaccine 25:8190–8197

Christopher WL, Adler B, Faine S (1982) Immunogenicity of leptospiral vaccines grown in protein-free medium. J Med Microbiol 15:493–501

Coutinho ML, Choy HA, Kelley MM, Matsunaga J, Babbitt JT, Lewis MS, Aleixo JA, Haake DA (2011) A LigA three-domain region protects hamsters from lethal infection by *Leptospira interrogans*. PLoS Negl Trop Dis 5:e1422

Cullen PA, Xu X, Matsunaga J, Sanchez Y, Ko AI, Haake DA, Adler B (2005) Surfaceome of *Leptospira* spp. Infect Immun 73:4853–4863

Dai B, Chen Z, Yan H, Zhao H, Li S (1997) PCR amplification, molecular cloning, DNA sequence analysis and immunoprotection in BALB/c mice of the 33 kDa endoflagellar protein of *L. interrogans* serovar Lai. Chin Med Sci J 12:15–21

Dai B, You Z, Chen Z, Yan H, Fang Z (2000) Protection against leptospirosis by immunization with plasmid DNA encoding 33 kDa endoflagellin of *L. interrogans* serovar Lai. Chin Med Sci J 15:14–19

Deveson Lucas DS, Cullen PA, Lo M, Srikram A, Sermswan RW, Adler B (2011) Recombinant LipL32 and LigA from *Leptospira* are unable to stimulate protective immunity against leptospirosis in the hamster model. Vaccine 29:3413–3418

Deveson Lucas DS, Lo M, Bulach DM, Quinsey NS, Murray GL, Allen A, Adler B (2014) Recombinant LipL32 stimulates gamma-interferon production in cattle vaccinated with a monovalent *Leptospira borgpetersenii* serovar Hardjo subtype Hardjobovis vaccine. Vet Microbiol 169:163–170

Faisal SM, Yan W, Chen CS, Palaniappan RU, McDonough SP, Chang YF (2008) Evaluation of protective immunity of *Leptospira* immunoglobulin like protein A (LigA) DNA vaccine against challenge in hamsters. Vaccine 26:277–287

Faisal SM, Yan W, McDonough SP, Chang CF, Pan MJ, Chang YF (2009) Leptosome-entrapped leptospiral antigens conferred significant higher levels of protection than those entrapped with PC-liposomes in a hamster model. Vaccine 27:6537–6545

Felix SR, Hartwig DD, Argondizzo AP, Silva EF, Seixas FK, Neto AC, Medeiros MA, Lilenbaum W, Dellagostin OA (2011) Subunit approach to evaluation of the immune protective potential of leptospiral antigens. Clin Vaccine Immunol 18:2026–2030

Flannery B, Costa D, Carvalho FP, Guerreiro H, Matsunaga J, Da Silva ED, Ferreira AGP, Riley LW, Reis MG, Haake DA, Ko AI (2001) Evaluation of recombinant *Leptospira* antigen-based enzyme-linked immunosorbent assays for the serodiagnosis of leptospirosis. J Clin Microbiol 39:3303–3310

Forster KM, Hartwig DD, Seixas FK, Bacelo KL, Amaral M, Hartleben CP, Dellagostin OA (2013) A conserved region of leptospiral immunoglobulin-like A and B proteins as a DNA vaccine elicits a prophylactic immune response against leptospirosis. Clin Vaccine Immunol 20:725–731

Fletcher W (1928) Recent work on leptospirosis, tsutsugamushi disease, and tropical typhus in the federated Malay States. Trans R Soc Trop Med Hyg 21:265–282

Grassmann AA, Felix SR, dos Santos CX, Amaral MG, Seixas Neto AC, Fagundes MQ, Seixas FK, da Silva EF, Conceicao FR, Dellagostin OA (2012) Protection against lethal leptospirosis after vaccination with LipL32 coupled or coadministered with the B subunit of *Escherichia coli* heat-labile enterotoxin. Clin Vaccine Immunol 19:740–745

Haake DA, Mazel MK, McCoy AM, Milward F, Chao G, Matsunaga J, Wagar EA (1999) Leptospiral outer membrane proteins OmpL1 and LipL41 exhibit synergistic immunoprotection. Infect Immun 67:6572–6582

Haake DA, Chao G, Zuerner RL, Barnett JK, Barnett D, Mazel M, Matsunaga J, Levett PN, Bolin
    CA (2000) The leptospiral major outer membrane protein LipL32 is a lipoprotein expressed
    during mammalian infection. Infect Immun 68:2276–2285
Hartwig DD, Forster KM, Oliveira TL, Amaral M, McBride AJ, Dellagostin OA (2013) A prime-
    boost strategy using the novel vaccine candidate, LemA, protects hamsters against
    leptospirosis. Clin Vaccine Immunol 20:747–752
Hashimoto VL, Abreu PAE, Carvalho E, Goncales AP, Morais ZM, Vasconcellos SA, Romero
    EC, Ho PL (2013) Evaluation of the elastinolytic activity and protective effect of Leptallo I, a
    protein composed by metalloprotease and FA5/8C domains, from *Leptospira interrogans*
    Copenhageni. Microb Pathog 61–62:29–36
He HJ, Wang WY, Wu Z, Lv Z, Li J, Tan L (2008) Protection of guinea pigs against *Leptospira
    interrogans* serovar Lai by LipL21 DNA vaccine. Cell Mol Immunol 5:385–891
Ido Y, Hoki R, Ito H, Wani H (1916) The prophylaxis of Weil's disease (Spirochaetosis
    icterohaemorrhagiae). J Exp Med 24:471–483
Jost BH, Adler B, Vinh T, Faine S (1986) A monoclonal antibody reacting with a determinant on
    leptospiral lipopolysaccharide protects guinea pigs against leptospirosis. J Med Microbiol
    22:269–275
Jost BH, Adler B, Faine S (1989) Experimental immunisation of hamsters with lipopolysaccharide
    antigens of *Leptospira interrogans*. J Med Microbiol 29:115–120
Kemenes F (1964) Cross-immunity studies on virulent strains of leptospires belonging to different
    serotypes. Zetschr Immun Allergieforsch 127:209–229
Koizumi N, Watanabe H (2004) Leptospiral immunoglobulin-like proteins elicit protective
    immunity. Vaccine 22:1545–1552
Li X, Wang Y, Yan J, Cheng D (2013) Prokaryotic expression of *Leptospira interrogans* groEL
    gene and immunoprotection of its products in hamsters. Zhejiang Da Xue Xue Bao Yi Xue Ban
    42:164–710
Lourdault K, Wang LC, Vieira A, Matsunaga J, Melo R, Lewis MS, Haake DA, Gomes-Solecki M
    (2014) Oral immunization with Escherichia coli expressing a lapidated form of LigA protects
    hamsters against challenge with *Leptospira interrogans* serovar Copenhageni. Infect Immun
    82:893–902
Luo D, Xue F, Ojcius DM, Zhao J, Mao Y, Li L, Lin X, Yan J (2010) Protein typing of major outer
    membrane lipoproteins from Chinese pathogenic *Leptospira* spp. and characterization of their
    immunogenicity. Vaccine 28:243–255
Maneewatch S, Tapchaisri P, Sakolvaree Y, Klaysing B, Tongtawe P, Chaisri U, Songserm T,
    Wongratanacheewin S, Srimanote P, Chongsa-nguanz M, Chaicumpa W (2007) OmpL1 DNA
    vaccine cross-protects against heterologous *Leptospira* spp. challenge. Asian Pac J Allergy
    Immunol 25:75–82
Maneewatch S, Sakolvaree Y, Saengjaruk P, Srimanote P, Tapchaisri P, Tongtawe P, Klaysing B,
    Wongratanacheewin S, Chongsa-Nguan M, Chaicumpa W (2008) Monoclonal antibodies to
    LipL32 protect against heterologous *Leptospira* spp. challenge. Hybridoma 27:453–465
Marcsisin RA, Bartpho T, Bulach DM, Srikram A, Sermswan RW, Adler B, Murray GL (2013)
    Use of a high-throughput screen to identify *Leptospira* mutants unable colonise the carrier host
    or cause disease in the acute model of infection. J Med Microbiol 62:1601–1608
Masuzawa T, Nakamura R, Shimizu T, Yanagihara Y (1990) Biological activities and endotoxic
    activities of protective antigens (PAgs) of *Leptospira interrogans*. Zentralbl Bakteriol
    274:109–117
Matsunaga J, Barocchi MA, Croda J, Young TA, Sanchez Y, Siqueira I, Bolin CA, Reis MG,
    Riley LW, Haake DA, Ko AI (2003) Pathogenic *Leptospira* species express surface-exposed
    proteins belonging to the bacterial immunoglobulin superfamily. Mol Microbiol 49:929–946
Matsunaga J, Sanchez Y, Xu X, Haake DA (2005) Osmolarity, a key environmental signal
    controlling expression of leptospiral proteins LigA and LigB and the extracellular release of
    LigA. Infect Immun 73:70–78

Matsuo K, Isogai E, Araki Y (2000) Control of immunologically crossreactive leptospiral infection by administration of lipopolysaccharides from a nonpathogenic strain of *Leptospira biflexa*. Microbiol Immunol 44:887–890

Midwinter A, Faine S, Adler B (1990) Vaccination of mice with lipopolysaccharide (LPS) and LPS-derived immuno-conjugates from *Leptospira interrogans*. J Med Microbiol 33:199–204

Midwinter A, Vinh T, Faine S, Adler B (1994) Characterization of an antigenic oligosaccharide from *Leptospira interrogans* serovar pomona and its role in immunity. Infect Immun 62:5477–5482

Murray GL, Srikram A, Hoke DE, Wunder EA Jr, Henry R, Lo M, Zhang K, Sermswan RW, Ko AI, Adler B (2009) Major surface protein LipL32 is not required for either acute or chronic infection with *Leptospira interrogans*. Infect Immun 77:952–958

Murray GL (2013) The lipoprotein LipL32, an enigma of leptospiral biology. Vet Microbiol 162:305–314

Murray GL, Lo M, Bulach DM, Srikram A, Seemann T, Quinsey NS, Sermswan RW, Allen A, Adler B (2013) Evaluation of 238 antigens of *Leptospira borgpetersenii* serovar Hardjo for protection against kidney colonisation. Vaccine 31:495–499

Naiman BM, Alt D, Bolin CA, Zuerner R, Baldwin CL (2001) Protective killed *Leptospira borgpetersenii* vaccine induces potent Th1 immunity comprising responses by CD4 and gammadelta T lymphocytes. Infect Immun 69:7550–7558

Nascimento A, Verjovski-Almeida S, Van Sluys M, Monteiro-Vitorell C, Camargo L, Digiampietri L, Harstkeerl R, Ho P, Marques M, Oliveira M, Setubal J, Haake D, Martins E (2004) Genome features of *Leptospira interrogans* serovar Copenhageni. Braz J Med Biol Res 37:459–477

Palaniappan RU, McDonough SP, Divers TJ, Chen CS, Pan MJ, Matsumoto M, Chang YF (2006) Immunoprotection of recombinant leptospiral immunoglobulin-like protein A against *Leptospira interrogans* serovar Pomona infection. Infect Immun 74:1745–1750

Pinne M, Haake DA (2013) LipL32 Is a subsurface lipoprotein of *Leptospira interrogans*: presentation of new data and reevaluation of previous studies. PLoS ONE 8:e51025

Plesko I, Lataste-Dorolle C (1970) Intertype immunity relations of *Leptospira* strains belonging to the "Australis" serogroup. Biologia (Bratisl) 25:402–411

Plesko I, Hlavata Z (1971) Cross immunity studies with lipase negative strains of leptospires. Biol (Brat) 26:689–693

Que-Gewirth NLS, Ribeiro AA, Kalb SR, Cotter RJ, Bulach DM, Adler B, Saint Girons I, Werts C, Raetz CRH (2004) A methylated phosphate group and four amide-linked acyl chains in *Leptospira interrogans* Lipid A: the membrane anchor of an unusual lipopolysaccharide that activates TLR2. J Biol Chem 279:25420–25429

Ricaldi J, Matthias M, Vinetz J, Lewis A (2012) Expression of sialic acids and other nonulosonic acids in *Leptospira*. BMC Microbiol 12:161

Rosario LA, Arencibia DF, Suarez YE, Infante JF, Valdes BY, Batista N (2012) Cross-protection among unrelated *Leptospira pathogens* serovars: an unfinished story. Adv Clin Exp Med 21:581–589

Rottini GD, Cinco M, Panizon F, Agosti E (1972) Comportamento dell Ig seriche nell'uomo dopo vaccinazione con *leptospira saprofita* (ceppo Patoc 1). G Mal Infett Parassit 24:879–885

Schoone GJ, Everard COR, Korver H, Carrington DG, Inniss VA, Baulu J, Terpstra WJ (1989) An immunoprotective monoclonal antibody directed against *Leptospira interrogans* serovar copenhageni. J Gen Microbiol 135:73–78

Seixas FK, da Silva EF, Hartwig DD, Cerqueira GM, Amaral M, Fagundes MQ, Dossa RG, Dellagostin OA (2007) Recombinant *Mycobacterium bovis* BCG expressing the LipL32 antigen of *Leptospira interrogans* protects hamsters from challenge. Vaccine 26:88–95

Shinagawa M, Yanagawa R (1972) Isolation and characterization of a leptospiral type-specific antigen. Infect Immun 5:12–19

Sonrier C, Branger C, Michel V, Ruvoen-Clouet N, Ganiere JP, Andre-Fontaine G (2000) Evidence of cross-protection within *Leptospira interrogans* in an experimental model. Vaccine 19:86–94

Silva EF, Medeiros MA, McBride AJ, Matsunaga J, Esteves GS, Ramos JG, Santos CS, Croda J, Homma A, Dellagostin OA, Haake DA, Reis MG, Ko AI (2007) The terminal portion of leptospiral immunoglobulin-like protein LigA confers protective immunity against lethal infection in the hamster model of leptospirosis. Vaccine 25:6277–6286

Srikram A, Zhang K, Bartpho T, Lo M, Hoke DE, Sermswan RW, Adler B, Murray GL (2010) Cross-protective immunity against leptospirosis elicited by a live, attenuated lipopolysaccharide mutant. J Infect Dis 203:870–879

Stalheim OH (1968) Vaccination of hamsters, swine, and cattle with viable, avirulent *Leptospira pomona*. Am J Vet Res 29:1463–1468

Stalheim OH (1971) Duration of immunity in cattle in response to a viable, avirulent *Leptospira pomona*vaccine. Am J Vet Res 32:851–854

Torten M, Shenberg E, Gerichter CB, Neuman P, Klingberg MA (1973) A new leptospiral vaccine for use in man. II. Clinical and serologic evaluation of a field trial with volunteers. J Infect Dis 128:647–651

Vinh T, Shi M-H, Adler B, Faine S (1989) Characterization and taxonomic significance of lipopolysaccharides of *Leptospira interrogans* serovar hardjo. J Gen Microbiol 135:2663–2673

Yan W, Faisal SM, McDonough SP, Divers TJ, Barr SC, Chang CF, Pan MJ, Chang YF (2009) Immunogenicity and protective efficacy of recombinant *Leptospira* immunoglobulin-like protein B (rLigB) in a hamster challenge model. Microbes Infect 11:230–237

Yan W, Faisal SM, McDonough SP, Chang CF, Pan MJ, Akey B, Chang YF (2010) Identification and characterization of OmpA-like proteins as novel vaccine candidates for leptospirosis. Vaccine 28:2277–2283

Zhang K, Murray GL, Seemann T, Srikram A, Bartpho T, Sermswan RW, Adler B, Hoke DE (2013) Leptospiral LruA is required for virulence and modulates an interaction with mammalian Apolipoprotein A-I. Infect Immun 81:3872–3879

The Role of Leptospirosis Reference Laboratories

Rudy A. Hartskeerl and Lee D. Smythe

Abstract The general goal of reference centres is to support the community, from diagnostic laboratories to research institutions, in the execution of their work by providing reference strains and reagents and giving instructions and recommendations to individual colleagues and national and international organisations on a wide variety of issues. There are different levels of reference centres, from local to international, with an increasing package of tasks and responsibilities. Local reference centres might limit activities to diagnostic confirmation by applying standard testing, while international reference centres cover a wider range of activities from design, validation and harmonisation of diagnostic and reference technologies to international monitoring associated with recommendations on the global burden and distribution of leptospirosis and its prevention and control to national and international health decision makers. This chapter focusses on four major pillars constituting reference tasks in addition to the obvious provision of reference substances, i.e. Research and training, Diagnosis, Identification of *Leptospira* and Surveillance. Due to financial and organisational constraints, reference centres are restricted in their capacity for basic research and consequently focus on applied research into various aspects of leptospirosis. They offer training, either individually or groupwise, that might vary from standard technologies to novel sophisticated methodologies, depending on the need and requests of the trainee. Most reference centres are involved in the confirmation of preliminary diagnosis obtained at peripheral levels, such as local hospitals and health centres, while other major activities involve the design and validation of diagnostics, their international harmonisation and quality assurance. Identification of causative *Leptospira* strains (or serovars) is key to the identification of infection sources and is critical for surveillance. Hence, reference

R.A. Hartskeerl (✉)
WHO/FAO/OIE and National Leptospirosis Reference Centre, Royal Tropical Institute,
KIT Biomedical Research, Meibergdreef 39, 1105 AZ Amsterdam, The Netherlands
e-mail: r.hartskeerl@kit.nl

L.D. Smythe
Health Support Queensland, WHO/FAO/OIE Collaborating Center for Reference
and Research on Leptospirosis, PO Box 594, Archerfield, QLD 4108, Australia
e-mail: Lee_Smythe@health.qld.gov.au

© Springer-Verlag Berlin Heidelberg 2015   273
B. Adler (ed.), *Leptospira and Leptospirosis*, Current Topics in Microbiology
and Immunology 387, DOI 10.1007/978-3-662-45059-8_11

centres also focus on the development, application and provision of methods that are required for unambiguous characterisation of new and recognised *Leptospira* strains and the maintenance of the integrity of strain collections. In line with their central role, reference centres are frequently associated with local, national and/or international surveillance activities linked to an advisory role and the production of guidelines. Such surveillance activities usually comprise collation of morbidity and mortality data, signalling of outbreaks and the investigation of infection sources and risks.

Contents

1 The Reference Centre

Although this term is used frequently, there is no such entity as "The Reference Centre". There are several levels of reference centres or reference laboratories with distinct packages of allocated tasks and responsibilities.

1.1 Levels of Reference Centres

The centres have responsibilities which may be at a local, national or international level. The local level laboratories tend to provide quite specific, but limited, services which target mainly a diagnostic level activity. These laboratories may have capacity only for providing screening testing, but additionally, may possess the capability to provide more complex diagnostics such as the microscopic agglutination test (MAT). The national level laboratories tend to provide not only diagnostic services but may also be charged with national surveillance activities, provide training and to some degree issue reference materials such as cultures and control sera, and in limited cases, execute the standard cross agglutinin adsorption testing (CAAT) for the serological identification of isolates. The international reference laboratories may fall under the scope of organisations such as the World Organization for Animal Health (OIE) and World Health Organisation (WHO) or Food and Agriculture Organisation (FAO) and have more defined terms of reference. They may form part of a network of laboratories to support the activities of the above organisations. The designations will be for defined periods of time and such designations generally are arranged in consultation with the respective government.

According to the minutes of the Subcommittee on the Taxonomy of *Leptospira* (TSC) (Anonymous 1984), it was agreed that laboratories should be recognised as reference laboratories only if they are designated by the Subcommittee. The list of reference laboratories has to be reviewed every 4 years. Internationally recognised reference centres are listed below in the section "Addresses of international expert centres on leptospirosis".

In general, a reference laboratory should be able to provide a higher level of service and expertise than local clinical and microbiological laboratories. Where designations are under organisations such as the WHO, FAO or OIE, and to a lesser extent when under a national flag, the centres generally are not financially supported by these organisations and largely depend on institutional and/or national governmental funding. Moreover, the need to avoid conflicts of interest often excludes centres from financial sources that are available to other research and educational institutions.

1.2 Terms of Reference

The formal definition by WHO for a collaborating centre is an institution designated by the Director—General to form part of an international collaborative network carrying out activities in support of the organisation's programme at all levels. A department or laboratory within an institution or a group of facilities for reference, research or training belonging to different institutions may be designated as a centre, one institution acting for them in relations with the organisation. An institution may be designated initially for a term of 4 years.

Examples of functions drawn from a WHO Programme Activity publication are:

- Collection, collation and dissemination of information
- Standardisation of terminology and nomenclature, of technology, of diagnostic, therapeutic and prophylactic substances, and of methods and procedures
- Development and application of appropriate technology
- Provision of reference substances and other services
- Participation in collaborative research developed under the organisation's leadership, including the planning, conduct, monitoring and evaluation of research, as well as promotion of the application of the results of research

- Training, including research training
- The coordination of activities carried out by several institutions within one country on a given subject.

To achieve designation at the various levels may mean that laboratories need to demonstrate their level of scientific expertise and recognition within the scientific community relating to the disease. This may be reflected by activity at the national and international levels and through the qualifications of the staff, publication records and any associated research activities.

Cited from World Organization for Animal Health (2013):

OIE Reference Laboratories are designated to pursue all the scientific and technical problems relating to a named disease or specific topic. The expert, responsible to the OIE and its members with regard to these issues, should be a leading and active researcher helping the Reference Laboratory to provide scientific and technical assistance and expert advice on topics linked to surveillance and control of the disease for which the Reference Laboratory is responsible. Reference Laboratories may also provide scientific and technical training for personnel from members, and coordinate scientific and technical studies in collaboration with other laboratories or organisations, including through OIE Laboratory Twinning (http://www.oie.int/our-scientific-expertise/reference-laboratories/introduction/).

The terms of reference which may be applied for an OIE laboratory as cited from http://www.oie.int/en/our-scientific-expertise/reference-laboratories/introduction/) are:

- To use, promote and disseminate diagnostic methods validated according to OIE Standards;
- To recommend the prescribed and alternative tests or vaccines as OIE Standards;
- To develop reference material in accordance with OIE requirements, and implement and promote the application of OIE Standards;
- To store and distribute to national laboratories biological reference products and any other reagents used in the diagnosis and control of the designated pathogens or diseases;
- To develop, standardise and validate according to OIE Standards new procedures for diagnosis and control of the designated pathogens or diseases;
- To provide diagnostic testing facilities, and, where appropriate, scientific and technical advice on disease control measures to OIE Member Countries;
- To carry out and/or coordinate scientific and technical studies in collaboration with other laboratories, centres or organisations;
- To collect, process, analyse, publish and disseminate epizootiological data relevant to the designated pathogens or diseases;
- To provide scientific and technical training for personnel from OIE Member Countries;
- To maintain a system of quality assurance, biosafety and biosecurity relevant for the pathogen and the disease concerned;
- To organise and participate in scientific meetings on behalf of the OIE;

- To establish and maintain a network with other OIE Reference Laboratories designated for the same pathogen or disease and organise regular inter-laboratory proficiency testing to ensure comparability of results;
- To organise inter-laboratory proficiency testing with laboratories other than OIE Reference Laboratories for the same pathogens and diseases to ensure equivalence of results;
- To place expert consultants at the disposal of the OIE.

This chapter will further deal with four main tasks of references centres, i.e. Research and training, Diagnosis and diagnostics, Identification of *Leptospira*, and Surveillance

2 Research and Training

2.1 Research Activities

Reference laboratories are frequently the source of collaborations in research and not necessarily the driver of the project. The inherent ability of reference laboratories to provide expert services in diagnosis, typing of isolates and interpretation of data means that they are valued collaborators. The limiting factors are increasingly funding and resources for research, frequently caused by prevailing terms of reference. Unless reference laboratories are able to access these additional to their baseline then collaborations will become more difficult in the future. The focus of reference laboratories may shift away from research and increasingly apply resources to supporting public or animal health investigations and supplying materials such as hyperimmune sera and cultures.

It is needless to say that reference centres have only limited possibilities to perform basic research. The majority of their research is in line with their reference tasks and thus consist of the translation of novel, innovate technologies to the improvement of the detection and characterization of *Leptospira,* with particular emphasis on their validation and harmonisation (Ahmed et al. 2006, 2009, 2011, 2012; Boonsilp et al. 2013; Herrmann et al. 1992; Salaun et al. 2006; Slack et al. 2005, 2006a, 2007a; Smythe et al. 2002; Thaipadungpanit et al. 2007, 2011). Increasingly sophisticated tools, like GIS and mathematical modelling, are implemented to improve the understanding of local and global epidemiological and socio-economic aspects of leptospirosis, although frequently in conjunction with internal or external epidemiological sections. It is clear that reference centres are increasingly involved as partners in multi-disciplinary studies; the age of individual action of reference centres is coming to an end.

Furthermore, the increasing costs of specimen transport, the underpinning regulatory requirements, licensing costs and compliance training are continuing to constrict the ability of reference laboratories to meet demands for supply of biologicals to other laboratories. This, coupled with the need to have higher levels of legal scrutiny across transfer agreements and quarantine issues, will begin to have an impact on the service levels that the centres are able to administer. Increasing costs associated with current trends of retreating governmental support endanger the execution of the role of reference centres and unfortunately force several centres to levy financial charges on their services in order to cover costs.

2.2 Transfer of Knowledge

Reference laboratories primarily provide training to facilitate development of the diagnostic capability of various institutions. The resources available to reference laboratories for training can be limited and in many cases 'bench fees' may apply to help cover the cost of consumables and reagents. The use of reference laboratories in training can be expanded to cover workshops and be broad enough to cover aspects of quality systems where (inter)nationally recognised accreditations may apply. The availability of websites managed by reference laboratories provides the opportunity for persons to access information, methods, standard operating procedures and contacts (*Leptospira* Library 2012; Leptospirosis Reference Centre 2012; Leptospirosis Reference Laboratory 2013; Biology of Spirochetes Unit 2013).

3 Diagnosis and Diagnostics

Diagnosis of human and animal leptospirosis, including appropriate tests and sample collection, has been detailed in chapters by D.A. Haake and P.N. Levett and W.A. Ellis, this volume.

Different levels of veterinary public health care require different levels of diagnostics. The 'reference centre' aims to identify gaps in available tests as compared to a distinct situation and, when needed act to provide the appropriate tools. The publication of two real-time PCRs by international reference centres, in conjunction with their validation provides a good example of this strategy (Ahmed et al. 2009; Smythe et al. 2002; Slack et al. 2006a, 2007a). The impetus for accurate early diagnosis has come mainly from western countries. The design of these two PCR tests was strongly promoted by national requests from health care providers to enable early, preferably 24/7, diagnostic services to support timely and adequate clinical support. On the other side of the spectrum, a lack of awareness can be attributed to the lack of easy, rapid point-of-care tests and also here, reference centres were among the first to develop such rapid diagnostic tests and to execute multi-centre evaluations (Blacksell et al. 2006; Goris et al. 2013a, b; McBride et al. 2007; Smits et al. 1999, 2000a, b, 2001).

The concern for local, regional or global harmonisation and quality of tests should be a pivotal role of reference centres. The MAT, which is the reference test for the diagnosis of leptospirosis, is subject to the subjectivity of the tester and its performance largely depends on the availability of local strains in the panel. For this reason, it is difficult to standardise the test and to provide a uniform laboratory case definition. To enable quality checks on the performance of the test, international and regional MAT proficiency tests, driven by international reference centres, are regularly issued (Chappel et al. 2004; Leptospirosis Reference Laboratory 2013). Furthermore, reference centres publish methodology and data on their own case definition so that these can serve as an example for others (Slack et al. 2006b, 2007b; Smythe et al. 2000; Victoriano et al. 2009).

Notably, a range of proposed rapid tests have shown varying diagnostic accuracy in distinct studies. There are several explanations for this observation, including varying quality in production processes and their quality checks, environmental factors that substantiate high infection pressures with several serovars or other, cross-reacting infectious agents, subjective judgment of test results, and last but not least, inexperience of the test performers. When confirming test results obtained with screening tests, at least some international reference centres are frequently confronted with negative results obtained with the reference tests associated with inconsistent results when performing the same rapid test. One way to overcome this drawback is the performance of targeted local or multi-centre evaluations. However, a solution for these inconsistencies that are continuously being observed would be to establish globally representative clinical samples at reference centres to enable comparative test validation. Indeed, at the time of writing this chapter, international efforts are being undertaken to achieve such globally relevant comparative evaluations.

4 Characterization of *Leptospira* Strains

There exist two classification schemes for *Leptospira*, with very little correlation between the two; one is based on serology with the serovar as the basic taxon and the other uses DNA similarity to identify species and sub-species, further denoted as strains (see chapter by P.N. Levett, this volume).

Characterization of serovars requires serological approaches. While several molecular methods have claimed the ability to identify strains at serovar level, these methods should be considered with caution. Often, these only have been applied to a small sample and thus might not be considered representatively or they lack acceptable levels of repeatability and reproducibility. All current molecular methods, however, share the fact that these are based on highly plastic general genomic features, whereas the serovar is determined by the LPS conformational characteristics. Hence, such general molecular methods actually reflect genome plasticity and do not define a serovar status. Pulsed field gel electrophoresis (PFGE) was claimed decades ago to largely coincide with serovar identities. However, because PFGE patterns are constituted by restriction enzyme generated DNA fragments, SNPs may easily alter the sequences that constitute the recognition sites of the enzymes resulting in changes of electrophoretic patterns without consequences for the serovar. Similarly, genome rearrangements can result in different patterns within the same serovar. For this reason, the TSC has presented in its minutes the need for care in attempting to deduce a serovar from a PFGE pattern, especially when locally circulating serovars are not well known (Anonymous 2012). The recent determination of the genome sequences of all leptospiral serovars presents the possibility of molecular tests targeting the unique LPS biosynthetic loci and thus a molecular basis for serovar specificity.

For serological typing, the CAAT is the standard test to determine the serovar. Other serological techniques are available. In addition, factor analysis and typing with monoclonal antibodies (mAbs) have been applied. It is stressed that repeated publications mention that MAT on serum samples should not be used to deduce the infecting serovar and at the best might give presumptive information at the serogroup level, all of course depending on the knowledge of locally circulating serovars.

International and, to some extent national, reference centres can assist in typing by offering reference materials and strains, typing protocols and guidelines, providing online information of strains and serovars and their characteristics (*Leptospira* Library 2012; Leptospirosis Reference Laboratory 2013; *Leptospira* MLST Database 2013), develop and publish on novel techniques (Ahmed et al. 2006, 2009, 2010, 2011; Boonsilp et al. 2013; Cerqueira et al. 2010; Da Silva et al. 2010; Herrmann et al. 1992; Salaun et al. 2006; Tanganachitcharnchai et al. 2012; Tulsiani et al. 2010a; Oliveira et al. 2003; Schreier et al. 2012; Slack et al. 2005, 2007a; Vijayachari et al. 2004), or by offering their services, notably when complex serological or molecular typing approaches are needed.

4.1 Serological Classification

4.1.1 Cross Agglutinin Absorption Test

The CAAT remains the serological gold standard for typing of *Leptospira* isolates and identification of serovars. The method is complex and rests in the domain of a small number of reference laboratories. The CAAT requires the use of hyperimmune sera produced in rabbits to conduct the test. This method is time consuming and takes 6–10 weeks before a suitable hyperimmune titre is achieved. The CAAT is different from the MAT which is the serological diagnostic tool for identifying cases of the disease in humans and animals. The preparation of rabbit hyperimmune sera should follow the method described in the minutes of the TSC (Anonymous 1984).

The CAAT allows reference laboratories to identify existing serovars as well as assign new serovars. The minutes of the above meeting have the following definition of a serovar. Two strains are considered to belong to different serovars if, after cross absorption with adequate amounts of heterologous antigen, 10 % or more of the homologous titre regularly remains in at least one of the two antisera in repeated tests.

The TSC advised that new serovars should be recognised if they are typed by the classical absorption method in at least one reference laboratory (Anonymous 1984).

4.1.2 Factor Serum Analysis

Typing with factor sera is a refinement of CAAT. Factor sera are rabbit-anti-*Leptospira* sera that through a complicated process of absorption with various reference strains have achieved a high degree of specificity. With factor sera, isolates can be quickly typed by MAT. The method is very complicated and is no longer in use.

4.1.3 Typing with Monoclonal Antibodies

Typing with mAbs uses panels of mAbs that agglutinate serovars in a characteristic way (Hartskeerl et al. 2004). It presents an alternative easy and rapid approach that is applicable on about 70 % of all isolates (Hartskeerl et al. 2006), but like the molecular approaches, requires some caution. mAbs recognise a small number of epitopes on the LPS and it cannot be excluded that these epitopes are shared by different serovars. Indeed distinct serovars with similar agglutination patterns with distinct panels of mAbs have been reported (Bourhy et al. 2012; Valverde et al. 2007).

4.1.4 Conclusions

CAAT and factor analysis are arduous methods, while mAbs typing is not applicable on all serovars. Moreover, the methods increasingly reach limitations in discriminative power. For example, several serovars in the serogroup Grippo-typhosa are not distinguishable by CAAT anymore (Hartskeerl et al. 2004). In addition, serological techniques are very expensive. Therefore, the use of this practice is declining. With the advent of faster nucleic acid-based technologies, typing to a species and subspecies level occurs more frequently.

4.2 Molecular Typing

Traditionally *Leptospira* species are based on percentages of DNA homology as determined by DNA hybridization experiments. The technique is arduous and executed only at CDC, Atlanta, USA. This makes reliance on the approach very fragile and the TSC is currently discussing the abandonment of this method as the standard for speciation and substituting it with one or more other phylogeny-based molecular methods (see chapter by P.N. Levett, this volume).

The increasing limitation in transporting pathogens across the world will greatly affect the choice of a new standard towards a technique that directly produces digital data that can be used for online comparisons.

4.2.1 Molecular Methods that Lack the Criteria of Easy Availability

Various methods, such as bacterial endonuclease DNA analysis (BRENDA), including PFGE, arbitrarily primed PCR (AP-PCR) IS-based PCR, low stringency single primer PCR (LSSP-PCR), and others, either have a poor reproducibility, require large quantities of good quality DNA and/or need the availability of live bacteria. Besides, they do not directly produce digital data, although transfer of patterns in a digital formal is often possible.

Notably, PFGE has been promoted as a standard test for genotyping, not only of *Leptospira*, but also for a variety of other prokaryotes. As indicated above, PFGE patterns generally coincide with the serovar status and provide a useful tool for molecular epidemiology and in very specific situations might serve to deduce to some level the serovar's identity.

4.2.2 Molecular Methods Generating Digital Data or Profiles

To date, a number of technologies have been described that allow the online availability of data or profiles for international comparison evading the need for shipments of pathogens. These include typing arrays, Multiple-Locus Variable Number of Tandem Repeat Analysis (MLVA), (Fluorescence) Amplified Fragment Length Polymorphism (F)AFLP and sequence-based characterization (Ahmed et al. 2006, 2010; Caimi et al. 2012; Nalam et al. 2010; Saito et al. 2013; Salaun et al. 2006; Slack et al. 2005, 2006; Tulsiani et al. 2010a, 2010b; Vijayachari et al. 2004).

Single strand conformational polymorphism (SSCP) has the potential for diagnosis or to type *Leptospira* isolates to sub-species level. The test is not complex and able to generate distinct profiles for detecting mutations and genotyping. This method is based on the principle of altered conformity of the single-stranded DNA due to single base changes, which subsequently affect the mobility of the DNA under specific electrophoresis conditions. (De Roy et al. 2012). The method has been used successfully over a number of years for typing a range of microorganisms (Mansano et al. 1997).

The *Leptospira* genome appears highly plastic and lateral DNA transfer has been reported (Bulach et al. 2006; Haake et al. 2004; Nascimento et al. 2004). Therefore, phylogenetic classification based on a single locus sequence holds the risk of erroneous results. Multilocus sequence genotyping overcomes this problem, as it can identify a putatively horizontally transferred locus. Currently, multilocus sequence typing (MLST) is the most robust, phylogeny-based typing method for *Leptospira* and offers the advantage of online analysis of new sequences (*Leptospira* MLST Database 2013). However, with the rapid accumulation of *Leptospira* genome sequences and decreasing costs for whole genome sequencing, it is anticipated that the method will be substituted by whole genome sequence typing in the future. This will be even more attractive as whole genome sequences might be used to also deduce serological features.

The availability of online data will have an increasing impact on the role of reference laboratories for the typing of isolates. The use of complex serological methods will be replaced by access to digitally-driven typing data which allow laboratories to more easily conduct their own typing outside the scope of the traditional reference laboratory role. The only limitations are the construction of libraries which carry sufficient data to allow profile comparisons and assigning of species and serovar.

5 Surveillance

The surveillance of communicable diseases and the knowledge gained from this activity is fundamental for disease prevention and control programmes. The information gained from surveillance is used for prioritising resource allocations, early detection of epidemics and evaluation of disease prevention strategies (Global Leptospirosis Environmental Action Network 2013; Hitoshi Oshitani, abstract from Leptospirosis in the Western Pacific and South—East Asia, January 21–22, 2000 Manila). Specific surveillance methods need to be engaged for specific diseases according to their individual characteristics and can be described as epidemiological, ecological, economic monitoring and with the specific training and education to implement and manage for the long to medium term (Dufour et al. 2008).

Leptospirosis reference laboratories are a primary resource for surveillance programmes, as they provide laboratory diagnostic and typing results which when combined with regional population and hospital data provide the greatest insight into disease trends and distribution. The ability of reference laboratories to engage in active surveillance relies significantly on the available resources and expertise. The type of surveillance quality will vary depending on the type of data to be gathered; this may be in the form of enhanced surveillance versus general surveillance. Those countries where leptospirosis is listed as a notifiable disease may find the quality of the surveillance data more accurate, due to mandatory reporting and scope of patient data collected (Bakoss et al. 2012; Baranton and Postic 2006; Goris et al. 2013a, b; Jansen et al. 2005, 2007). The use of suitable or standardised case definitions is important for the collection and evaluation of surveillance data. This issue is also further impacted by the various methods now available for the detection of the disease in humans and animals. The use of nucleic acid-based methods can now provide more detailed and timely information on the types of circulating leptospires (Nalam et al. 2010; Slack et al. 2010; Thaipadungpanit et al. 2007, 2011; Vijayachari et al. 2004).

The issue of climate change has placed considerable importance on surveillance data. In the case of leptospirosis, more enhanced surveillance will assist to better inform on the potential for changing transmission dynamics created by climate change; this at the local, regional and global levels. This has other implications where there is value in monitoring post disasters where the long-term effects need to be understood (Cann et al. 2013; Lau et al. 2010, 2012).

Surveillance can relate to monitoring, whereby during an outbreak leptospirosis reference laboratories are able to establish serological profiles of emerging cases and in collaboration with health authorities determine the volatility and progression of an outbreak and assist with the implementation of prevention and control programmes. The selection of vaccines for use or development can be influenced through the use of surveillance data.

The surveillance (and associated databases) provided by reference laboratories has significant value in relation to the review of historical data. These data, when aligned with more recent surveillance data, can inform health authorities of a changing serovar landscape and any notable changes in clinical presentations and mortality. The absence of surveillance data can impact on regional health planning; in some countries this may affect how authorities manage animal vaccination programmes, developing or maintaining diagnostic capabilities and infrastructure.

Surveillance and the associated data need to be readily available to assist with health response planning, research or general access by the public. This is now achieved electronically through the provision of websites which facilitate access to a broad range of information. For leptospirosis this has been achieved through sites operated by the World Health Organisation, International Leptospirosis Society, individual reference laboratories and various government agencies. The surveillance activities of leptospirosis reference laboratories are also available through peer review publications in journals.

Surveillance, together with diagnostics, case definition and epidemiological thresholds are amongst the key factors addressed by the current international effort of the Global Leptospirosis Environmental Action Network (GLEAN). GLEAN is a consortium comprising several international organisations, including WHO and a number of WHO Collaborating Centres, aimed at the understanding of outbreaks to facilitate their prediction, prevention and control (Global Leptospirosis Environmental Action Network 2013).

Addresses of international expert centres on leptospirosis

WHO Collaborating Centres

WHO/FAO Collaborating Centre for Reference and Research on Leptospirosis, Health Support Queensland, PO Box 594, Archerfield, Queensland 4108, Australia. www.health.qld.gov.au/qhcss/lepto.asp.
Current head, Dr. LD Smythe. e-mail: Lee_Smythe@health.qld.gov.au

WHO/FAO Collaborating Centre for Reference and Research on Leptospirosis, KIT Biomedical Research, Meibergdreef 39, 1105 AZ Amsterdam, The Netherlands. www.kit.nl/Leptospirosis-Reference-Centre.
Current head, Dr. RA Hartskeerl. e-mail: r.hartskeerl@kit.nl

WHO Collaborating Centre for Reference and Research on Leptospirosis, Institut Pasteur, 28 rue du Docteur Roux, F-75724 Cedex 15, Paris, France. www.pasteur. fr/sante/clre/cadrecnr/lepto-index.html.
Current head, Dr. M. Picardeau. e-mail: mpicard@pasteur.fr

WHO Collaborating Centre for Diagnosis, Research, Reference and Training in Leptospirosis, Regional Medical Research Centre, PO Box 13 Dollygunj, Port Blair-744101, India. www.rmrc.res.in.
Current head, Dr. P Vijayachari. e-mail: pblicmr@sanchar.net,
vijayacharip@yahoo.com

WHO Collaborating Centre for Leptospirosis, Instituto Oswaldo Cruz (FIOCRUZ), Avenida Brasil, 4365, 21045-900, Rio de Janeiro, Bazil. http://www.fiocruz.br.
Current head, Dr. Martha Maria Pereira. e-mail: mpereira@ioc.fiocruz.br

OIE Reference Laboratories

Leptospirosis Reference laboratory, Health Support Queensland, PO Box 594, Archerfield, Queensland 4108, Australia.
www.health.qld.gov.au/qhcss/lepto.asp.
Current head, Dr LD Smythe. e-mail: Lee_Smythe@health.qld.gov.au

Reference Laboratory for Leptospirosis, KIT Biomedical Research, Meibergdreef 39, 1105AZ Amsterdam, The Netherlands.
www.kit.nl/Leptospirosis-Reference-Centre.
Current head, Dr RA Hartskeerl. e-mail: r.hartskeerl@kit.nl

Leptospira Reference Laboratory, Veterinary Sciences Division, AFBI, Stoney Road, Stormont, Belfast, Northern Ireland, United Kingdom, BT23 6RW. http:// www.afbini.gov.uk/index/services/services-diagnostic-and-analytical/leptospirosis. htm.
Current head, Dr Z Arent. e-mail: zbigniew.arent@afbini.gov.uk

Instituto de Bacteriología, CICV, INTA, Castelar, Casilla de Correo 77, Morón 1708, Pcia de Buenos Aires, Argentina.
Current head, Dr L Samartino. e-mail: lsanma@cnia.inta.gov.ar

Laboratorio de Leptospirosis, Dirección General de Laboratorios y Control Técnico, Servicio Nacional de Sanidad y Calidad Agroalimentaria (SENASA), Avenida Talcahuano N°1660 (1640), Martínez, Pcia de Buenos Aires, Argentina.
Current head, Sra. J Petrakovsky. e-mail: jpetrako@senasa.gov.ar

National Veterinary Services Laboratories, USDA, APHIS, Veterinary Services, PO Box 844, Ames, Iowa 50010, United States of America.
Current head, Dr M Wilson. e-mail: mark.a.wilson@aphis.usda.gov

References

Ahmed A, Engelberts MF, Boer KR et al (2009) Development and validation of a real-time PCR for detection of pathogenic *Leptospira* species in clinical materials. PLoS ONE 4:e7093

Ahmed A, Anthony RM, Hartskeerl RA (2010) Array Tube: A simple and rapid molecular method for *Leptospira* species identification. Infect Genet Evol 10:955–962

Ahmed A, Thaipadngpanit J, Boonsilp S et al (2011) Comparison of two multilocus sequence based genotyping schemes for *Leptospira* species. PLoS Negl Trop Dis 5:e1374

Ahmed A, Klaasen HLBM, Van der Veen M et al (2012) Evaluation of real-time PCR and culturing for the detection of leptospires in canine samples. Adv Microbiol 2:162–170

Ahmed N, Devi SM, de Valverde ML et al (2006) Multilocus sequence typing method for identification and genotypic classification of pathogenic *Leptospira* species. Ann Clin Microbiol Antimicrob 5:28

Anonymous (1984). International committee on systematic bacteriology, subcommittee on the taxonomy of *Leptospira*; minutes of the meeting, 6 to 10 August 1982, Boston, Massachusetts. Int J Syst Bacteriol 34:258–259

Anonymous (2012). International committee on systematics of prokaryotes, subcommittee on the taxonomy of *Leptospiraceae*; minutes of the closed meeting, 20 September 2011, Mérida, Mexico. Int J Syst Evol Microbiol 62:2810–2811

Bakoss P, Macháčova E, Jareková J (2012) Long-term trends in the epidemiology of human leptospirosis (Slovak Republic, 1954–2006). Eur J Clin Microbiol Infect Dis 31:2167–2176

Baranton G, Postic D (2006) Trends in leptospirosis epidemiology in France. Sixty-six years of passive serological surveillance from 1920 to 2003. Int J Infect Dis 10:162–170

Biology of Spirochetes unit (2013). Institute Pasteur, Paris. http://www.pasteur.fr/ip/easysite/ pasteur/en/research/scientific-departments/microbiology/units-and-groups/biology-of-spirochetes/index. Accessed 17 Aug 2013

Blacksell SD, Smythe L, Phetsouvanh R et al (2006) Limited diagnostic capacities of two commercial assays for the detection of *Leptospira* immunoglobulin M antibodies in Laos. Clin Vac Immunol 13:1166–1169

Boonsilp S, Thaipadungpanit J, Amornchai P et al (2013) A single multilocus sequence typing (MLST) scheme for seven pathogenic *Leptospira* species. PLoS Negl Trop Dis 7:e1954

Bourhy P, Collet L, Lernout T et al (2012) Human *Leptospira* isolates circulating in Mayotte (Indian Ocean) have unique serological and molecular features. J Clin Microbiol 50:307–311

Bulach DM, Zuerner RL, Wilson P et al (2006) Genome reduction in *Leptospira* borgpetersenii reflects limited transmission potential. Proc Nat Acad Sci 103:14560–14565

Caimi K, Varni V, Melendez Y et al (2012) A combined approach of VNTR and MLST analysis: improving molecular typing of Argentinean isolates of *Leptospira interrogans*. Mem Inst Oswaldo Cruz 107:644–651

Cann KF, Thomas D, Salmon R et al (2013) Extreme water-related weather events and waterborne disease. Epidemiol Infect 141:671–686

Cerqueira GM, McBride AJA, Hartskeerl RA et al (2010) Bioinformatics describes novel loci for high resolution discrimination of *Leptospira* isolates. PLoS ONE 5:e15335

Chappel RJ, Goris M, Palmer MF et al (2004) Impact of proficiency testing on results of the microscopic agglutination test for the diagnosis of leptospirosis. J Clin Microbiol 42:5484–5488

Da Silva JB, Carvalho E, Hartskeerl RA et al (2010) Evaluation of the use of selective PCR amplification of LPS biosynthesis genes for molecular typing of *Leptospira* at the serovar level. Current Microbiol 62:518–524

De Roy M, Thavachelvam K, Batra HV et al (2012) PCR–SSCP: a tool for molecular diagnosis of leptospirosis. Int J Pharm Bio Sci 3:179–186

Dufour B, Moutou F, Hattenberger AM et al (2008) Global change: impact, management, risk approach and health measures—the case of Europe. Rev Sci Tech Int Epiz 27:541–550

Global Leptospirosis Environmental Action Network (2013). GLEAN. http://glean-lepto.org/. Accessed 14 Aug 2013

Goris MGA, Leeflang MMG, Loden M et al (2013a) Prospective evaluation of three rapid diagnostic tests for diagnosis of human leptospirosis. PLoS Negl Trop Dis 7:e2290

Goris MGA, Boer KR, Duarte TATE et al (2013b) Human leptospirosis trends, the Netherlands, 1925–2008. Emerg Infect Dis 19:371–378

Haake DA, Suchard MA, Kelley MM et al (2004) Molecular evolution and mosaicism of leptospiral outer membrane proteins involves horizontal DNA transfer. J Bacteriol 186:2818–2828

Hartskeerl RA, Goris MGA, Brem S et al (2004) Classification of *Leptospira* from the eyes of horses suffering from recurrent uveitis. J Vet Med Series B 51:110–115

Hartskeerl RA, Smits HL, Korver H et al (2006) International course on laboratory methods for the diagnosis of leptospirosis. Royal Tropical Institute, Amsterdam

Herrmann JL, Bellenger E, Perolat P et al (1992) Pulsed-field gel electrophoresis of NotI digests of leptospiral DNA: a new rapid method of serovar identification. J Clin Microbiol 30:1696–1702

Jansen A, Schoneberg I, Frank C et al (2005) Leptospirosis in Germany, 1962–2003. Emerg Infect Dis 11:1048–1054

Jansen A, Stark K, Schneider T et al (2007) Sex differences in clinical leptospirosis in Germany: 1997–2005. Clin Infect Dis 44:e69–72

Lau CL, Smythe LD, Craig SB et al (2010) Climate change, flooding, urbanisation and leptospirosis: fuelling the fire? Trans R Soc Trop Med Hyg 104:631–638

Lau C, Skelly C, Craig S et al (2012) Emergence of new leptospiral serovars in American Samoa —ascertainment or ecological change? BMC Infect Dis 12:19

Leptospira Library (2012) KIT Biomedical Research, Amsterdam. http://www.kit.nl/Leptospira-Library. Accessed 14 August 2013

Leptospira MLST Database (2013) Imperial College London. http://leptospira.mlst.net. Accessed 14 Aug 2013

Leptospirosis Reference Centre (2012) KIT Biomedical Research, Amsterdam. http://www.kit.nl/Leptospirosis-Reference-Centre. Accessed 14 Aug 2013

Leptospirosis Reference Laboratory (2013) Health Services Support Agency, Coopers Plains. http://www.health.qld.gov.au/qhcss/lepto.asp. Accessed 14 August 2013

Manzano M, Cocolin L, Pipan C et al (1997) Single-strand conformation polymorphism (SSCP) analysis of *Listeria monocytogenes* iap gene as tool to detect different serogroups. Mol Cell Probes 11:459–462

McBride AJA, Santos BL, Queirox A et al (2007) Evaluation of four whole-cell *Leptospira*-based serological tests for the diagnosis of urban leptospirosis. Clin Vac Immunol 14:1245–1248

Nascimento ALTO, Ko AI, Martins EAL et al (2004) Comparative genomics of two *Leptospira interrogans* serovars reveals novel insights into physiology and pathogenesis. J Bacteriol 186:2164–2172

Nalam K, Ahmed A, Devi SM et al (2010) Genetic affinities within a large global collection of pathogenic *Leptospira*: implications for strain identification and molecular epidemiology. PLoS ONE 5:e12637

Oliveira MA, Caballero OL, Vago AR et al (2003) Low-stringency single specific primer PCR for identification *Leptospira*. J Med Microbiol 52:127–135

Saito M, Villaneuva S, Chakraborty A et al (2013) Comparative analysis of *Leptospira* strains isolated from environmental soil and water in the Philippines and Japan. Appl Environ Microbiol 79:601–609

Salaun L, Merien F, Gurianova S et al (2006) Application of multilocus variable-number tandem-repeat analysis for molecular typing of the agent of leptospirosis. J Clin Microbiol 44:3954–3962

Schreier S, Doungchaweeb G, Triampoc D et al (2012) Development of a magnetic bead fluorescence microscopy immunoassay to detect and quantify *Leptospira* in environmental water samples. Acta Trop 22:119–125

Slack AT, Dohnt MF, Symonds ML et al (2005) Development of a multiple-locus variable number of tandem repeat analysis (MLVA) for *Leptospira interrogans* and its application to *Leptospira interrogans* serovar Australis isolates from Far North Queensland. Ann Clin Microbiol Antimicrob, Australia 4

Slack A, Symonds M, Dohnt M et al (2006a) Identification of pathogenic *Leptospira* species by conventional or real-time PCR and sequencing of the DNA gyrase subunitB encoding gene. BMC Microbiol 6:95

Slack AT, Symonds ML, Dohnt MF et al (2006b) The epidemiology of leptospirosis and the emergence of *Leptospira borgpetersenii* serovar Arborea in Queensland, Australia, 1998–2004. Epidemiol Infect 11:1–9

Slack A, Symonds M, Dohnt M et al (2007a) Evaluation of a modified Taqman assay detecting pathogenic *Leptospira* spp. against culture and *Leptospira*-specific IgM enzyme-linked immunosorbent assay in a clinical environment. Diagn Microbiol Infect Dis 57:361–366

Slack A, Symonds M, Dohnt M et al (2007b) Epidemiology of *Leptospira weilii* serovar Topaz infections in Australia. Comm Dis Intel 31:216–222

Slack AT, Symonds ML, Dohnt MF et al (2010) Molecular epidemiology of *Leptospira borgpetersenii* serovar Arborea, Queensland, Australia, 1998–2005. Am J Trop Med Hyg 83:820–821

Smits HL, Chee HD, Eapen CK et al (2001) Latex based, rapid and easy assay for human leptospirosis in a single test format. Trop Med Int Health 6:114–118

Smits HL, Ananyina YV, Chereshsky A et al (1999) International multicenter evaluation of the clinical utility of a dipstick assay for the detection of *Leptospira*-specific immunoglobulin M antibodies in human serum specimens. J Clin Microbiol 37:2904–2909

Smits HL, Hartskeerl RA, Terpstra WJ (2000a) An international multicentre evaluation of a dipstick assay for human leptospirosis, a quick and easy test for the serodiagnosis of acute human leptospirosis. Trop Med Intl Hlth 5:124–128

Smits HL, Van der Hoorn MAWG, Goris MGA et al (2000b) Simple latex agglutination assay for rapid diagnosis of human leptospirosis. J Clin Microbiol 38:1272–1275

Smythe L, Dohnt M, Symonds M et al (2000) Review of leptospirosis notifications in Queensland and Australia: January 1998—June 1999. Comm Dis Intel 24:153–157

Smythe L, Smith I, Smith G et al (2002) A quantitative PCR (TaqMan) assay for pathogenic *Leptospira* spp. BMC Infect Dis 2:13

Tanganuchitcharnchai A, Smythe L, Dohnt M et al (2012) Evaluation of the standard diagnostics *Leptospira* IgM ELISA for diagnosis of acute leptospirosis in Lao PDR. Trans R Soc Trop Med Hyg 106:563–566

Tulsiani SM, Craig SB, Graham GC et al (2010a) High-resolution melt-curve analysis of random amplified polymorphic DNA (RAPD-HRM) for the characterisation of pathogenic leptospires: intra-serovar divergence, inter-serovar convergence, and evidence of attenuation in *Leptospira* reference collections. Ann Trop Med Parasitol 104:427–437

Tulsiani SM, Craig SB, Graham GC et al (2010b) High-resolution melt-curve analysis of random-amplified-polymorphic-DNA markers, for the characterisation of pathogenic *Leptospira*. Ann Trop Med Parasitol 104:151–161

Thaipadungpanit J, Wuthiekanun V, Chierakul W et al (2007) A dominant clone of *Leptospira interrogans* associated with an outbreak of human leptospirosis in Thailand. PLoS Negl Trop Dis 1:e56

Thaipadungpanit J, Chierakul W, Wuthiekanun V et al (2011) Diagnostic accuracy of real-time PCR assays targeting 16S rRNA and lipL32 genes for human leptospirosis in Thailand: a case-control study. PLoS ONE 6:e16236

Valverde MA de los A, Ramirez JM, Montes de Oca LG et al (2007) Arenal, a new *Leptospira* serovar of serogroup Javanica, isolated from a patient in Costa Rica. Infect Genet Evol 8:529–533

Victoriano AF, Smythe LD, Gloriani-Barzaga N et al (2009) Leptospirosis in the Asia Pacific region. BMC Infect Dis 9:147

Vijayachari P, Ahmed N, Sugunan AP et al (2004) Use of fluorescent amplified fragment length polymorphism for molecular epidemiology of leptospirosis in India. J Clin Microbiol 42:3575–3580. doi:10.1128/JCM.42.8.3575-3580

World Organisation for Animal Health (2013) OIE Paris. http://www.oie.int/our-scientific-expertise/reference-laboratories/introduction/. Accessed 17 Aug 2013

Index

B. Adler (ed.), *Leptospira and Leptospirosis*, Current Topics in Microbiology
and Immunology 387, DOI 10.1007/978-3-662-45059-8